DSM-5-TR®
Self-Exam Questions

Test Questions for the Diagnostic Criteria

DSM-5-TR®
Self-Exam Questions

Test Questions for the Diagnostic Criteria

Edited by

Philip R. Muskin, M.D., M.A., DLFAPA, LFACLP
Professor of Psychiatry and Senior Consultant in Consultation-Liaison Psychiatry,
Columbia University Irving Medical Center, New York, New York

Anna Dickerman, M.D., FAPA, FACLP
Chief, Consultation-Liaison Psychiatry Service, Program Director, Consultation-Liaison Psychiatry Fellowship, and Associate Attending Psychiatrist,
New York-Presbyterian Hospital; Associate Professor of Clinical Psychiatry,
Weill Cornell Medical College, New York, New York

Andrew T. Drysdale, M.D., Ph.D.
Assistant in Clinical, Department of Psychiatry, Columbia University Irving Medical Center;
Postdoctoral Clinical Fellow, Department of Psychiatry,
Columbia University Irving Medical Center; Fellow,
New York State Psychiatric Institute/Columbia University, New York, New York

Claire Holderness, M.D., DFAPA
Associate Clinical Professor of Psychiatry, Columbia University Vagelos College of Physicians and Surgeons; Attending Psychiatrist, New York State Psychiatric Institute, New York, New York

Maalobeeka Gangopadhyay, M.D.
Associate Professor of Psychiatry, Columbia University Irving Medical Center;
Director of Acute Services, Child and Adolescent Psychiatry,
New York-Presbyterian Morgan Stanley Children's Hospital;
Medical Director, Quality and Patient Safety NYP-Columbia,
Department of Psychiatry, New York-Presbyterian, New York, New York

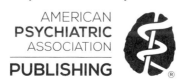

AMERICAN
PSYCHIATRIC
ASSOCIATION
PUBLISHING

If you wish to buy 50 or more copies of the same title, please go to www.appi.org/specialdiscounts for more information.

First Edition

Manufactured in the United States of America on acid-free paper
27 26 25 24 23   5 4 3 2 1

American Psychiatric Association Publishing
800 Maine Avenue SW, Suite 900
Washington, DC 20024-2812
www.appi.org

Library of Congress Cataloging-in-Publication Data
A CIP record is available from the Library of Congress.
ISBN: 798-1-61537-509-7 (pb), 978-1-61537-510-3 (eb)

British Library Cataloguing in Publication Data
A CIP record is available from the British Library.

Contents

PART I: Questions

PART II: Answer Guide

Preface

This edition of the DSM-5 self-examination guide incorporates the changes made since DSM-5 was released in 2013 (American Psychiatric Association 2013). The guide is a companion to, but not a replacement for, a thorough reading of DSM-5-TR (American Psychiatric Association 2022). The most recent edition of the diagnostic manual brings new diagnoses and revisions to the text of many of the DSM-5 diagnoses. There are new approaches to diagnosis in DSM-5-TR. Our framework in preparing this self-examination guide was to challenge the reader, hopefully in an engaging way, to learn about the criteria for previous and new diagnoses, to review revisions made in DSM-5-TR, and to self-educate about new approaches to the diagnostic endeavor. Some questions will seem obvious or easy and some questions will be quite difficult. As you work through the book, let it guide you to diagnostic sections where you would like to learn more as well as reassure you about those areas in which you feel you are well versed. The editors prepared a variety of clinical vignettes in order to allow the typical process we use to engage diagnostic considerations. The editors of this book are a diverse group of clinicians, educators, and researchers who undertook the task of learning about DSM-5-TR in order to help others self-educate. There are no commentary or political statements about diagnosis in the 475 questions contained in this study guide. All author proceeds from this book are donated to charitable foundations.

Anna Dickerman, M.D., FAPA, FACLP

Andrew T. Drysdale, M.D., Ph.D.

Claire Holderness, M.D., DFAPA

Maalobeeka Gangopadhyay, M.D.

Philip R. Muskin, M.D., M.A., DLFAPA, LFACLP

References

American Psychiatric Association: Diagnostic and Statistical Manual of Mental Disorders, 5th Edition. Arlington, VA, American Psychiatric Association, 2013

American Psychiatric Association: Diagnostic and Statistical Manual of Mental Disorders, 5th Edition, Text Revision. Washington, DC, American Psychiatric Association, 2022

PART I

Questions

DSM-5-TR Introduction

I.1 Which of the following differentiates the vetting process of contributors to DSM-5 from previous editions of DSM?

  A. Only clinicians were on the task force.
  B. Only researchers were on the task force.
  C. Disclosure of all income for members of the task force.
  D. Only physicians were on the task force.

I.2 Which of the following was not a principle guiding the DSM-5 draft revision process?

  A. DSM-5 was primarily intended to be a manual to be used by clinicians, and revisions must be feasible for routine clinical practice.
  B. Recommendations for revisions should be guided by research evidence.
  C. There were no considerations for maintaining continuity with previous editions of DSM.
  D. No a priori constraints should be placed on the degree of change between DSM-IV and DSM-5.

I.3 Which of the following best describes the use of DSM-5-TR in forensic settings?

  A. Anyone involved in forensic cases can use DSM-5-TR to arrive at a psychiatric diagnosis.
  B. A person who meets criteria of a diagnosis will also meet the standard for having a mental illness as defined by law.
  C. There is a risk that the diagnoses will be misused or misunderstood.
  D. A diagnosis carries implications regarding the etiology of the person's mental disorder.

CHAPTER 1

Neurodevelopmental Disorders

1.1 Which of the following is *not* required for a DSM-5-TR diagnosis of intellectual developmental disorder (intellectual disability)?

   A. Full-scale IQ below 70.
   B. Deficits in intellectual functions confirmed by clinical assessment and individualized, standardized intelligence testing.
   C. Deficits in adaptive functioning that result in failure to meet developmental and sociocultural standards for personal independence and social responsibility.
   D. Symptom onset during the developmental period.

1.2 A 7-year-old boy in second grade displays significant delays in his ability to reason, solve problems, and learn from experiences. He has been slow to develop skills in reading, writing, and mathematics. These skills have lagged behind peers throughout the child's development, although he is making slow progress. The deficits significantly impair his ability to play in an age-appropriate manner with peers and to begin to acquire independent skills at home. He requires ongoing assistance with basic skills (dressing, feeding, bathing, and doing any type of schoolwork) on a daily basis. Which of the following diagnoses best fits this presentation?

   A. Childhood-onset major neurocognitive disorder.
   B. Intellectual developmental disorder (intellectual disability).
   C. Communication disorder.
   D. Autism spectrum disorder.

1.3 A 7-year-old boy in second grade displays significant delays in his ability to reason, solve problems, and learn from his experiences. He has been slow to develop reading, writing, and mathematics skills in school. All through development, these skills lagged behind peers, although he is making slow progress. These deficits significantly impair his ability to play in an age-appropriate manner with peers and to begin to acquire independent skills at home. He requires ongoing assistance with basic skills (dressing, feeding, bathing, and doing any type of schoolwork) on a daily basis. What is the appropriate severity rating for this patient's current presentation?

A. Mild.
B. Moderate.
C. Severe.
D. Cannot be determined without an IQ score.

1.4   What can lead to an invalid assessment of overall mental abilities and adaptive functioning in individuals with intellectual developmental disorder?

A. Comparing the individual with age- and gender-matched peers from the same linguistic and sociocultural group.
B. A full-scale IQ score with highly discrepant subtest scores.
C. Using multiple IQ or other cognitive tests to create a profile.
D. Accounting for factors that may limit performance, such as sociocultural background, native language, associated communication/language disorder, and motor or sensory handicap.

1.5   A 15-year-old patient is enrolled in the eighth grade in a special education setting. She has an IQ of 70 and has trouble keeping track of time, although she is able to read a digital watch. It has taken considerable time for her family to teach her how to do simple tasks in the kitchen, and she continues to need supervision with the stove. She is able to socialize with other peers in her class but is no longer friends with other kids of similar age in the neighborhood. She attends a social skills group, but her parents must keep track of the appointments. What is the specifier for her current severity of intellectual developmental disorder (intellectual disability)?

A. Normal variation.
B. Mild.
C. Moderate.
D. Severe

1.6   Which of the following is *not* a diagnostic feature of intellectual developmental disorder (intellectual disability)?

A. Repetitive, seemingly driven, and apparently purposeless motor behavior (e.g., hand shaking, body rocking).
B. Inability to perform complex daily living tasks (e.g., money management, medical decision-making) without support.
C. Gullibility, with naiveté in social situations and a tendency to be easily led by others.
D. Lack of age-appropriate communication skills for social and interpersonal functioning.

1.7   How is adaptive functioning related to the diagnosis of intellectual develop-
       mental disorder (intellectual disability)?

       A. Adaptive functioning is based on an individual's IQ score.
       B. Impairment in at least two domains of adaptive functioning must be pres-
          ent to meet Criterion B for the diagnosis of intellectual developmental dis-
          order.
       C. Adaptive functioning in intellectual developmental disorder tends to im-
          prove over time, although the threshold of cognitive capacities and associ-
          ated developmental disorders can limit it.
       D. Individuals diagnosed with intellectual developmental disorder in child-
          hood will typically continue to meet criteria in adulthood even if their
          adaptive functioning improves.

1.8   In which of the following clinical scenarios could comorbid intellectual devel-
       opmental disorder (intellectual disability) occur as an acquired disorder?

       A. Lesch-Nyhan syndrome.
       B. Prader-Willi syndrome.
       C. Head trauma occurring during the developmental period.
       D. Rett syndrome.

1.9   Which of the following is a true statement about the developmental course of
       iintellectual developmental disorder (intellectual disability)?

       A. Delayed motor, language, and social milestones are not identifiable until af-
          ter the first 2 years of life.
       B. Intellectual disability caused by an illness (e.g., encephalitis) or by head
          trauma occurring during the developmental period would be diagnosed as
          a neurocognitive disorder, not as intellectual developmental disorder (intel-
          lectual disability).
       C. Major neurocognitive disorder may co-occur with intellectual developmen-
          tal disorder.
       D. Even if early and ongoing interventions throughout childhood and adult-
          hood lead to improved adaptive and intellectual functioning, the diagnosis
          of intellectual developmental disorder (intellectual disability) would con-
          tinue to apply.

1.10   The DSM-5-TR diagnosis of intellectual developmental disorder (intellectual
       disability) includes severity specifiers—mild, moderate, severe, and pro-
       found—to indicate the level of support required in various domains of adap-
       tive functioning. Which of the following features would be characteristic of an
       individual with a *mild* level of impairment?

       A. The individual generally has little understanding of written language or of
          concepts involving numbers, quantity, time, and money.

B. The individual's spoken language is quite limited in terms of vocabulary and grammar.

C. The individual requires support for all activities of daily living, including meals, dressing, bathing, and toileting.

D. In adulthood, the individual may be able to sustain competitive employment in a job that does not emphasize conceptual skills.

1.11 A 10-year-old boy with a history of dyslexia, who is otherwise developmentally normal, is in a skateboarding accident in which he experiences severe traumatic brain injury. This results in significant global intellectual impairment (with a persistent reading deficit that is more pronounced than his other newly acquired but stable deficits, along with a full-scale IQ of 75). There is mild impairment in his adaptive functioning such that he requires support in some areas of functioning. He is also displaying anxious and depressive symptoms in response to the accident and hospitalization. What is the *least likely* diagnosis?

A. Intellectual developmental disorder (intellectual disability).

B. Traumatic brain injury.

C. Major neurocognitive disorder due to traumatic brain injury.

D. Adjustment disorder.

1.12 In which of the following situations would a diagnosis of global developmental delay be *inappropriate*?

A. The patient is a child who is too young to fully manifest specific symptoms or to complete requisite assessments.

B. The patient, a 7-year-old child, has a full-scale IQ of 65 and severe impairment in adaptive functioning.

C. The patient's scores on psychometric tests suggest intellectual developmental disorder (intellectual disability), but there is insufficient information about the patient's adaptive functional skills.

D. The patient's impaired adaptive functioning suggests intellectual developmental disorder, but there is insufficient information about the level of cognitive impairment measured by standardized instruments.

1.13 For whom should a clinician consider the diagnosis of global developmental delay?

A. Children younger than age 5 years.

B. Children who can undergo systematic assessments.

C. Children with a full-scale IQ <65.

D. Children with a diagnosis of intellectual developmental disorder (intellectual disability), severe.

1.14 A 3½-year-old girl with a history of lead exposure and a seizure disorder demonstrates substantial delays across multiple domains of functioning, including communication, learning, attention, and motor development, which limit her ability to interact with same-age peers and require substantial support in all activities of daily living at home. Unfortunately, her parents are extremely poor historians, and the child has received no formal psychological or learning evaluation to date. She is about to be evaluated for readiness to attend preschool. What is the most appropriate diagnosis?

A. Major neurocognitive disorder.
B. Autism spectrum disorder.
C. Global developmental delay.
D. Specific learning disorder.

1.15 A 5-year-old boy has difficulty making friends and has problems with initiating and sustaining back-and-forth conversation, reading social cues, and sharing his feelings with others. He makes good eye contact, has normal speech intonation, displays facial gestures, and has a range of affect that generally seems appropriate to the situation. He demonstrates an interest in trains that seems abnormal in intensity and focus, and he engages in little imaginative or symbolic play. Which of the following diagnostic requirements for autism spectrum disorder are *not* met in this case?

A. Deficits in social-emotional reciprocity.
B. Deficits in nonverbal communicative behaviors used for social interaction.
C. Deficits in developing and maintaining relationships.
D. Restricted, repetitive patterns of behavior, interests, or activities as manifested by symptoms in two of the specified four categories.

1.16 Which of the following statements about the development and course of autism spectrum disorder is *false*?

A. Symptoms of autism spectrum disorder are usually not noticeable until ages 5–6 years or later.
B. First symptoms frequently involve delayed language development, often accompanied by lack of social interest or unusual social interactions.
C. Autism spectrum disorder is not a degenerative disorder, and it is typical for learning and compensation to continue throughout life.
D. Because many normally developing young children have strong preferences and enjoy repetition, distinguishing restricted and repetitive behaviors that are diagnostic of autism spectrum disorder can be difficult in preschoolers.

1.17 Which of the following was a criterion symptom for autistic disorder in DSM-IV that was eliminated from the diagnostic criteria for autism spectrum disorder in DSM-5-TR?

A. Stereotyped or restricted patterns of interest.
B. Stereotyped and repetitive motor mannerisms.
C. Inflexible adherence to routines.
D. Persistent preoccupation with parts of objects.

1.18   A 7-year-old girl presents with a history of normal language skills (vocabulary and grammar intact) but is unable to use language in a socially pragmatic manner to share ideas and feelings. She has never made good eye contact and has difficulty reading social cues. Consequently, she has had difficulty making friends, which is further complicated by her obsession with cartoon characters, which she repetitively scripts. She tends to excessively smell objects. Because she insists on wearing the same shirt and shorts every day, regardless of the season, getting dressed is a difficult activity. These symptoms date from early childhood and cause significant impairment in her functioning. What diagnosis best fits this child's presentation?

   A. Asperger's disorder.
   B. Autism spectrum disorder.
   C. Social (pragmatic) communication disorder.
   D. Rett syndrome.

1.19   A 15-year-old teenager has a long history of nonverbal communication deficits. As an infant, he was unable to shift his gaze in the direction someone else pointed. As a toddler, he was not interested in social events, discussing feelings, or playing games with others, including his own family. From school age into adolescence, his speech was odd in tonality and phrasing, and his body language was awkward. What do these symptoms represent?

   A. Restricted range of interests.
   B. Developmental regression.
   C. Prodromal schizophreniform symptoms.
   D. Deficits in nonverbal communicative behaviors.

1.20   A 10-year-old boy demonstrates hand-flapping and finger flicking. He repetitively flips coins and lines up his trucks. He tends to "echo" the last several words of a question posed to him before answering, mixes up his pronouns (refers to himself in the second person), tends to repeat phrases in a perseverative fashion, and is quite fixated on routines related to dress, eating, travel, and play. He spends hours in the garage playing with his father's tools. What do these behaviors represent?

   A. Restricted, repetitive patterns of behaviors, interests, or activities characteristic of autism spectrum disorder.
   B. Symptoms of obsessive-compulsive disorder.
   C. Prototypical manifestations of obsessive-compulsive personality.
   D. Complex tics.

1.21   A 25-year-old man presents with long-standing nonverbal communication deficits, inability to have a back-and-forth conversation or share interests in an appropriate fashion, and a complete lack of interest in having relationships with others. His speech reflects awkward phrasing and intonation and is mechanical in nature. He has a history of sequential fixations and obsessions with various games and objects throughout childhood; however, this is not currently a major issue for him. He is living in an assisted living residence and follows the same routine daily. He works at the register in the store in the residence because he enjoys math, and his wages are managed by a guardian. When the store is closed for holidays, he has a hard time adjusting to the change. What is the appropriate diagnosis?

A. Intellectual developmental disorder (intellectual disability), moderate.
B. Intellectual developmental disorder (intellectual disability), severe.
C. Autism spectrum disorder, level 1 ("requiring support").
D. Autism spectrum disorder, level 2 ("requiring substantial support").

1.22   A 9-year-old girl presents with a history of intellectual impairment, a structural language impairment, nonverbal communication deficits, disinterest in peers, and inability to use language in a social manner. She has extreme food and tactile sensitivities. She is obsessed with one particular computer game that she plays for hours each day, scripting and imitating the characters. She is clumsy, has an odd gait, and walks on her tiptoes. In the past year, she developed a seizure disorder and has begun to bang her wrists against the wall repetitively, causing bruising. On the other hand, she plays several musical instruments in an extremely precocious manner. Which feature of this child's clinical presentation fulfills a criterion symptom for DSM-5-TR autism spectrum disorder?

A. Motor abnormalities.
B. Structural language impairment.
C. Intellectual impairment.
D. Nonverbal communicative deficits.

1.23   An 11-year-old girl with autism spectrum disorder displays no spoken language and is minimally responsive to overtures from others. She can be somewhat inflexible, which interferes with her ability to travel, do schoolwork, and be managed in the home. She has difficulty planning, organizing, and transitioning activities. These problems can usually be managed with incentives and reinforcers. What severity levels should be specified in the DSM-5-TR diagnosis?

A. Level 3 (requiring very substantial support) for social communication and level 1 (requiring support) for restricted, repetitive behaviors.
B. Level 1 (requiring support) for social communication and level 3 (requiring very substantial support) for restricted, repetitive behaviors.
C. Level 1 (requiring support) for social communication and level 1 (requiring support) for restricted, repetitive behaviors.
D. Level 2 (requiring substantial support) for social communication and level 1 (requiring support) for restricted, repetitive behaviors.

1.24   Which of the following is *not* a specifier included in the diagnostic criteria for autism spectrum disorder?

A. With or without accompanying intellectual impairment.
B. With or without associated dementia.

C. Associated with a known medical or genetic condition or environmental factor.

D. Associated with another neurodevelopmental, mental, or behavioral disorder.

1.25   Which of the following is *not* typical for the developmental course of children diagnosed with autism spectrum disorder?

A. Developmental gains in later childhood.

B. Early, prominent lack of interest in social interaction.

C. Regression across multiple domains occurring after age 2–3 years.

D. First symptoms that often include delayed language development.

1.26   A 4-year-old girl has some food aversions. She enjoys having the same book read to her at night but does not become terribly upset if her mother asks her to choose a different book. She spins around repeatedly when her favorite show is on television. She generally likes her toys neatly arranged in bins and complains when her sister leaves them on the floor. With which of the following diagnoses are these behaviors consistent?

A. Obsessive-compulsive disorder.

B. Autism spectrum disorder.

C. Attention-deficit/hyperactivity disorder.

D. Typical development.

1.27   Which of the following is typical for the developmental course for autism spectrum disorder?

A. Lack of degenerative course.

B. Behavioral deterioration during adolescence.

C. Reduction in learning throughout life.

D. Absence of symptoms in early childhood and early school years, with developmental losses in later childhood in areas such as social interaction.

1.28   A 21-year-old patient, who was not previously diagnosed with a developmental disorder, presents for evaluation after taking a leave from college for psychological reasons. He makes little eye contact, does not appear to pick up on social cues, has become disinterested in friends, spends hours each day on the computer surfing the internet and playing games, and has become so sensitive to smells that he keeps multiple air fresheners in all locations of the home. He reports that he has had long-standing friendships dating from childhood and high school (corroborated by his parents). He reports making many friends in his social club at college. His parents report good social and communication skills in childhood, although he was quite shy and somewhat inflexible and ritualistic at home. What is the *least likely* diagnosis?

A. Depression.

B. Schizophreniform disorder or schizophrenia.

C. Autism spectrum disorder.

D. Social anxiety disorder (social phobia).

1.29   Which of the following characteristics is generally *not* associated with autism spectrum disorder?

A. Anxiety, depression, and isolation as an adult.

B. Catatonia.

C. Insistence on routines and aversion to change.

D. Successful adaptation in regular school settings.

1.30   Which of the following disorders is generally *not* comorbid with autism spectrum disorder?

A. Attention-deficit/hyperactivity disorder (ADHD).

B. Selective mutism.

C. Intellectual developmental disorder (intellectual disability).

D. Stereotypic movement disorder.

1.31   Which of the following is *not* a criterion for the DSM-5-TR diagnosis of attention-deficit/hyperactivity disorder (ADHD)?

A. Onset of several inattentive or hyperactive-impulsive symptoms prior to age 12 years.

B. Manifestation of several inattentive or hyperactive-impulsive symptoms in two or more settings (e.g., at home, school, or work; with friends or relatives; in other activities).

C. Persistence of symptoms for at least 12 months.

D. Inability to explain symptoms as a manifestation of another mental disorder (e.g., mood disorder, anxiety disorder, dissociative disorder, personality disorder, substance intoxication or withdrawal).

1.32   The parents of a 15-year-old tenth grader believe that she should be doing better in high school, given how bright she seems and the fact that she received mostly As through eighth grade. However, her papers are frequently handed in late, and she makes careless mistakes on examinations. On formal testing, her Wechsler Adult Intelligence Scale, 4th Edition (WAIS-IV) results are as follows: Verbal IQ, 125; Perceptual Reasoning Index, 122; Full-Scale IQ, 123; Working Memory Index, 55th percentile; Processing Speed Index, 50th percentile. Weaknesses in executive function are noted. During a psychiatric evaluation, the teenager reports a long history of failing to give close attention to details; difficulty sustaining attention while in class or doing homework; failing to finish chores and tasks; and significant difficulties with time management, planning, and organization. She is forgetful, often loses things, and is easily distracted. She has no history of restlessness or impulsivity and is well liked by peers. What is the most likely diagnosis?

A. Adjustment disorder with anxiety.

B. Specific learning disorder.

C. Attention-deficit/hyperactivity disorder, predominantly inattentive.

D. Major depressive disorder.

1.33 A 7-year-old boy is having behavioral and social difficulties in his second-grade class. Although he seems to be able to pay attention and is doing "well" from an academic standpoint (although seemingly not up to his assumed capabilities), he is constantly interrupting, fidgeting, talking excessively, and getting out of his seat. He has friends but sometimes annoys his peers because of difficulty sharing and taking turns and frequently talking over others. Although he seeks out play dates, he exhausts his friends by wanting to play sports nonstop. At home, he can barely stay in his seat for a meal and is unable to play quietly. Although he shows remorse when the consequences of his behavior are pointed out to him, he can become angry in response and nevertheless is unable to inhibit himself. What is the most likely diagnosis?

A. Autism spectrum disorder.

B. Generalized anxiety disorder.

C. Attention-deficit/hyperactivity disorder, predominantly hyperactive/impulsive.

D. Specific learning disorder.

1.34 A 37-year-old stock trader schedules a visit after his 8-year-old son is diagnosed with attention-deficit/hyperactivity disorder (ADHD), combined inattentive and hyperactive. Although the patient does not currently note motor restlessness like his son, he recalls being that way as a child, along with being quite inattentive, being impulsive, talking excessively, interrupting, and having problems waiting his turn. He was an underachiever in high school and college, when he did his work inconsistently and had difficulty following rules. Nevertheless, he never failed any classes and was never evaluated by a psychologist or psychiatrist. Currently, he works about 60–80 hours a week and often gets insufficient sleep. He tends to make impulsive business decisions, can be impatient and short-tempered, and notes that his mind tends to wander both in one-on-one interactions with associates and his wife and during business meetings, for which he is often late; he is forgetful and disorganized. Overall, he tends to perform fairly well and is quite successful, but he frequently feels overwhelmed and demoralized. What is the most likely diagnosis?

A. Major depressive disorder.

B. Generalized anxiety disorder.

C. Specific learning disorder.

D. ADHD, in partial remission.

1.35 A hyperactive, impulsive, and inattentive 5-year-old boy presents with hypertelorism, highly arched palate, and low-set ears. He is uncoordinated and clumsy, has no sense of time, and constantly leaves toys and clothes strewn all over the house. He recently developed what appears to be a motor tic involving blinking. He enjoys playing with peers, who tend to like him, although he seems to willfully defy all requests from parents and teachers, which does not seem to be due simply to inattention. He is delayed in beginning to learn how to read. What is the *least likely* diagnosis?

A. Autism spectrum disorder.
B. Developmental coordination disorder.
C. Oppositional defiant disorder (ODD).
D. Attention-deficit/hyperactivity disorder (ADHD).

1.36   What is the prevalence of attention-deficit/hyperactivity disorder (ADHD) in children?

A. 2%.
B. 7%.
C. 10%.
D. 12%.

1.37   What is the prevalence of attention-deficit/hyperactivity disorder (ADHD) in adults?

A. 0.5%.
B. 2.5%.
C. 5%.
D. 8%.

1.38   What is the gender ratio of attention-deficit/hyperactivity disorder (ADHD) in children?

A. Male:female ratio of 2:1.
B. Male:female ratio of 3:2.
C. Male:female ratio of 5:1.
D. Male:female ratio of 1:2.

1.39   A child is born with very low birth weight and had prenatal exposure to smoking. He is currently being treated for encephalitis. Which neurodevelopmental disorder should the parents consider as a possibility for their child?

A. Attention deficit/hyperactivity disorder (ADHD).
B. Specific learning disorder.
C. Stereotypic movement disorder.
D. Childhood-onset fluency disorder.

1.40   Which of the following is *not* associated with attention-deficit/hyperactivity disorder (ADHD)?

A. Reduced school performance.

B. Higher probability of unemployment.

C. Elevated interpersonal conflict.

D. Reduced risk of substance use disorders.

1.41   Which of the following is *not* associated with attention-deficit/hyperactivity disorder (ADHD)?

A. Social rejection.

B. Increased risk of developing conduct disorder in childhood and antisocial personality disorder in adulthood.

C. Increased risk of Alzheimer's disease.

D. Increased risk of accidental injury.

1.42   A 15-year-old has developed concentration problems in school that have been associated with a significant decline in grades. When interviewed, he explains that his mind is occupied with worrying about his mother, who has a serious autoimmune disease. As his grades falter, he becomes increasingly demoralized and sad and notices that his energy levels drop, further compromising his ability to pay attention in school. At the same time, he complains of feeling restless and unable to sleep. What is the most likely diagnosis?

A. Specific learning disorder.

B. Attention-deficit/hyperactivity disorder (ADHD).

C. Adjustment disorder with mixed anxiety and depressed mood.

D. Separation anxiety disorder.

1.43   A 5-year-old boy is consistently moody, irritable, and intolerant of frustration. In addition, he is pervasively and chronically restless, impulsive, and inattentive. Which diagnosis best fits the clinical picture?

A. Attention-deficit/hyperactivity disorder (ADHD).

B. ADHD and disruptive mood dysregulation disorder (DMDD).

C. Bipolar disorder.

D. Oppositional defiant disorder (ODD).

1.44   Which comorbidity is found in a minority of children with attention-deficit/hyperactivity disorder (ADHD)?

A. Oppositional defiant disorder (ODD).

B. Disruptive mood dysregulation disorder (DMDD).

C. Intermittent explosive disorder.

D. Specific learning disorder.

1.45   What are the characteristics of specific learning disorder?

A. It is part of a more general learning impairment as manifested in intellectual developmental disorder (intellectual disability).

B. It usually can be attributed to a sensory, physical, or neurological disorder.

C. It involves pervasive and wide-ranging deficits across multiple domains of information processing.

D. It consists of persistent difficulties learning keystone academic skills with onset during the years of formal schooling.

1.46 DSM-5-TR classifies all learning disorders under the diagnosis of specific learning disorder, along with the requirement to "specify all academic domains and subskills that are impaired" at the time of assessment. What is *not* characteristic of specific learning disorder?

A. The persistent learning difficulties manifest as restricted progress in learning for at least 6 months despite the provision of extra help at home or school.

B. Current skills in one or more of these academic areas are well below the average range for the individual's age, gender, cultural group, and level of education.

C. There usually is a discrepancy of more than 3 standard deviations (SDs) between achievement and IQ.

D. The learning difficulties significantly interfere with academic achievement, occupational performance, or activities of daily living that require these academic skills.

1.47 What is associated with the diagnosis of specific learning disorder?

A. A neurodegenerative cognitive disorder.
B. An uneven profile of abilities.
C. Lack of educational opportunity.
D. There are four formal subtypes of specific learning disorder.

1.48 What is associated with prevalence rates for specific learning disorder?

A. Prevalence rates range from 1% to 5% among school-age children across languages and cultures.

B. Specific learning disorder is equally common among males and females.

C. Prevalence rates vary according to the range of ages in the sample, selection criteria, severity of specific learning disorder, and academic domains investigated.

D. Gender ratios can be attributed to factors such as ascertainment bias, definitional or measurement variation, language, race, or socioeconomic status.

1.49 What disorder(s) is/are typically comorbid with specific learning disorders?

A. Attention-deficit/hyperactivity disorder (ADHD).
B. Speech sound disorder.
C. Developmental coordination disorder.
D. All of the above.

1.50   Which of the following is *not* associated with developmental coordination disorder (DCD)?

A. Additional (usually suppressed) motor activity, such as choreiform movements of unsupported limbs or mirror movements.
B. Improvement in learning new tasks involving complex/automatic motor skills, including driving and using tools.
C. Prenatal exposure to alcohol.
D. Impairments in underlying neurodevelopmental processes affecting visuomotor skills.

1.51   Which of the following statements about developmental coordination disorder (DCD) is *true*?

A. Symptoms have usually improved significantly at 1-year follow-up.
B. In most cases, symptoms are no longer evident by adolescence.
C. DCD has no clear relationship with prenatal alcohol exposure, preterm birth, or low birth weight.
D. Cerebellar dysfunction is hypothesized to play a role in DCD.

1.52   Which of the following is *not* a criterion for the DSM-5-TR diagnosis of stereotypic movement disorder?

A. Repetitive, seemingly driven, and apparently purposeless movements are present.
B. Onset occurs during the early developmental period.
C. Behaviors result in self-inflicted bodily injury.
D. Behaviors are not attributable to the effects of a substance or neurological condition.

1.53   Which of the following is *not* consistent with stereotypic movement disorder?

A. The presence of stereotypic movements may indicate an undetected neurodevelopmental problem, especially in children ages 1–3 years.
B. Among typically developing children, the repetitive movements may be stopped when attention is directed to them or when the child is distracted from performing them.
C. In some children, the stereotypic movements would result in self-injury if protective measures were not used.
D. Stereotypic movements typically begin within the first year of life.

1.54   Which of the following is a DSM-5-TR diagnostic criterion for Tourette's disorder?

A. Tics occur throughout a period of more than 1 year without a tic-free period of more than 3 consecutive months.
B. Onset is before age 5 years.

C. Tics may wax and wane in frequency but have persisted for more than 1 year since first tic onset.

D. Motor tics must precede vocal tics.

1.55 At an 8-year-old boy's third office visit, his mother describes a 6-month history of excessive eye blinking and intermittent chirping, noting that these characteristics have also been accompanied by grunting sounds since the recent start of a new school term. What is the most likely diagnosis?

A. Tourette's disorder.

B. Provisional tic disorder.

C. Persistent (chronic) vocal tic disorder.

D. Transient tic disorder, recurrent.

1.56 A 5-year-old girl is referred to your care with a DSM-IV diagnosis of chronic motor or vocal tic disorder. She has had motor tics only since a year ago, and there were 2 months when there were no tics. Which diagnosis is consistent under DSM-5-TR criteria?

A. Tourette's disorder.

B. Provisional tic disorder.

C. Persistent (chronic) motor tic disorder.

D. Other specified tic disorder.

1.57 A highly functional 20-year-old college student with a history of anxiety symptoms and attention-deficit/hyperactivity disorder, for which she is prescribed lisdexamfetamine (Vyvanse), tells her psychiatrist that she has been researching the side effects of her medication for one of her class projects. In addition, she says that for the past week she has been feeling stressed by her schoolwork, and her friends have been asking her why she intermittently bobs her head up and down multiple times a day. What is the most likely diagnosis?

A. Provisional tic disorder.

B. Unspecified tic disorder.

C. Unspecified stimulant use disorder.

D. Unspecified stimulant-induced disorder.

1.58 Which of the following is *not* a DSM-5-TR diagnostic criterion for language disorder?

A. Persistent difficulties in the acquisition and use of language across modalities due to deficits in comprehension or production.

B. Language abilities that are substantially and quantifiably below those expected for age.

C. Inability to attribute difficulties to hearing or other sensory impairment, motor dysfunction, or another medical or neurological condition.

D. Failure to meet criteria for mixed receptive-expressive language disorder or a pervasive developmental disorder.

1.59   Which of the following statements about speech sound disorder is *true*?

   A. Speech sound production must be present by age 2 years.
   B. "Failure to use developmentally expected speech sounds" is assessed by comparison of a child with their peers of the same age and dialect.
   C. The difficulties in speech sound production need not result in functional impairment to meet diagnostic criteria.
   D. Symptom onset is in the early developmental period.

1.60   A parent brings a 4-year-old child to you for an evaluation with concerns that he has struggled with speech articulation since early development. He has not sustained any head injuries, is otherwise healthy, and has a normal IQ. His preschool teacher reports that it is difficult to understand what the boy is saying and that other children tease him by calling him a "baby" because of his difficulty with communication. He does not have trouble relating to other people or understanding nonverbal social cues. What is the most likely diagnosis?

   A. Selective mutism.
   B. Global developmental delay.
   C. Speech sound disorder.
   D. Unspecified anxiety disorder.

1.61   A 6-year-old boy is failing school and continues to struggle significantly with grammar, sentence construction, and vocabulary. He also interjects "and" in between all words when speaking. He is generally quiet and does not cause trouble otherwise. He is playful with peers and enjoys playing soccer at recess. He switches between music class and lunch easily. Which of the following diagnoses would be on your differential?

   A. Language disorder.
   B. Expressive language disorder.
   C. Childhood-onset fluency disorder.
   D. Autism spectrum disorder.

1.62   Which of the following types of disturbance in speech is *not* included in the DSM-5-TR criteria for childhood-onset fluency disorder (stuttering)?

   A. Sound prolongation.
   B. Reduced vocabulary.
   C. Circumlocutions.
   D. Sound and syllable repetitions.

1.63   A 14-year-old in regular education tells you that he believes a classmate likes him. His mother is surprised to hear this because, since a young age, he has often struggled with making inferences or understanding nuances from what other people say. His teacher has also noticed that he sometimes misses nonverbal cues. He tends to get along better with adults, perhaps because they are not as likely to be put off by a stilted speech pattern. When he makes jokes, his peers do not always find the humor appropriate. Although he enjoys spending time with his best friend engaging in a wide range of activities, he can be talkative and struggles with taking turns in conversation. What is the most likely diagnosis?

A. Social (pragmatic) communication disorder.
B. Autism spectrum disorder.
C. Social anxiety disorder.
D. Language disorder.

1.64   A 15-year-old with a prior diagnosis of Tourette's disorder is referred to your care. His mother tells you that during middle school, he was teased for having vocal and motor tics. Since he started ninth grade, his tics have become less frequent. Currently, only mild motor tics remain. What is the appropriate DSM-5-TR diagnosis?

A. Tourette's disorder.
B. Persistent (chronic) motor tic disorder.
C. Provisional tic disorder.
D. Unspecified tic disorder.

1.65   The onset of tics typically occurs for the first time during which developmental stage?

A. Prepuberty.
B. Latency.
C. Adolescence.
D. Adulthood.

1.66   A 7-year-old boy with a history of speech delay presents with long-standing repetitive hand waving, arm flapping, and finger wiggling. His mother reports that these symptoms first appeared when he was a toddler and wonders whether they could represent tics. She reports that he tends to flap more when he is engrossed in activities, such as while watching a favorite television program, but will stop when called or distracted. On the basis of the mother's report, which of the following conditions would be highest on your list of possible diagnoses?

A. Persistent (chronic) motor or vocal tic disorder.
B. Chorea.
C. Dystonia.
D. Motor stereotypies.

1.67   Assessment of co-occurring conditions is important for understanding the overall functional consequence of tics on an individual. Which of the following conditions has been associated with tic disorders?

A. Attention-deficit/hyperactivity disorder (ADHD).
B. Obsessive-compulsive and related disorders.
C. Depressive disorders.
D. All of the above.

1.68　By what age should most children have acquired adequate speech and language ability to understand and follow social rules of verbal and nonverbal communication, follow rules for conversation and storytelling, and change language according to the needs of the listener or situation?

A. Age 3–4 years.
B. Age 4–5 years.
C. Age 5–6 years.
D. Age 6–7 years.

1.69　Having a family history of which of the following psychiatric disorders increases an individual's risk of social (pragmatic) communication disorder?

A. Social anxiety disorder (social phobia).
B. Autism spectrum disorder.
C. Attention-deficit/hyperactivity disorder (ADHD).
D. Intellectual developmental disorder (intellectual disability)

1.70　A 6-year-old boy with a history of mild language delay is brought to your office by his mother, who is concerned that the boy is being teased in school because he misinterprets nonverbal cues and speaks in overly formal language with his peers. She tells you that her son was in an early intervention program, but his written and spoken language is now at grade level. The boy does not have a history of repetitive movements, sensory issues, or ritualized behaviors. Although he prefers constancy, he adapts fairly well to new situations. Additionally, he has a long-standing interest in trains and cars and is able to recite for you all the car models he memorized from a book on the history of transportation. Which of the following disorders would be a primary consideration in the differential diagnosis?

A. Social (pragmatic) communication disorder.
B. Autism spectrum disorder.
C. Global developmental delay.
D. Language disorder.

1.71　Below what age is it difficult to distinguish a language disorder from normal developmental variations?

A. <3 years.
B. <4 years.
C. <5 years.
D. <6 years.

1.72   Which of the following psychiatric diagnoses is strongly associated with language disorder?

A. Attention-deficit/hyperactivity disorder (ADHD).
B. Diurnal enuresis.
C. Generalized anxiety disorder.
D. Disruptive mood dysregulation disorder.

1.73   Which of the following statements about the development of speech as it applies to speech sound disorder is *false*?

A. Most children with speech sound disorder respond well to treatment.
B. Speech sound production should be mostly intelligible by age 3 years.
C. Most speech sounds should be pronounced clearly and accurately according to age and community norms before age 10 years.
D. It is abnormal for children to shorten words when they are learning to talk.

1.74   Which of the following would likely *not* be an important condition to rule out in the differential diagnosis of speech sound disorder?

A. Normal variations in speech.
B. Hearing or other sensory impairment.
C. Dysarthria.
D. Depression.

1.75   Which of the following statements about the development of childhood-onset fluency disorder (stuttering) is *true*?

A. Stuttering occurs by age 6 for 80%–90% of affected individuals.
B. Stuttering always begins abruptly and is noticeable to everyone.
C. Stress and anxiety do not exacerbate disfluency.
D. Motor movements are not associated with this disorder.

1.76   An 18-year-old who moved from Mexico to the United States when he was 8 years old is now entering college. He has been able to arrange financial aid and a work study schedule. He wants academic support in college, and the Office of Academic Support has referred him to you. In the process of completing an evaluation, you contact the student's high school teachers, who share that he struggled with essay writing in all social studies and literature classes. In his last 6 months of high school, he used study hall and tutoring sessions to work on grammar and organization and needed extra time to complete written assignments. With these supports, he was able to pass these courses with a 75% average. What is the most likely diagnosis?

A. Expressive language disorder.
B. Specific learning disorder with impairment in written expression.
C. Social (pragmatic) communication disorder.
D. Intellectual developmental disorder (intellectual disability), mild.

CHAPTER 2

Schizophrenia Spectrum and Other Psychotic Disorders

2.1   Criterion A for schizoaffective disorder requires an uninterrupted period of illness during which Criterion A for schizophrenia is met. Which of the following additional symptoms must be present to fulfill diagnostic criteria for schizoaffective disorder?

   A. An anxiety episode—either panic or general anxiety.
   B. Rapid eye movement (REM) sleep behavior disorder.
   C. A major depressive or manic episode.
   D. Cyclothymia.

2.2   In order to differentiate schizoaffective disorder from depressive or bipolar disorder with psychotic features, which of the following symptoms must be present for at least 2 weeks in the absence of a major mood episode at some point during the lifetime duration of the illness?

   A. Delusions or hallucinations.
   B. Delusions or paranoia.
   C. Regressed behavior.
   D. Projective identification.

2.3   A 27-year-old unmarried truck driver has a 5-year history of active and residual symptoms of schizophrenia. He develops symptoms of depression, including depressed mood and anhedonia. These symptoms last 4 months and resolve with treatment but do not meet criteria for major depression. Which diagnosis best fits this clinical presentation?

   A. Schizoaffective disorder.
   B. Unspecified schizophrenia spectrum and other psychotic disorder.
   C. Unspecified depressive disorder.
   D. Schizophrenia and unspecified depressive disorder.

2.4   How common is schizoaffective disorder relative to schizophrenia?

A. Twice as common.
B. Equally common.
C. One-half as common.
D. One-third as common.

2.5   A 30-year-old single woman reports having experienced auditory and perse-
       cutory delusions for 2 months, followed by a full major depressive episode
       with sad mood, anhedonia, and suicidal ideation lasting 3 months. Although
       the depressive episode resolves with pharmacotherapy and psychotherapy,
       the psychotic symptoms persist for another month before resolving. What di-
       agnosis best fits this clinical picture?

       A. Brief psychotic disorder.
       B. Schizoaffective disorder.
       C. Major depressive disorder.
       D. Major depressive disorder with psychotic features.

2.6   Which of the following statements about the incidence of schizoaffective disor-
       der is *true*?

       A. The incidence is equal in women and men.
       B. The incidence is higher in men.
       C. The incidence is higher in women.
       D. The incidence rates vary based on seasonality of birth.

2.7   Substance/medication-induced psychotic disorder cannot be diagnosed if the
       disturbance is better explained by an independent psychotic disorder that is
       not induced by a substance or medication. Which of the following psychotic
       symptom presentations would *not* be evidence of an independent psychotic
       disorder?

       A. Psychotic symptoms that meet full criteria for a psychotic disorder and that
          persist for a substantial period after cessation of severe intoxication or acute
          withdrawal.
       B. Psychotic symptoms that are substantially in excess of what would be ex-
          pected given the type or amount of the substance used or the duration of use.
       C. Psychotic symptoms that occur during a period of sustained substance ab-
          stinence.
       D. Psychotic symptoms that occur during a medical admission for substance
          withdrawal.

2.8   A 55-year-old man with a known history of alcohol dependence and schizo-
       phrenia is brought to the emergency department because of frank delusions
       and visual hallucinations. Which of the following would *not* be a diagnostic
       possibility for inclusion in the differential diagnosis?

       A. Substance/medication-induced psychotic disorder.
       B. Alcohol dependence.

C. Psychotic disorder due to another medical condition.

D. Borderline personality disorder with psychotic features.

2.9   Which of the following sets of specifiers is included in the DSM-5-TR diagnostic criteria for substance/medication-induced psychotic disorder?

A. *With onset before intoxication* and *with onset before withdrawal*.

B. *With onset during intoxication* and *with onset during withdrawal*.

C. *With good prognostic features* and *without good prognostic features*.

D. *With catatonia* and *without catatonia*.

2.10   A 65-year-old man with systemic lupus erythematosus, who is being treated with corticosteroids, witnesses a serious motor vehicle accident. He begins to have disorganized speech, which lasts for several days before resolving. What diagnosis best fits this clinical picture?

A. Psychotic disorder associated with systemic lupus erythematosus.

B. Steroid-induced psychosis.

C. Brief psychotic disorder, with marked stressor.

D. Schizoaffective disorder.

2.11   Which of the following psychotic symptom presentations would *not* be appropriately diagnosed as *other specified schizophrenia spectrum and other psychotic disorder*?

A. Psychotic symptoms that have lasted for less than 1 month but have not yet remitted, so the criteria for brief psychotic disorder are not met.

B. Persistent auditory hallucinations occurring in the absence of any other features.

C. Postpartum psychosis that does not meet criteria for a depressive or bipolar disorder with psychotic features, brief psychotic disorder, psychotic disorder due to another medical condition, or substance/medication-induced psychotic disorder.

D. Psychotic symptoms that are temporally related to use of a substance.

2.12   Which of the following patient presentations would *not* be classified as psychotic for the purpose of diagnosing schizophrenia?

A. A patient is hearing a voice that tells him he is a special person.

B. A patient believes he is being followed by a secret police organization that is focused exclusively on him.

C. A patient has a flashback to a war experience that feels like it is happening again.

D. A patient cannot organize his thoughts and stops responding in the middle of an interview.

2.13   Which of the following would rule out a diagnosis of brief psychotic disorder?

A. Continuation of symptoms for 6 weeks, followed by complete resolution.

B. Visions of a religious figure occurring in several individuals during a religious ceremony.

C. Severe impairment from the symptoms that requires nutritional support.

D. A suicide attempt.

2.14 A 32-year-old man presents to the emergency department distressed and agitated. He reports that his sister has been killed in a car accident on a trip to South America. When asked how he found out, he says that he and his sister were very close and he "just knows it." After being put on the phone with his sister, who was comfortably staying with friends while on her trip, the man expressed relief that she was alive. Which of the following descriptions best fits this presentation?

A. He did not have a delusional belief because it changed in light of new evidence.

B. He had a grandiose delusion because he believed he could know things happening far away.

C. He had a nihilistic delusion because it involved an untrue, imagined catastrophe.

D. He did not have a delusion because in some cultures people believe they can know things about family members outside ordinary communications.

2.15 Which of the following is *not* a commonly recognized type of delusion?

A. Persecutory.

B. Alien abduction.

C. Somatic.

D. Grandiose.

2.16 A 64-year-old man who had been a widower for 3 months presents to the emergency department on the advice of his primary care physician after he reports to the doctor that he hears his deceased wife's voice calling his name when he looks through old photos and sometimes as he is trying to fall asleep. His primary care physician tells him he is having a psychotic episode and needs to get a psychiatric evaluation. Which of the following statements correctly explains why these experiences should not be considered to be psychotic?

A. The experience occurs as he is falling asleep.

B. He can invoke her voice with certain activities.

C. The voice calls his name.

D. Both A and B.

2.17 Which of the following does *not* represent a negative symptom of schizophrenia?

A. Affective flattening.

B. Decreased motivation.

C. Impoverished thought processes.

D. Sadness over loss of functionality.

2.18 Schizophrenia spectrum and other psychotic disorders are defined by abnormalities in one or more of five domains, four of which are also considered psychotic symptoms. Which of the following is *not* considered a psychotic symptom?

A. Delusions.
B. Hallucinations.
C. Disorganized thinking.
D. Avolition.

2.19 What is the most common type of delusion?

A. Somatic delusion of distorted body appearance.
B. Grandiose delusion.
C. Thought insertion.
D. Persecutory delusion.

2.20 Which of the following presentations would *not* be classified as disorganized behavior for the purpose of diagnosing schizophrenia spectrum and other psychotic disorders?

A. Masturbating in public.
B. Wearing slacks on one's head.
C. Speaking in tongues during a religious retreat.
D. Turning to face 180 degrees away from the interviewer when answering questions.

2.21 Which of the following statements about catatonic motor behaviors is *false*?

A. Catatonic motor behavior is a type of grossly disorganized behavior that has historically been associated with schizophrenia spectrum and other psychotic disorders.
B. Catatonic motor behaviors may occur in many mental disorders (such as mood disorders) and in other medical conditions.
C. A behavior is considered catatonic only if it involves motoric slowing or rigidity, such as mutism, posturing, or waxy flexibility.
D. Catatonia can be diagnosed independently of another psychiatric disorder.

2.22 Which of the following statements about negative symptoms of schizophrenia is *false*?

A. Negative symptoms are easily distinguished from medication side effects such as sedation.
B. Negative symptoms include diminished emotional expression.
C. Negative symptoms can be difficult to distinguish from medication side effects such as sedation.
D. Negative symptoms include reduced peer or social interaction.

2.23   Which of the following statements correctly describes a way in which schizoaffective disorder may be differentiated from bipolar disorder?

A. In bipolar disorder, psychotic symptoms do not last longer than 1 month.
B. In bipolar disorder, psychotic symptoms always co-occur with mood symptoms.
C. Schizoaffective disorder never includes full-blown episodes of major depression.
D. In bipolar disorder, psychotic symptoms are always mood congruent.

2.24   Which of the following symptom combinations, if present for 1 month, would meet Criterion A for schizophrenia?

A. Prominent auditory and visual hallucinations.
B. Grossly disorganized behavior and avolition.
C. Disorganized speech and diminished emotional expression.
D. Paranoid and grandiose delusions.

2.25   Which of the following statements about violent or suicidal behavior in schizophrenia is *false*?

A. About 5%–6% of individuals with schizophrenia die by suicide.
B. Persons with schizophrenia frequently assault strangers in a random fashion.
C. Compared with the general population, persons with schizophrenia are more frequently victims of violence.
D. Youth, male sex, and substance abuse are factors that increase the risk for suicide among persons with schizophrenia.

2.26   Which of the following statements about childhood-onset schizophrenia is *true*?

A. Childhood-onset schizophrenia tends to resemble poor-outcome adult schizophrenia, with gradual onset and prominent negative symptoms.
B. Disorganized speech patterns in childhood are usually indicative of schizophrenia.
C. Because of the childhood capacity for imagination, delusions and hallucinations in childhood-onset schizophrenia are more elaborate than those in adult-onset schizophrenia.
D. In a child presenting with disorganized behavior, schizophrenia should be ruled out before other childhood diagnoses are considered.

2.27   Which of the following statements about sex differences in schizophrenia is *true*?

A. Women with schizophrenia tend to have fewer psychotic symptoms than do men over the course of the illness.
B. A first onset of schizophrenia after age 40 is more likely in women than in men.

C. Psychotic symptoms in women tend to burn out with age to a greater extent than they do in men.

D. Negative symptoms and affective flattening are more frequently observed in women with schizophrenia than in men with the disorder.

2.28 A 19-year-old college student is brought to the emergency department by her family over her objection. Three months ago, she suddenly started feeling "odd," and she came home from college because she could not concentrate. Two weeks after she came home, she began hearing voices telling her that she is "a sinner" and must repent. Although never a religious person, she now believes she must repent, but she does not know how, and she feels confused. She is managing her activities of daily living despite the ongoing auditory hallucinations and delusions, and she is affectively reactive on examination. Which diagnosis best fits this presentation?

A. Schizophreniform disorder, with good prognostic features, provisional.

B. Schizophreniform disorder, without good prognostic features, provisional.

C. Schizophreniform disorder, with good prognostic features.

D. Schizophreniform disorder, without good prognostic features.

2.29 A 24-year-old college student is brought to the emergency department by the college health service team. A few weeks ago, he was involved in a car accident in which one of his friends was critically injured and died in his arms. The man has not come out of his room or showered for the last 2 weeks. He has eaten only minimally, claimed that aliens have targeted him for abduction, and asserted that he could hear their radio transmissions. Nothing seems to convince him that this abduction will not happen or that the transmissions are not real. Which of the following diagnoses (and justifications) is most appropriate?

A. Brief psychotic disorder with a marked stressor because the symptoms began after the tragic car accident.

B. Brief psychotic disorder without a marked stressor because the content of the psychosis is unrelated to the accident.

C. Unspecified schizophrenia spectrum and other psychotic disorder because more information is needed.

D. Schizophreniform disorder because there are psychotic symptoms but not yet a full-blown schizophrenia picture.

CHAPTER 3

Bipolar and Related Disorders

3.1 A 32-year-old patient reports 1 week of feeling unusually irritable. During this time, he has increased energy and activity, sleeps less, and finds it difficult to sit still. He also is more talkative than usual and is easily distractible, to the point of finding it difficult to complete his work assignments. A physical examination and laboratory workup are negative for any medical cause of his symptoms, and he takes no medications. What diagnosis best fits this clinical picture?

A. Manic episode.
B. Hypomanic episode.
C. Bipolar I disorder, with mixed features.
D. Cyclothymic disorder.

3.2 A 28-year-old patient reports 1 week of increased activity associated with an elevated mood, a decreased need for sleep, and inflated self-esteem. She does not object to her current state ("I'm getting more work done than ever before!"). A physical examination and laboratory work are unrevealing for any medical cause of her symptoms. She had taken fluoxetine for a major depressive episode but self-discontinued it 2 months ago because she felt that her mood was stable. Which diagnosis best fits this clinical picture?

A. Bipolar I disorder.
B. Bipolar II disorder.
C. Cyclothymic disorder.
D. Substance/medication-induced bipolar disorder.

3.3 Approximately what percentage of individuals who experience a single manic episode will go on to have recurrent mood episodes?

A. 90%.
B. 50%.
C. 25%.
D. 10%.

3.4 Which of the following factors is most associated with manic relapse in bipolar I disorder?

    A. Childhood adversity.
    B. Recent life stress.
    C. Initial episode of manic polarity.
    D. Suicide attempt.

3.5 Which of the following is more common in men than women with bipolar I disorder?

    A. Rapid cycling.
    B. Lethal suicide.
    C. Earlier onset.
    D. Mixed symptoms.

3.6 A patient with a history of bipolar I disorder presents with a new-onset manic episode and is successfully treated with medication adjustment. He notes chronic depressive symptoms that, on reflection, long preceded the manic episodes. He describes these symptoms as "feeling down," having decreased energy, and more often than not having no motivation. He does not endorse other depressive symptoms; however, the current symptoms have been sufficient to negatively affect his marriage. Which diagnosis best fits this presentation?

    A. Other specified bipolar and related disorder.
    B. Bipolar I disorder, current or most recent episode depressed.
    C. Cyclothymic disorder.
    D. Bipolar I disorder and persistent depressive disorder (dysthymia).

3.7 In which of the following ways do manic episodes differ from attention-deficit/hyperactivity disorder (ADHD)?

    A. Manic episodes are more strongly associated with impulsivity.
    B. Manic episodes have clearer symptomatic onsets and offsets.
    C. Manic episodes are more likely to show a chronic course.
    D. Manic episodes first appear at an earlier age.

3.8 A patient with a history of bipolar disorder reports experiencing 1 week of elevated and expansive mood. Evidence of which of the following would suggest that the patient is experiencing a hypomanic, rather than manic, episode?

    A. Prominent irritability.
    B. Increased productivity at work.
    C. Psychotic symptoms.
    D. Good insight into the illness.

3.9   A 25-year-old graduate student presents to a psychiatrist complaining of feeling down and "not enjoying anything." Her symptoms began about a month ago, along with insomnia and poor appetite. She has little interest in activities and is having difficulty attending to her schoolwork. She recalls a similar episode 1 year ago that lasted about 2 months before improving without treatment. She also reports several episodes of increased energy over the past 2 years. The episodes usually last 1–2 weeks, during which time she is very productive, feels more social and outgoing, tends to sleep less, and still feels energetic during the day. Friends tell her that she speaks more rapidly during these episodes but that they do not see it as off-putting. They tell her that she seems more outgoing and clever. She has no medical problems, does not take any medications, and denies using drugs or alcohol. What is the most likely diagnosis?

A. Bipolar I disorder, current episode depressed.
B. Cyclothymic disorder.
C. Bipolar II disorder, current episode depressed.
D. Major depressive disorder.

3.10 How do the depressive episodes associated with bipolar II disorder differ from those associated with bipolar I disorder?

A. They are lengthier than those associated with bipolar I disorder.
B. They are less disabling than those associated with bipolar I disorder.
C. They are less severe than those associated with bipolar I disorder.
D. They are rarely a reason for the patient to seek treatment.

3.11 How does the course of bipolar II disorder differ from the course of bipolar I disorder?

A. It is less episodic than the course of bipolar I disorder.
B. It is more chronic than the course of bipolar I disorder.
C. It involves longer asymptomatic periods than the course of bipolar I disorder.
D. It involves a much lower number of lifetime mood episodes than the course of bipolar I disorder.

3.12 Which of the following features confers a worse prognosis for a patient with bipolar II disorder?

A. Younger age.
B. Higher educational level.
C. Rapid-cycling pattern.
D. Married marital status.

3.13 Women with bipolar II disorder are more likely than men to experience which of the following?

A. More severe illness course.

B. Hypomania with mixed depressive features.

C. More manic episodes.

D. Onset with depressive symptoms.

3.14   Which of the following is associated with postpartum hypomania?

A. The late postpartum period.

B. Preserved sleep.

C. Postpartum depression.

D. Infanticide.

3.15   A 42-year-old woman with a history of panic disorder presents to the emergency department, brought in by her family after 2 days of abnormal behavior. They report that she has not slept for the past 2 days, is speaking unusually rapidly, and has been irritable. The patient reports feeling "incredible" despite running out of her long-term benzodiazepine prescription 3 days ago. On exam she repeatedly paces back and forth while demanding immediate discharge from the emergency department. What is the most likely diagnosis?

A. Panic disorder.

B. Bipolar II disorder.

C. Benzodiazepine intoxication.

D. Substance/medication-induced bipolar and related disorder.

3.16   A 36-year-old man presents to a psychiatry clinic for intake. He describes a history of several months-long periods throughout his lifetime with sustained low mood, increased sleep, decreased appetite, poor energy, and worsening ability to concentrate at work. He also notes that he has had many periods of uncharacteristically happy moods with excellent energy despite sleeping only 2–4 hours. These periods have never lasted longer than 3 days and typically last only 1–2 days before his mood returns to normal. What is the appropriate diagnosis for this patient?

A. Bipolar I disorder.

B. Other specified bipolar and related disorder.

C. Cyclothymia.

D. Bipolar II disorder.

3.17   In which of the following aspects does cyclothymic disorder differ from bipolar I disorder?

A. Duration.

B. Severity.

C. Age at onset.

D. Pervasiveness.

CHAPTER 4

Depressive Disorders

4.1 A 41-year-old patient without any previous mood disorder history reports two recent periods of sustained sadness, lack of interest in her hobbies, worsened concentration, increased fatigue, and decreased productivity at work. She notes that each of these periods began after a cocaine binge. The mood episodes persisted almost 2 weeks after the cocaine use stopped. After each period, the patient returned to her typical euthymic state without treatment. What is the most appropriate diagnosis?

A. Substance/medication-induced depressive disorder.
B. Premenstrual dysphoric disorder.
C. Major depressive disorder.
D. Unspecified bipolar disorder.

4.2 A 47-year-old woman with diagnosed major depressive disorder (MDD) presents to your office with new psychiatric complaints. Women are more likely to experience which of the following comorbid disorders?

A. Substance/medication-induced depressive disorder.
B. Generalized anxiety disorder.
C. Alcohol use disorder.
D. Cocaine use disorder.

4.3 What diagnostic provision is made for depressive symptoms following the death of a loved one?

A. Depressive symptoms lasting less than 2 months after the loss of a loved one are excluded from receiving a diagnosis of major depressive episode (MDE).
B. To qualify for a diagnosis of MDE, the depression must start no less than 12 weeks following the loss.
C. To qualify for a diagnosis of MDE, the depressive symptoms in such individuals must include suicidal ideation.
D. Depressive symptoms following the loss of a loved one are not excluded from receiving an MDE diagnosis if the symptoms otherwise fulfill the diagnostic criteria.

4.4   How does grief differ from a major depressive episode (MDE)?

     A. Grief is often characterized by an inability to experience happiness or pleasure.
     B. In grief, dysphoria is typically constant, whereas in an MDE sadness commonly comes as "pangs" that come in waves over days or weeks.
     C. The thought content associated with grief is generally self-critical or pessimistic ruminations.
     D. In grief, when the bereaved individual thinks about death and dying, such thoughts are generally focused on the deceased and possibly about "joining" the deceased, whereas in MDE such thoughts are focused on ending one's own life because of feeling worthless, undeserving of life, or unable to cope with the pain of depression.

4.5   Which of the following is a risk factor for developing substance/medication-induced depressive disorder?

     A. Female sex.
     B. High socioeconomic status.
     C. Recent life stressors.
     D. Remission from substance abuse.

4.6   A 50-year-old man presents with persistently depressed mood lasting for several weeks that interferes with his ability to work. He has insomnia and fatigue, feels guilty, has thoughts he would be better off dead, and has begun researching ways to die without anyone knowing it was a suicide. His wife informs you that on most days during this period he has also displayed odd behaviors, including speaking rapidly, requesting sex several times a day, and writing extensively about ideas for a "better internet." These behaviors are marked changes from his typical behavior. Which diagnosis best fits this patient?

     A. Manic episode, with mixed features.
     B. Major depressive episode.
     C. Major depressive episode, with mixed features.
     D. Major depressive episode, with atypical features.

4.7   A 45-year-old woman with classic features of schizophrenia has experienced chronic, co-occurring symptoms of feeling "down in the dumps," having a poor appetite, and hopelessness during her episodes of active psychosis. These depressive symptoms occured only during her psychotic episodes and only during the 4-year period when she was experiencing active symptoms of schizophrenia. After her psychotic episodes were successfully controlled by medication, no further symptoms of depression were present. At no time has the patient met full criteria for major depressive episode. What is the appropriate DSM-5-TR diagnosis?

     A. Schizophrenia.
     B. Schizoaffective disorder.

C. Persistent depressive disorder (dysthymia).

D. Schizophrenia and persistent depressive disorder (dysthymia).

4.8 Which depressive disorder diagnoses were new to DSM-5 and continued in DSM-5-TR?

A. Subsyndromal depressive disorder, premenstrual dysphoric disorder, and mixed anxiety and depressive disorder.

B. Disruptive mood dysregulation disorder, premenstrual dysphoric disorder, and persistent depressive disorder.

C. Disruptive mood dysregulation disorder, premenstrual dysphoric disorder, and subsyndromal depressive disorder.

D. Disruptive mood dysregulation disorder, postmenopausal dysphoric disorder, and persistent depressive disorder.

4.9 A patient in a current major depressive episode reports experiencing no pleasure from positive everyday experiences that would usually be enjoyable. He also notes waking up early in the morning with terminal insomnia, feeling worse in the morning than at other times of the day, and having excessive guilt over minor mistakes. Which of the following is the appropriate diagnosis and specifier for this patient?

A. Major depressive disorder, with anxious distress.

B. Major depressive disorder, with atypical features.

C. Major depressive disorder, with melancholic features.

D. Major depressive disorder, with mixed features.

4.10 A 39-year-old woman describes becoming quite depressed in the winter last year when her company closed for the season and then experiencing spontaneous remission without treatment in the following spring. She recalls experiencing multiple other major depressive episodes (MDEs) over the past decade during spring and summer months, although none were related to her occupation. Would this patient be eligible for a diagnosis of major depressive disorder, *with seasonal pattern*?

A. The patient *does not* qualify for this diagnosis because this specifier requires that depressive episode with seasonal features must start in the fall.

B. The patient *does not* qualify for this diagnosis because this specifier requires onset and remission over at least a 2-year period without any nonseasonal episodes during this period.

C. The patient *does* qualify for this diagnosis because she experienced a spontaneous remission of a depressive episode with a seasonal relationship.

D. The patient *does* qualify for this diagnosis because her symptoms are related to a specific psychosocial stressor.

4.11 Which of the following demographic groups has the highest depression prevalence?

A. Reproductive age females.
B. Reproductive age males.
C. Elderly males.
D. Female children.

4.12 Which of the following statements is associated with an increased risk of recurrence in major depressive disorder?

A. Older age.
B. Severe symptoms.
C. Recent first episode.
D. Longer duration of remission.

4.13 Which of the following is an accurate diagnostic marker for major depressive disorder (MDD)?

A. Pro-inflammatory cytokine levels.
B. Neurotrophic factor genetic variants.
C. Hypothalamic-pituitary-gonadal hyperactivity.
D. None of the above.

4.14 In major depressive disorder, which of the following is more common in men than women?

A. Suicide completion.
B. Associated gastrointestinal symptoms.
C. Hypersomnia.
D. Treatment responsiveness.

4.15 A 12-year-old youth has been experiencing episodes of temper outbursts that are out of proportion to the situation several times per week over the past year. She frequently screams at anyone in her vicinity and occasionally breaks nearby objects during these episodes. Which of the following aspects of this patient's presentation precludes a diagnosis of disruptive mood dysregulation disorder (DMDD)?

A. Outburst frequency.
B. Aggression toward others.
C. Age at symptom onset.
D. Age at diagnosis.

4.16 Which of the following features distinguishes disruptive mood dysregulation disorder (DMDD) from bipolar disorder in children?

A. Age at onset.
B. Chronicity.

C. Irritability.

D. Severity.

4.17 Children with disruptive mood dysregulation disorder are most likely to develop which of the following disorders in adulthood?

A. Bipolar I disorder.

B. Unipolar depressive disorders.

C. Antisocial personality disorder.

D. Borderline personality disorder.

4.18 An irritable 8-year-old child has a history of nearly daily temper outbursts both at home and at school over the past 2 years. These outbursts are age-inappropriate and severe. Between outbursts, what characteristic mood is required to qualify this child for a diagnosis of disruptive mood dysregulation disorder?

A. Irritability.

B. Depression.

C. Euthymia.

D. Lability.

4.19 According to DSM-5-TR diagnostic criteria, disruptive mood dysregulation disorder (DMDD) can be assigned in combination with which of the following diagnoses?

A. Oppositional defiant disorder (ODD).

B. Bipolar II disorder.

C. Intermittent explosive disorder (IED).

D. Attention-deficit/hyperactivity disorder (ADHD).

4.20 Which of the following factors is associated with a decreased risk of death by suicide?

A. Marriage.

B. Firearm ownership.

C. Impaired cognition.

D. Anhedonia.

4.21 A 9-year-old boy is brought in for evaluation because of explosive outbursts when he is frustrated with schoolwork. The parents report that their son is well behaved and pleasant at other times. Which diagnosis best fits this clinical picture?

A. Disruptive mood dysregulation disorder (DMDD).

B. Bipolar disorder.

C. Intermittent explosive disorder (IED).

D. Major depressive disorder.

4.22 A 14-year-old boy describes himself as feeling irritable the vast majority of the time for the past year. He remembers feeling better while he was at camp for 4 weeks during the summer; however, his mood complaints returned when he came home and have continued since. He reports poor concentration and feelings of hopelessness but denies suicidal ideation or changes in his appetite or sleep. What is the most appropriate diagnosis?

    A. Major depressive disorder.
    B. Disruptive mood dysregulation disorder.
    C. Depressive episodes with short-duration hypomania.
    D. Persistent depressive disorder, with early onset.

4.23 A 30-year-old woman reports 3 years of ongoing depressed mood, accompanied by loss of pleasure in all activities, ruminations that she would be better off dead, feelings of guilt about "bad things" she has done, and thoughts about quitting work because of her inability to focus. Although she has never been treated for depression, she feels so distressed at times that she wonders if she should be hospitalized. She denies drug or alcohol use, and her medical workup is completely normal, including laboratory tests for vitamins. The consultation was prompted by further worsening of her mood over the past several weeks. What is the most appropriate diagnosis?

    A. Major depressive disorder (MDD).
    B. Persistent depressive disorder, with persistent major depressive episode.
    C. Cyclothymia.
    D. MDD, with melancholic features.

4.24 A 67-year-old woman presents with new depressive symptoms that began approximately 3 weeks after she experienced a cerebrovascular accident (CVA). The symptoms have continued for 2 months. Along with daily depressed mood, she reports middle insomnia, poor appetite, trouble concentrating, and lack of interest in sex. Per her neurologist, she has very limited residual symptoms from her CVA. Despite the lack of residual deficits, she describes frequent absence from and poor performance at work. She denies any active plans to attempt suicide but admits that she "wishes for death" as her mood has worsened. The patient and her husband both deny that she had any previous history of even a mild depressive episode. What is the most likely diagnosis?

    A. Major depressive disorder.
    B. Persistent depressive disorder.
    C. Depressive disorder due to another medical condition.
    D. Substance/medication-induced depressive disorder.

4.25 A 17-year-old high school senior complains to her gynecologist about periods of pronounced irritability, sadness, conflicts with her classmates, increased appetite, decreased energy, feeling bloated, and decreased concentration. She feels that these symptoms generally start about 3–4 days prior to the onset of menses and disappear within a week. She cannot recall many menstrual cycles without these symptoms since menarche at age 12, but she has never kept any notes or records about them. Her gynecologist asks you to consult on the case. On the basis of her symptoms, which is the most appropriate diagnosis for this patient?

A. Premenstrual syndrome.
B. Major depressive disorder.
C. Premenstrual dysphoric disorder, provisional.
D. The patient has no DSM-5 diagnosis.

4.26 The presence of which of the following excludes a diagnosis of premenstrual dysphoric disorder?

A. Labile affect.
B. Continuous symptoms.
C. Physical pain.
D. Delusions.

4.27 A 29-year-old woman complains of sad mood every month in anticipation of her very painful menses. The pain begins with the start of her flow and continues for several days. She does not experience pain during other times of the month. She has tried a variety of treatments, none of which have given her relief. What is the appropriate diagnosis?

A. Premenstrual dysphoric disorder.
B. Premenstrual syndrome.
C. Dysmenorrhea.
D. Persistent depressive disorder.

4.28 A 23-year-old woman reports that during every menstrual cycle she experiences breast swelling, bloating, hypersomnia, an increased craving for sweets, poor concentration, and a feeling that she cannot handle her normal responsibilities. She notes that she also feels somewhat more sensitive emotionally and may become tearful when hearing a sad story. She takes no oral medication but does use a drospirenone/ethinyl estradiol patch. What diagnosis best fits this clinical picture?

A. Premenstrual dysphoric disorder (PMDD).
B. Dysthymia.
C. Premenstrual syndrome.
D. Substance/medication-induced depressive disorder.

4.29 Which of the following is an established risk factor for the development of persistent depressive disorder?

A. Older age.
B. Borderline personality disorder.
C. Schizophrenia.
D. College degree.

4.30   A 31-year-old woman with no history of mood symptoms reports that she experiences distressing mood lability and irritability starting about 4 days before the onset of menses. She feels "on edge," cannot concentrate, has little enjoyment from any of her activities, experiences bloating, and notes swelling of her breasts. The patient reports that these symptoms started 6 months ago when she began taking oral contraceptives for the first time. If she stops the oral contraceptives and her symptoms remit, what would the diagnosis be?

A. Premenstrual dysphoric disorder.
B. Premenstrual syndrome.
C. Major depressive episode.
D. Substance/medication-induced depressive disorder.

4.31   A 37-year-old woman describes a several year history of episodic sadness. Each individual period lasts no longer than 10 days and is accompanied by pronounced anhedonia, insomnia, a loss of appetite, and profound hopelessness. She denies any other psychiatric symptoms. She cannot identify any related life events or stressors. A comprehensive laboratory evaluation is normal. Which of the following would be the most appropriate diagnosis?

A. Cyclothymia.
B. Major depressive disorder.
C. Other specified depressive disorder, recurrent brief depression.
D. Premenstrual dysphoric disorder.

CHAPTER 5

Anxiety Disorders

5.1   Which of the following disorders is included in the "Anxiety Disorders" chapter of DSM-5-TR?

   A. Obsessive-compulsive disorder.
   B. Posttraumatic stress disorder.
   C. Acute stress disorder.
   D. Separation anxiety disorder.

5.2   A 9-year-old boy cannot go to sleep without having a parent in his room. While falling asleep, he frequently awakens to check that a parent is still there. One parent usually stays until the boy falls asleep. If he wakes up alone during the night, he starts to panic and gets up to find his parents. He also reports frequent nightmares in which he or his parents are harmed. He occasionally calls out that he saw a strange figure peering into his dark room. The parents usually wake in the morning to find the boy asleep on the floor of their room. They once tried to leave him with a relative so they could go on a vacation; however, he became so distressed in anticipation of this that they canceled their plans. What is the most likely diagnosis?

   A. Specific phobia.
   B. Nightmare disorder.
   C. Delusional disorder.
   D. Separation anxiety disorder.

5.3   Which of the following is considered a culture-specific symptom of panic attacks?

   A. Derealization.
   B. Headaches.
   C. Fear of going crazy.
   D. Shortness of breath.

5.4   Which of the following statements best describes how panic attacks differ from panic disorder?

   A. Panic attacks require fewer symptoms for a definitive diagnosis.
   B. Panic attacks are discrete, occur suddenly, and are usually less severe.

C. Panic attacks are invariably unexpected.

D. Panic attacks represent symptoms that can occur with a variety of other disorders.

5.5   The determination of whether a panic attack is expected or unexpected is ultimately best made by which of the following?

A. Careful clinical judgment.

B. Whether the patient associates it with external stress.

C. The presence or absence of nocturnal panic attacks.

D. Ruling out possible culture-specific syndromes.

5.6   Which of the following forms of panic disorder can be triggered by interpersonal arguments?

A. *Khyâl* attacks.

B. *Trúng gió* attacks.

C. *Ataque de nervios*.

D. Soul loss.

5.7   A 50-year-old man reports occasional episodes in which he suddenly and unexpectedly awakens from sleep feeling a surge of intense fear that peaks within minutes. He feels short of breath and experiences heart palpitations and sweating. His medical history is significant only for hypertension, which is well controlled with hydrochlorothiazide. As a result of these symptoms, he has begun to have anticipatory anxiety associated with going to sleep. What is the most likely explanation for his symptoms?

A. Anxiety disorder due to another medical condition (hypertension).

B. Substance/medication-induced anxiety disorder.

C. Nocturnal panic attacks.

D. Sleep terrors.

5.8   Which of the following is predictive of suicidal behavior in patients with panic disorder?

A. Derealization.

B. Nausea.

C. Anxiety due to another medical condition.

D. Illness anxiety disorder.

5.9   A 65-year-old woman reports being housebound despite being in good physical health. She fell several years ago while shopping but was not injured. Physical examination reveals no problems with mobility or balance. She experiences panic every time she leaves her house unaccompanied. Her distress is absent when she is home; however, she avoids taking the bus to shop for groceries without a companion. What is the most likely diagnosis?

A. Specific phobia, situational type.
B. Social anxiety disorder (social phobia).
C. Posttraumatic stress disorder.
D. Agoraphobia.

5.10   A 32-year-old man has regularly experienced panic attacks with palpitations, nausea, headaches, shortness of breath, dizziness, derealization, and fear of dying when out of his home alone. These episodes occur when he stands in line to take the bus and while he is on the bus. He now works only from home for fear of experiencing these attacks, despite loss of income due to remote work. What is the most appropriate diagnosis?

A. Panic disorder with agoraphobia.
B. Agoraphobia with panic attacks.
C. Specific phobia, situational type.
D. Two separate disorders: panic disorder and agoraphobia.

5.11   A 35-year-old man lost a high-paying job because it required frequent long-range traveling. Two years earlier he had been on a particularly turbulent flight. He was convinced that the pilot minimized the risk and that the plane almost crashed. His coworker repeatedly told him that her experience of the flight was that it was only mildly uncomfortable. He flew again 1 month later, and despite having a smooth flight, the anticipation of turbulence was so distressing that he experienced overwhelming anxiety during the flight. He has not flown since and becomes extremely anxious when the possibility of flying is raised. What is the most appropriate diagnosis?

A. Agoraphobia.
B. Posttraumatic stress disorder (PTSD).
C. Specific phobia, situational type.
D. Social anxiety disorder (social phobia).

5.12   Which of the following types of specific phobia is most likely to be associated with vasovagal fainting?

A. Animal type.
B. Natural environment type.
C. Blood-injection-injury type.
D. Situational type.

5.13   Although onset of a specific phobia can occur at any age, specific phobias most typically develop during which age period?

A. Childhood.
B. Late adolescence to early adulthood.
C. Middle age.
D. Old age.

5.14   In social anxiety disorder, the object of an individual's fear is the potential for which of the following?

   A. Social or occupational impairment.
   B. Harm to self or others.
   C. Scrutiny by others.
   D. Separation from objects of attachment.

5.15   When called on at school, a 7-year-old boy will only nod or write in response. The family of the child is surprised to hear this from the teacher because the boy speaks normally when at home with his parents. The child has achieved appropriate developmental milestones, and a medical evaluation indicates that he is healthy. The boy is unable to give any explanation for his behavior, but the parents are concerned that it will affect his school performance. What diagnosis best fits this child's symptoms?

   A. Separation anxiety disorder.
   B. Autism spectrum disorder.
   C. Agoraphobia.
   D. Selective mutism.

5.16   Social anxiety disorder differs from normative shyness in that the disorder leads to which of the following?

   A. Social or occupational dysfunction.
   B. Higher probability of long-term relationships.
   C. Higher probability of being associated with immigrant status.
   D. Anxiety at home but not in school for children.

5.17   In addition to anxiety and worry, individuals with generalized anxiety disorder are most likely to experience which of the following symptoms?

   A. Dizziness.
   B. Tachycardia.
   C. Muscle tension.
   D. Shortness of breath.

5.18   Which of the following characteristics is suggestive of generalized anxiety disorder in children who have the disorder?

   A. Complaining of feeling restless.
   B. Being lax with schoolwork.
   C. Often being late for appointments.
   D. Seeking frequent reassurance from others.

5.19   What is the primary difference in the clinical expression of generalized anxiety disorder across age groups?

A. Content of worry.

B. Degree of worry.

C. Patterns of comorbidity.

D. Predominance of cognitive versus somatic symptoms.

5.20 In what aspect of generalized anxiety disorder do men and women most commonly differ?

A. Course.

B. Symptom profile.

C. Degree of impairment.

D. Patterns of comorbidity.

5.21 Which of the following is more suggestive of nonpathological anxiety as opposed to anxiety that qualifies for a diagnosis of generalized anxiety disorder?

A. Anxiety and worry that interfere significantly with functioning.

B. Anxiety and worry that last for months to years.

C. Anxiety and worry in response to a clear precipitant.

D. Anxiety and worry focused on a wide range of life circumstances.

5.22 A 26-year-old man is brought to the emergency department suffering from a sudden, severe surge of panic. He has no history of panic disorder, but he reports taking several doses of an over-the-counter cold medication earlier that day. Which of the following clinical features, if present in this case, would help to confirm a diagnosis of substance/medication-induced anxiety disorder?

A. Symptoms that are mild and do not impair functioning.

B. Symptoms that do not develop for a long time after the substance or medication use.

C. Symptoms that are in excess of what would be expected for the substance or medication.

D. Lack of any prior history of anxiety disorder or panic symptoms.

5.23 In which of the following circumstances would a diagnosis of substance/medication-induced anxiety disorder be appropriate rather than a diagnosis of substance withdrawal?

A. Significant anxiety symptoms are present.

B. Anxiety was not present prior to stopping the medication.

C. Anxiety is present that is sufficiently severe to warrant independent clinical attention.

D. Anxiety is present only during bouts of delirium.

5.24 A 60-year-old man has just been diagnosed with congestive heart failure and pulmonary edema. He describes himself as intensely anxious and reports feeling as if he cannot breathe, which he describes as "a panic attack." Which of the following features would support a diagnosis of anxiety disorder due to another medical condition rather than adjustment disorder with anxiety?

    A. The patient says he does not know why he is anxious because knowing his diagnosis does not worry him.
    B. The patient has no anxiety-associated physical symptoms.
    C. The patient is focused on what it means that he has a cardiac disorder.
    D. The patient is delirious.

5.25   Which of the following anxiety disorders is most associated with a transition from suicidal thoughts to suicide attempts?

    A. Separation anxiety disorder.
    B. Agoraphobia.
    C. Selective mutism.
    D. Generalized anxiety disorder.

CHAPTER 6

Obsessive-Compulsive and Related Disorders

6.1 How are compulsions defined in obsessive-compulsive disorder (OCD)?

A. Compulsions in OCD are typically goal-directed, fulfilling a realistic purpose.
B. Compulsions include paraphilias (sexual compulsions) and addictive behaviors such as gambling or substance use.
C. Compulsions involve repetitive and persistent thoughts, images, or urges.
D. Compulsions in OCD are aimed at reducing the distress triggered by obsessions.

6.2 A 52-year-old man with raw, chapped hands is referred to a psychiatrist by his primary care doctor. The man reports that he washes his hands repeatedly, spending up to 4 hours a day, using abrasive cleansers and scalding hot water. Although he admits that his hands are uncomfortable, he is entirely convinced that unless he washes in this manner he will become gravely ill. A medical workup is unrevealing, and the man takes no medications. What is the most appropriate diagnosis?

A. Delusional disorder, somatic type.
B. Illness anxiety disorder.
C. Obsessive-compulsive disorder (OCD), with absent insight.
D. Factitious disorder.

6.3 In obsessive-compulsive disorder (OCD), which of the following is more likely to be seen in men than women?

A. Comorbid tics.
B. Later age of onset.
C. Obsession with cleaning.
D. Hormonal symptom associations.

6.4 A 63-year-old woman has been saving financial documents and records for decades, placing papers in piles throughout her apartment to the point where it has become unsafe. She acknowledges that the piles are a concern; however, she says that the papers include important documents and she is afraid to throw them away. She recalls a previous instance when her taxes were audited and she needed certain documents to avoid a penalty. She describes repetitive worries about a new audit with an inability to ignore these worries. She feels somewhat reassured by her growing pile of legal paperwork but notes concern because her landlord is threatening to evict her unless she removes the piles of papers. What is the most likely diagnosis?

A. Nonpathological collecting behavior.
B. Hoarding disorder.
C. Obsessive-compulsive disorder (OCD).
D. Dementia (major neurocognitive disorder).

6.5   Which of the following is a protective factor for suicide risk associated with obsessive-compulsive disorder (OCD)?

A. Male gender.
B. Religious obsessions.
C. Substance abuse.
D. Comorbid anxiety disorder.

6.6   Which of the following is required for a diagnosis of body dysmorphic disorder (BDD)?

A. An apparent physical defect noticeable by a physician.
B. Repetitive behaviors or thoughts related to concerns about one's appearance.
C. Unhealthy weight loss with the goal of improving one's appearance.
D. Preservation of baseline social, occupational, and general function.

6.7   A 25-year-old man is concerned that he looks "weak" and "puny" despite the fact that to neutral observers he appears very muscular. When confronted about his belief, he thinks he is being humored and that people are in fact making fun of his small size behind his back. He has tried a number of strategies to increase muscle mass, including exercising excessively and using anabolic steroids; however, he remains dissatisfied with his appearance. What is the most likely diagnosis?

A. Delusional disorder, somatic type.
B. Body dysmorphic disorder (BDD), with muscle dysmorphia.
C. Body identity integrity disorder.
D. *Koro*.

6.8   A 19-year-old woman is referred to a psychiatrist by her internist after she admits to him that she recurrently pulls hair from her eyebrows to the point that she has scarring and there is little or no eyebrow hair left. She states that her natural eyebrows are "bushy" and "repulsive" and that she "looks like a caveman." A photograph of the woman before she began pulling her eyebrow hair shows a normal-looking teenager. What is the most appropriate diagnosis?

A. Trichotillomania (hair-pulling disorder).

B. Delusional disorder, somatic type.

C. Body dysmorphic disorder (BDD).

D. Obsessive-compulsive disorder (OCD).

6.9   A 48-year-old man presents to a psychiatrist along with his husband, stating that he pressured him to seek help. He explains that he likes to collect wine, and he does not see a problem with this; he claims that many of the wines are quite valuable and a potential investment. On further questioning, he admits that he rarely drinks the wines because it "never seems the right time." He has never sold or given away any wine because he finds it hard to part with the bottles. He has filled multiple rooms of his house for storage of the wine, which, along with the financial hardship, is his husband's primary concern. The husband notes that when the patient attempts to discard or sell any of the wine, he bursts into tears. The patient admits that many of the wine bottles have probably spoiled because he cannot afford to properly store the wine and the bottles have sat for years on shelves. What is the most appropriate diagnosis?

A. Narcissistic personality disorder .

B. Obsessive-compulsive disorder (OCD).

C. Delusional disorder.

D. Hoarding disorder, excessive acquisition type.

6.10   A diagnosis of hoarding disorder can still be given even if which of the following is suspected to contribute to the presentation?

A. Prader-Willi syndrome.

B. Focal brain damage.

C. Neurocognitive dysfunction.

D. Family history.

6.11   Hoarding disorder has the highest prevalence in which population?

A. Men.

B. Adolescents.

C. Elderly adults.

D. Reproductive age women.

6.12   Which of the following would be inconsistent with a diagnosis of trichotillomania (hair-pulling disorder)?

A. Acceptance of hair-pulling behavior as normative.

B. Episodic hair pulling.

C. Failed attempts to reduce hair pulling.

D. Hair pulling in areas covered by clothing.

6.13   Which of the following is *not* associated with trichotillomania (hair-pulling disorder)?

A. Broken hair follicles.
B. Alopecia.
C. Dental damage.
D. Bezoar.

6.14   A 25-year-old man is referred to a psychiatrist by his primary care doctor after mentioning to the doctor that he routinely spends a lot of time pulling out facial hair with tweezers, even after carefully shaving. On evaluation, he admits to frequent pulling of his facial hair, consuming a significant amount of time; he explains that he becomes anxious when looking at himself because his mustache, hairline, and sideburns are asymmetrical. He pulls out hairs in an effort to make his facial hair more symmetrical but is rarely satisfied with the results. He finds this very upsetting but cannot resist the urge to try to "fix" his facial hair. What is the most appropriate diagnosis?

A. Trichotillomania (hair-pulling disorder).
B. Body dysmorphic disorder (BDD).
C. Delusional disorder, somatic type.
D. Obsessive-compulsive disorder (OCD).

6.15   A 17-year-old girl is brought to a child and adolescent psychiatry clinic for evaluation. Her parents report that over the past 3 years she has developed a worsening habit of digging into her forearms and shins with her fingernails. The patient describes a bothersome feeling, almost like an itch, that is relieved on scratching. She finds it deeply relieving in the moment but is embarrassed about the residual scars, wearing long sleeves in the summer and staying home more often to avoid others seeing her resulting lesions. Despite support from parents, a school counselor, and friends, the habit has only gotten worse in the past year. Laboratory testing is all within normal limits. What is the appropriate diagnosis for this patient?

A. Delusional parasitosis.
B. Dermatitis artefacta.
C. Obsessive-compulsive disorder (OCD).
D. Excoriation (skin-picking) disorder.

6.16   Which of the following is a common comorbid condition with trichotillomania (hair-pulling) disorder?

A. Borderline personality disorder.
B. Bipolar disorder.
C. Excoriation (skin-picking) disorder.
D. Generalized anxiety disorder.

6.17   In excoriation (skin-picking) disorder, which of the following is the most typi-
        cal motivation for the skin-picking behavior?

        A. Inducing pain.
        B. Symmetry concerns.
        C. Boredom.
        D. Fear of infection.

6.18   A 55-year-old retail worker believes that he has "chronic halitosis" and fears
        that his bad breath is "scaring away shoppers." He is in danger of losing his job
        because he so frequently absents himself from the sales floor to brush his teeth
        and use mouthwash. He constantly chews mint gum, even though his em-
        ployer has asked him not to. His coworkers regularly reassure him that his
        breath is fine, but he is convinced that they are just being polite. Although the
        possibility of losing his job causes him concern, he finds his worries about his
        breath to be intolerable. He has seen his doctor and dentist, both of whom tell
        him that he is healthy and does not have malodorous breath. What is the most
        appropriate diagnosis?

        A. Social anxiety disorder (social phobia).
        B. Other specified obsessive-compulsive and related disorder
        C. Body dysmorphic disorder.
        D. Illness anxiety disorder.

6.19   A 44-year-old woman goes to the emergency department with excoriations
        down her forearms bilaterally. She describes an overwhelming concern that
        she has a skin infection based on "itchy" feelings in her arms and states that
        she finds some relief in repetitive scratching. She is convinced that the scratch-
        ing and resulting excoriations are helping prevent spread of infection through-
        out her body. She does not want medical care, but a companion brought her
        into the emergency department, concerned that her thinking was out of char-
        acter and concerning. Laboratory testing is positive for amphetamines, and the
        patient reports last use approximately 4 hours ago. What is the most appropri-
        ate diagnosis for this patient?

        A. Substance/medication-induced obsessive compulsive and related disorder.
        B. Amphetamine withdrawal.
        C. Obsessive-compulsive disorder.
        D. Delusional disorder.

CHAPTER 7

Trauma- and Stressor-Related Disorders

7.1   How does DSM-5-TR differ from DSM-5 in the diagnoses included in the trauma- and stressor-related disorders category?

    A. In DSM-5-TR, prolonged grief disorder is included as a trauma- and stressor-related disorder diagnosis.
    B. In DSM-5-TR, posttraumatic stress disorder (PTSD) has been placed with the depressive disorders.
    C. In DSM-5-TR, PTSD has been placed in a newly created chapter.
    D. In DSM-5-TR, prolonged grief disorder has been placed with "Other Conditions That May Be a Focus of Clinical Attention."

7.2   Which two trauma- and stressor-related disorders require social neglect as a criterion?

    A. Posttraumatic stress disorder and panic disorder.
    B. Acute stress disorder and posttraumatic stress disorder.
    C. Reactive attachment disorder and disinhibited social engagement disorder.
    D. Prolonged grief disorder and reactive attachment disorder.

7.3   Which of the following statements about reactive attachment disorder is *true?*

    A. It occurs only in children who lack healthy attachments.
    B. It occurs only in children who have secure attachments.
    C. It occurs only in children who have impaired communication.
    D. It occurs in children without a history of severe social neglect.

7.4   A 4-year-old boy in day care often displays fear that does not seem to be related to any of his activities. Although frequently distressed, he does not seek contact with any of the staff and does not respond when a staff member tries to comfort him. What additional caregiver-obtained information about this child would be important in deciding whether his symptoms represent reactive attachment disorder or autism spectrum disorder?

A. Age at first appearance of the behavior.
B. Family history about his siblings.
C. History of language delay.
D. Indications that he has experienced severe social neglect.

7.5 Which of the following situations would qualify for a disorder specifier of *severe* in a child diagnosed with reactive attachment disorder?

A. The child has been in five foster homes.
B. The child never expresses positive emotions when interacting with caregivers.
C. The disorder has been present for 18 months.
D. The child meets all symptoms of the disorder, with each symptom manifesting at relatively high levels.

7.6 A 6-year-old girl has repeatedly approached strangers while in the park with her class. The teacher requests an evaluation of the behavior. The girl has a history of being placed in several different foster homes over the past 3 years. Which diagnosis is suggested from this history?

A. Attention-deficit/hyperactivity disorder (ADHD).
B. Disinhibited social engagement disorder.
C. Autism spectrum disorder.
D. Bipolar I disorder.

7.7 A 25-year-old woman presents with a history of being accosted on her way home approximately 2 months ago. The attacker told her he had a gun, was going to rape her, and would shoot her if she resisted. He walked her toward an alley. She was sure he would kill her afterward no matter what she did, and therefore she pushed away from him, aware that she might be shot. She was able to escape unharmed. She describes not being able to fall asleep or walk down that street the day after the incident. Subsequently, she resumed her usual activity, with normalization of her sleep, and was able to walk down that street without anxiety. Now, 4 months after the incident, she says she feels highly anxious all of the time, is often tearful, and feels uncomfortable leaving the house but can walk down that street on her way to work. She denies flashbacks or intrusive thoughts about the incident. What is the most likely diagnosis?

A. Posttraumatic stress disorder (PTSD).
B. Acute stress disorder.
C. Adjustment disorder.
D. Dissociative amnesia.

7.8 After a routine chest X-ray, a 53-year-old man with a history of heavy cigarette use is told that he has a suspicious lesion on his lung. A bronchoscopy leads to a diagnosis of a benign tumor that needs to be resected. The man delays scheduling a follow-up appointment with the surgeon for more than a month and describes feeling as if "all of this is not real." He is tearful and is afraid he will die. He feels intense guilt that his smoking caused the tumor and expresses the thought that he "deserves" to have cancer. What diagnosis best fits this clinical picture?

A. Acute stress disorder.
B. Posttraumatic stress disorder (PTSD).
C. Adjustment disorder.
D. Major depressive disorder.

7.9 Criterion B for acute stress disorder requires the presence of 9 (or more) of 12 symptoms from any of five categories of response. Which of the following is *not* one of these five categories?

A. Intrusion.
B. Dissociation.
C. Confusion.
D. Avoidance.

7.10 Which of the following stressful situations would meet Criterion A for the diagnosis of acute stress disorder?

A. Finding out that one's spouse has been fired.
B. Failing an important final examination.
C. Receiving a serious medical diagnosis.
D. Being in the crossfire of a police shootout but not being harmed.

7.11 Following discharge from the hospital, a 22-year-old man describes vivid and intrusive memories of his stay in the ICU. During the ICU stay, he was extremely agitated, requiring antipsychotic treatment for a few days. Now at home, he states that he has memories of people being tortured in the ICU. He dreams of this every night, waking from sleep in a terror. He talks about not feeling like himself after the experience, finding little pleasure in life after what happened to him, and being easily angered by his family; in addition, he avoids his physician out of fear that he will be told he needs to return to the ICU. What is the most likely explanation for this patient's symptoms?

A. He has acute stress disorder because his life was in danger during the ICU stay.
B. He has posttraumatic stress disorder because his life was in danger during the ICU stay.
C. He has a delirium persisting from the ICU stay.
D. He had a delirium in the ICU and now has an adjustment disorder.

7.12 Which of the following experiences would *not* qualify as exposure to a traumatic event (Criterion A) in the diagnosis of acute stress disorder or posttraumatic stress disorder?

A. Hearing that one's brother was killed in combat.
B. Hearing that one's close childhood friend survived a motor vehicle accident but is paralyzed.
C. Hearing that one's child has been kidnapped.
D. Hearing that one's company has suddenly closed.

7.13   A 31-year-old man narrowly escapes (without injury) from a house fire caused when he dropped a lighter while trying to light his crack pipe. Six weeks later, while smoking crack, he thinks he smells smoke and runs from the building in a panic, shouting, "It's on fire!" Which of the following symptoms or circumstances would rule out a diagnosis of posttraumatic stress disorder (PTSD) for this patient?

A. Having difficulty falling asleep.
B. Being uninterested in going back to work.
C. Inappropriately getting angry at family members.
D. Experiencing symptoms only when smoking crack cocaine.

7.14   Criterion A4 of posttraumatic stress disorder (PTSD) requires "Experiencing repeated or extreme exposure to aversive details of the traumatic event." Which of the following would *not* qualify as experiencing trauma under this criterion?

A. A police officer reviewing surveillance videotapes of homicides to identify perpetrators.
B. A social worker interviewing children who have been sexually abused and obtaining the details of the abuse.
C. A soldier sifting through the rubble of a collapsed building to retrieve remains of comrades.
D. A college student at a film festival watching a series of violent movies that contain scenes of graphic violence.

7.15   Which of the following is *true* about the risk of developing posttraumatic stress disorder (PTSD) in women and men?

A. The risk is lower in females in preschool-age populations.
B. The risk is higher in females across the life span.
C. The risk is higher in males in elderly populations.
D. The risk is lower in middle-age females than in middle-age males.

7.16   A 5-year-old child was present when her babysitter was sexually assaulted. Which of the following symptoms would be most suggestive of posttraumatic stress disorder (PTSD) in this child?

A. Playing normally with toys.
B. Having dreams about princesses and castles.
C. Taking the clothing off her dolls while playing.
D. Expressing no fear when talking about the event.

7.17 Which of the following statements about risk factors for developing posttraumatic stress disorder (PTSD) is *true*?

A. Sustaining personal injury does not affect the risk of developing PTSD.
B. Severity of the trauma influences the risk of developing PTSD.
C. Dissociation has no impact on the risk of developing PTSD.
D. Perceived life threat is the only risk factor for developing PTSD.

7.18 A woman complains of sad mood and feeling hopeless 3 months after her husband files for divorce. She finds it difficult to take care of her home or make meals for her family but has continued to fulfill her responsibilities. She denies suicidal ideation, feels she was a good wife who has "nothing to feel guilty about," and wishes she could "forget about the whole thing." She cannot stop thinking about her situation. Which diagnosis best fits this symptom picture?

A. Adjustment disorder, with depressed mood.
B. Adjustment disorder, with disturbance of conduct.
C. Adjustment disorder, with anxiety.
D. Adjustment disorder, with mixed disturbance of emotions and conduct.

7.19 Twelve months after the death of her husband, a 70-year-old woman is seen for symptoms of overwhelming sadness, anger regarding her husband's unexpected death from a heart attack, intense yearning for him to come back, and repeated unsuccessful attempts to begin moving out of her large home (which she can no longer afford) due to inability to sort through and dispose of her husband's belongings. She cannot believe that he has died and expresses the feeling that "a part of me died that day." What is the most appropriate diagnosis?

A. Major depressive disorder.
B. Posttraumatic stress disorder.
C. Adjustment disorder, with depressed mood.
D. Prolonged grief disorder

7.20 A 25-year-old woman with asthma becomes extremely anxious when she gets an upper respiratory infection. She presents to the emergency department with complaints of being unable to breathe. While there, she begins to hyperventilate and then reports feeling extremely dizzy. Her hyperventilation causes her to become fatigued, and when the medical evaluation indicates that she is retaining carbon dioxide, it becomes necessary to admit her. The woman denies any other symptoms beyond anxiety. What is the most appropriate diagnosis?

A. Acute stress disorder.
B. Generalized anxiety disorder.
C. Adjustment disorder with anxiety.
D. Psychological factors affecting other medical conditions.

7.21 How many Criterion B symptoms are required to be present for the diagnosis of acute stress disorder?

A. One.
B. Three.
C. Five.
D. Nine.

7.22 Criterion B in the DSM-5-TR diagnostic criteria for acute stress disorder requires the presence of symptoms from five different categories: *intrusion*, *negative mood*, *dissociative*, *avoidance*, and *arousal*. Match each of the following symptoms to the appropriate category (each symptom may be placed into only one category).

A. Recurrent, involuntary, and intrusive distressing memories of the traumatic event(s).
B. Problems with concentration.
C. Persistent inability to experience positive emotions (e.g., inability to experience happiness, satisfaction, or loving feelings).
D. An altered sense of the reality of one's surroundings or oneself (e.g., seeing oneself from another's perspective, being in a daze, time slowing).
E. Efforts to avoid external reminders (people, places, conversations, activities, objects, situations) that arouse distressing memories, thoughts, or feelings about or closely associated with the traumatic event(s).
F. Irritable behavior and angry outbursts (with little or no provocation), typically expressed as verbal or physical aggression toward people or objects.
G. Inability to remember an important aspect of the traumatic event(s) (typically due to dissociative amnesia and not other factors such as head injury, alcohol, or drugs).
H. Recurrent distressing dreams in which the content and/or affect of the dream is related to the event(s).
I. Hypervigilance.
J. Dissociative reactions (e.g., flashbacks) in which the individual feels or acts as if the traumatic event(s) were recurring.
K. Exaggerated startle response.
L. Efforts to avoid distressing memories, thoughts, or feelings about or closely associated with the traumatic event(s).
M. Sleep disturbance (e.g., difficulty falling or staying asleep, restless sleep).
N. Intense or prolonged psychological distress or marked physiological reactions in response to internal or external cues that symbolize or resemble an aspect of the traumatic event(s).

7.23 Two months following the death of her son, a 49-year-old woman consults you for psychotherapy. She reports that her son died following a skiing accident on a trip that she gave him as a gift for his 17th birthday. She is preoccupied with the death and blames herself for providing the gift of the trip, but she does not experience yearning for her son. Although she denies any overt suicidal plans, she describes sadness and anxiety related to his death. She has not entered her son's room since his death and has difficulty relating to her husband, feeling anger toward him for agreeing to allow their son to go on the ski trip. She was treated with a selective serotonin reuptake inhibitor at full dose for 3 months after her son's death but reports that the medication had no impact on her symptoms. What is the most appropriate diagnosis?

A. Major depressive disorder.
B. Normal grief.
C. Prolonged grief disorder.
D. Adjustment disorder.

CHAPTER 8

Dissociative Disorders

8.1   Which of the following disorders can be comorbid with dissociative identity disorder?

   A. Bipolar disorder.
   B. Schizophrenia.
   C. Posttraumatic stress disorder (PTSD).
   D. Factitious disorder.

8.2   Which of the following is considered a dissociative disorder?

   A. Acute stress disorder.
   B. Posttraumatic stress disorder (PTSD).
   C. Traumatic brain injury.
   D. Depersonalization/derealization disorder.

8.3   Which of the following statements correctly describes the adjectives *positive* and *negative* when applied to dissociative symptoms?

   A. Negative dissociative symptoms involve loss of continuity in subjective experience.
   B. Positive dissociative symptoms include amnesia.
   C. Negative dissociative symptoms refer to the inability to access information or to control mental functions in a normal fashion.
   D. Negative dissociative symptoms include division of identity.

8.4   Which of the following is a *true* statement about depersonalization/derealization disorder?

   A. The 12-month prevalence of depersonalization/derealization disorder is thought to be markedly less than the prevalence of transient depersonalization/derealization symptoms.
   B. The mean age at onset of depersonalization/derealization disorder is 25 years.
   C. During depersonalization or derealization experiences, individuals typically lose reality testing.
   D. Sexual abuse is the most common childhood interpersonal trauma in individuals with depersonalization/derealization disorder.

8.5   Which of the following symptom presentations is the most common manifestation of Criterion A for non-possession-form dissociative identity disorder?

A. Elaborate personality states with different names, wardrobes, hairstyles, handwritings, and accents.
B. Ego-syntonic abrupt inhibition of speech and action.
C. Alterations in sense of self and agency that the individual experiences as under their control.
D. Experience of the self as multiple simultaneously overlapping and interfering states.

8.6   Which of the following statements best characterizes Criterion B (dissociative amnesia) in dissociative identity disorder?

A. Dissociative amnesia is not typically apparent to others.
B. Minimization or rationalization of amnesia is common.
C. Amnesia is limited to stressful or traumatic events.
D. Dissociative fugues are uncommon.

8.7   Which of the following is the most common type of dissociative amnesia?

A. Continuous amnesia.
B. Irreversible amnesia.
C. Localized or selective amnesia.
D. Generalized amnesia.

8.8   Which of the following presentations can be specified using the *other specified dissociative disorder* designation?

A. Symptoms characteristic of a dissociative disorder that do not meet the full criteria for any of the disorders in the dissociative disorders diagnostic class.
B. Chronic and recurrent syndromes of mixed dissociative symptoms.
C. Presentations for which there is insufficient information to make a more specific diagnosis.
D. The clinician chooses *not* to specify the reason that the criteria are not met for a specific dissociative disorder.

CHAPTER 9

Somatic Symptom and Related Disorders

9.1 Somatoform disorders in DSM-IV are referred to as somatic symptom and related disorders in DSM-5-TR. Which of the following features characterizes the major diagnosis in this class, somatic symptom disorder?

   A. Absence of a medical explanation for somatic symptoms.
   B. Initial presentation mainly in mental health care rather than medical settings.
   C. Lack of medical comorbidity.
   D. Distressing somatic symptoms plus abnormal thoughts, feelings, and behaviors in response to these symptoms.

9.2 In DSM-IV, a patient with a high level of anxiety about having a disease and many associated somatic symptoms would have been given the diagnosis of hypochondriasis. What DSM-5-TR diagnosis would apply to this patient?

   A. Psychological factors affecting other medical condition.
   B. Illness anxiety disorder.
   C. Somatic symptom disorder.
   D. Functional neurologic symptom disorder.

9.3 In DSM-III and DSM-IV, a large number of somatic symptoms were needed to qualify for the diagnosis of somatization disorder. How many somatic symptoms are needed to meet symptom criteria for the DSM-5-TR diagnosis of somatic symptom disorder?

   A. None.
   B. Two or more.
   C. One.
   D. Any number of symptoms that are continuously present.

9.4 After an airplane flight, a 60-year-old woman with a history of chronic anxiety develops deep vein thrombophlebitis and a subsequent pulmonary embolism. Over the next year, she focuses relentlessly on sensations of pleuritic chest pain and repeatedly seeks medical attention for this symptom, with concern that it is due to recurrent pulmonary emboli, despite negative test results. Review of systems reveals the presence of chronic back pain and multiple prior consultations for symptoms of culture-negative cystitis. What diagnosis best fits this clinical picture?

A. Illness anxiety disorder.
B. Panic disorder.
C. Generalized anxiety disorder.
D. Somatic symptom disorder.

9.5 Illness anxiety disorder involves a preoccupation with having or acquiring a serious illness. How severe are the accompanying somatic symptoms?

A. Moderate.
B. Severe.
C. Somatic symptoms are not present.
D. Mild.

9.6 Over a period of several years, a 50-year-old woman visits her dermatologist's office every few weeks to be evaluated for skin cancer, showing the dermatologist various freckles, nevi, and patches of dry skin. None of the skin findings have ever been abnormal, and the dermatologist has provided repeated reassurance. The patient has no pain, itching, bleeding, or other somatic symptoms. What is the most likely diagnosis?

A. Adjustment disorder.
B. Illness anxiety disorder.
C. Obsessive-compulsive disorder (OCD).
D. Somatic symptom disorder.

9.7 A 45-year-old man with a family history of early-onset coronary artery disease avoids climbing stairs, eschews exercise, and abstains from sexual activity for fear of provoking a heart attack. He frequently checks his pulse, reads extensively about preventive cardiology, and tries many health food supplements alleged to be good for the heart. When experiencing an occasional twinge of chest discomfort, he rests in bed for 24 hours; however, he does not go to doctors because of fear about hearing bad news. What diagnosis best fits this clinical picture?

A. Generalized anxiety disorder.
B. Major depressive disorder.
C. Illness anxiety disorder.
D. Other medical condition.

9.8 A 25-year-old woman is hospitalized for evaluation of witnessed episodes that include loss of consciousness, rocking of the head from side to side, and nonsynchronous, bicycling movements of the arms and legs. Per family report, the episodes occur a few times per day and last for 2–5 minutes. Electroencephalography during the episodes does not reveal any ictal activity. Immediately after a fit, the sensorium appears clear. What is the most likely diagnosis?

A. Factitious disorder.
B. Malingering.
C. Somatic symptom disorder.
D. Conversion disorder (functional neurological symptom disorder), with attacks or seizures.

9.9 Which of the following presentations is most suggestive of a diagnosis of conversion disorder (functional neurological symptom disorder)?

A. Absence of Hoover's sign.
B. Chronic dystonic movements.
C. Tunnel vision.
D. Tremor with consistent direction and frequency.

9.10 Why is *la belle indifférence* (apparent lack of concern about the symptom) not included as a diagnostic criterion for conversion disorder (functional neurological symptom disorder)?

A. It is often associated with dissociative symptoms.
B. It has poor specificity.
C. It may be absent in up to 50% of individuals.
D. It is present only at symptom onset or during attacks.

9.11 A 20-year-old man presents with the complaint of acute onset of decreased visual acuity in the left eye. Physical, neurological, and laboratory examinations are entirely normal, including stereopsis testing, fogging test, and brain magnetic resonance imaging. The remainder of the history is negative except for the patient's perseverative focus on facial asymmetry with plans to have plastic surgery soon. Which of the following diagnoses is suggested?

A. Somatic symptom disorder and panic disorder.
B. Factitious disorder and malingering.
C. Body dysmorphic disorder and conversion disorder (functional neurological symptom disorder).
D. Depressive disorder.

9.12 A 50-year-old man with hard-to-control hypertension admits regularly "taking a break" from medications because he was brought up with the belief that pills are bad and natural remedies are better. He is well aware that his blood pressure can become dangerously high when he is not taking his medications. Which diagnosis best fits this case?

A. Somatic symptom disorder.
B. Illness anxiety disorder.

C. Adjustment disorder.

D. Psychological factors affecting other medical conditions.

9.13 A 60-year-old man with prostate cancer has bony metastases that cause persistent pain. He is being treated with antiandrogen medications that result in hot flashes. Although (by his own assessment) his pain is well controlled with analgesics, he states that he is unable to work because of his symptoms. Despite reassurance that his medications are controlling his metastatic disease, every instance of pain leads him to worry that he has new bony lesions and is about to die, and he continually expresses fears about his impending death to his wife and children. Which diagnosis best fits this patient's presentation?

A. Panic disorder.

B. Illness anxiety disorder.

C. Somatic symptom disorder.

D. Psychological factors affecting other medical conditions.

9.14 What is the essential diagnostic feature of factitious disorder?

A. Motivation to assume the sick role.

B. Falsification of medical or psychological signs and symptoms.

C. Obvious external rewards.

D. Absence of a preexisting medical condition.

9.15 When a parent knowingly and deceptively reports signs and symptoms of illness in her preschool-age child, resulting in the child's hospitalization and subjection to numerous tests and procedures, what diagnosis should be recorded for the child?

A. Deception to avoid legal liability.

B. Educational deficits or disabilities.

C. No diagnosis is made for the child.

D. Factitious disorder imposed on another.

9.16 A 25-year-old woman with a history of intravenous heroin abuse is admitted to the hospital with infective endocarditis. Blood cultures are positive for several fungal species. Search of the patient's belongings discloses hidden syringes and needles and a small bag of dirt, which, when cultured, yields the same fungal species. Which of the following diagnoses apply?

A. Opioid use disorder and borderline personality disorder.

B. Opioid use disorder and malingering.

C. Opioid use disorder and factitious disorder.

D. Malingering and borderline personality disorder.

9.17 After finding a breast lump, a 50-year-old woman with a family history of breast cancer is overwhelmed by feelings of anxiety. Consultation with a breast surgeon, mammogram, and biopsy show the lump to be benign. The surgeon tells her that she requires no treatment; however, she continues to ruminate about the possibility of cancer and surgery that will result in disfigurement. Her sleep is restless, and she is having trouble concentrating at work. After 6 weeks of these symptoms, her primary physician refers her for psychiatric consultation. Her medical and psychiatric history is otherwise negative. Which diagnosis best fits this presentation?

A. Somatic symptom disorder.
B. Illness anxiety disorder.
C. Unspecified somatic symptom and related disorder.
D. Other specified somatic symptom and related disorder.

9.18 After finding a breast lump, a 53-year-old woman with a family history of breast cancer is overwhelmed by feelings of anxiety. Consultation with a breast surgeon, mammogram, and biopsy show the lump to be benign. The surgeon indicates that she requires no treatment; however, she continues to ruminate about the possibility of cancer and surgery that will result in disfigurement. Her sleep is restless, and she is having trouble concentrating at work. After 6 weeks in this state, her primary physician requests that she consult a psychiatrist. On initial evaluation the patient weeps throughout the interview and is so distraught that the evaluator is unable to elicit details of her medical and psychiatric history beyond reviewing the current "crisis." Which diagnosis best fits this presentation?

A. Somatic symptom disorder.
B. Illness anxiety disorder.
C. Unspecified somatic symptom and related disorder.
D. Other specified somatic symptom and related disorder.

CHAPTER 10

Feeding and Eating Disorders

10.1   A 27-year-old pregnant woman in her first trimester is joined at her OB-GYN appointment by her partner. The partner informs the physician that the patient has been eating odd items such as pieces of paper and cloth over the past 2 months. The patient admits this behavior, noting that it disturbs her. She is upset at having lost weight and denies any desire to do so. What is the most appropriate diagnosis?

   A. Anorexia nervosa.
   B. Unspecified feeding or eating disorder.
   C. Pica
   D. Factitious disorder.

10.2   Which of the following is a common comorbid diagnosis with rumination disorder?

   A. Anorexia nervosa.
   B. Intellectual disability.
   C. Bulimia nervosa.
   D. Avoidant/restrictive food intake disorder.

10.3   Which of the following distinguishes anorexia nervosa from bulimia nervosa?

   A. Binge eating.
   B. Intense fear of gaining weight.
   C. Abnormally low body weight.
   D. Compensatory behaviors.

10.4   Which of the following distinguishes binge-eating disorder from bulimia nervosa?

   A. Compensatory behaviors.
   B. Binge-eating frequency.
   C. Binge-eating quantity.
   D. Frequent dieting.

10.5 According to DSM-5-TR criteria, which of the following precludes a diagnosis of avoidant/restrictive food intake disorder (ARFID)?

   A. A lifetime anorexia nervosa diagnosis.
   B. Significant weight loss.
   C. Dependence on enteral feeding.
   D. Distorted body image.

10.6 Which specific pattern of avoidant/restrictive food intake disorder (ARFID) is most likely to appear during infancy?

   A. ARFID based on food characteristics.
   B. ARFID related to aversive experiences.
   C. ARFID with lack of interest in food.
   D. ARFID affecting social functioning.

10.7 A 45-year-old woman had a choking episode 3 years ago after eating salad. Since that time she has been afraid to eat a wide range of foods, fearing that she will choke. This fear has affected her functionality and her ability to go to restaurants with friends and has contributed to weight loss. Which diagnosis best fits this clinical picture?

   A. Anorexia nervosa.
   B. Avoidant/restrictive food intake disorder.
   C. Specific phobia.
   D. Adjustment disorder.

10.8 What are the two subtypes of anorexia nervosa?

   A. Restricting type and binge-eating/purging type.
   B. Energy-sparing type and binge-eating/purging type.
   C. Low-calorie/low-carbohydrate type and restricting type.
   D. Restricting type and low-weight type.

10.9 Which of the following is required for the diagnosis of anorexia nervosa?

   A. Inability to gain weight despite normal intake.
   B. Social, occupational, or functional disturbance.
   C. Compensatory purging behaviors.
   D. Disturbed body image.

10.10 Which of the following laboratory abnormalities is commonly found in individuals with anorexia nervosa?

   A. Elevated thyroxine (T_4).
   B. Elevated blood urea nitrogen (BUN).

C. Elevated bone density.

D. Elevated phosphate.

10.11   Which of the following is commonly comorbid with anorexia nervosa?

A. Major depressive disorder.

B. Narcissistic personality disorder.

C. Schizophrenia.

D. Intellectual disability.

10.12   In which developmental period does bulimia nervosa most commonly begin?

A. Middle adulthood.

B. Early childhood.

C. Adolescence.

D. It is equally distributed across the life cycle.

10.13   Which of the following is a common comorbid diagnosis in patients with bulimia nervosa?

A. Stimulant use disorder.

B. Antisocial personality disorder.

C. Avoidant personality disorder.

D. Binge-eating disorder.

10.14   To meet criteria for a diagnosis of binge-eating disorder, which of the following accurately characterizes an episode of binge eating?

A. It is independent of cultural context.

B. It can go on for up to 6 hours.

C. It occurs at least once a week for 3 months.

D. It may consist of continual snacking.

CHAPTER 11

Elimination Disorders

11.1   A 7-year-old boy with moderate developmental delay presents with a chronic history of wetting his clothes during the day about once weekly, even during school. He is now refusing to go to school for fear of wetting his pants and being ridiculed by his classmates. Which of the following statements accurately describes the diagnostic options regarding enuresis in this case?

    A. He should not be diagnosed with enuresis because the frequency is less than twice per week.
    B. He should be diagnosed with enuresis because the incontinence is resulting in impairment of age-appropriate role functioning.
    C. He should not be diagnosed with enuresis because his mental age is likely less than 5 years.
    D. He should be diagnosed with enuresis, diurnal-only subtype.

11.2   What is more common in children with enuresis?

    A. High self-esteem.
    B. Being socially oppressed.
    C. Persistence of urinary incontinence into adulthood.
    D. Older age.

11.3   What is associated with the diurnal-only subtype of enuresis?

    A. Male sex.
    B. Age >9 years old.
    C. Monosymptomatic enuresis.
    D. *Voiding postponement*, in which micturition is consciously deferred because of a social reluctance to use the bathroom or to interrupt a play activity.

11.4   Which of the following statements correctly identifies a distinction between primary enuresis and secondary enuresis?

    A. Children with secondary enuresis have higher rates of psychiatric comorbidity than do children with primary enuresis.
    B. Primary enuresis has a typical onset at age 10, much later than the onset of secondary enuresis.

C. Primary enuresis is never preceded by a period of continence, whereas secondary enuresis is always preceded by a period of continence.
D. Unlike primary enuresis, secondary enuresis tends to persist into late adolescence.

11.5 Which of the following statements correctly describes factors related to the etiology and/or onset of enuresis?

A. Enuresis has been shown to be heritable, with a child being at least twice as likely to have the diagnosis if either parent has had it.
B. Mode of toilet training or its neglect can affect rates of enuresis, as shown by high rates seen in orphanages.
C. In girls with enuresis, nocturnal enuresis is the more common form.
D. Rates of enuresis are much higher in European countries than in developing countries.

11.6 A 4-year-old boy with moderate developmental delay presents with a history of accidentally passing feces into his underwear during the day about once every 2 weeks, even during school. He is now refusing to go to school for fear of soiling his pants and being ridiculed by classmates. Which of the following statements accurately describes the diagnostic options regarding encopresis in this case?

A. Encopresis diagnosis is incorrect because the frequency is less than twice per week.
B. Encopresis diagnosis is incorrect because the incontinence is unintentional.
C. Encopresis diagnosis is incorrect because the patient's mental age is likely less than 4 years old.
D. Encopresis diagnosis is correct.

11.7 Which of the following statements about encopresis is *true*?

A. When oppositional defiant disorder or conduct disorder is present, one cannot diagnose encopresis.
B. When constipation is present, one cannot diagnose encopresis.
C. Urinary tract infections can be comorbid with encopresis.
D. Although it is embarrassing, encopresis has no effect on children's self-esteem.

11.8 Which of the following statements about the encopresis specifier *with constipation and overflow incontinence* is accurate?

A. Encopresis with constipation and overflow incontinence is often involuntary.
B. Encopresis with constipation and overflow incontinence usually involves well-formed stool.

C. Encopresis with constipation and overflow incontinence cannot be diagnosed if the behavior results from psychologically motivated avoidance of defecation.
D. Encopresis with constipation and overflow incontinence rarely resolves after treatment of the constipation.

11.9   When enuresis persists into late childhood or adolescence, the incontinence may resolve. What else is known about enuresis for this population?

A. Urinary frequency generally persists over time.
B. The diurnal form is more likely to persist into adolescence.
C. Incontinence is highly unlikely to recur later in adulthood in women.
D. Cognitive and behavioral problems are less likely.

11.10 What are comorbidities associated with nocturnal enuresis?

A. Gastrointestinal infections.
B. Restless legs syndrome.
C. Depression.
D. Insomnia.

CHAPTER 12

Sleep-Wake Disorders

12.1   Which of the following is a diagnostic criterion for insomnia disorder?

A. The sleep difficulty occurs at least 1 night per week.
B. A prominent complaint of dissatisfaction with sleep quantity or quality.
C. The sleep difficulty is present for at least 6 months.
D. The sleep difficulty may be related to inadequate opportunity to sleep.

12.2   Which of the following is necessary to make a diagnosis of insomnia disorder?

A. Absence of a coexisting medical condition.
B. Difficulty with initiating or maintaining sleep or early morning awakening with inability to return to sleep.
C. Absence of a coexisting mental disorder.
D. Absence of a coexisting sleep disorder.

12.3   An 80-year-old man has a history of myocardial infarction and had coronary artery bypass graft surgery 8 years ago. He plays tennis three times a week, takes care of his grandchildren two afternoons each week, generally enjoys life, and manages all of his activities of daily living independently; however, he complains of excessively early morning awakening. He goes to sleep at 9:00 P.M. and sleeps well, with nocturia once nightly, but wakes at 3:30 A.M. although he would like to rise at 5:00 A.M. He does not endorse daytime sleepiness as a problem. His physical examination, mental status, and cognitive function are normal. What is the most likely sleep-wake disorder diagnosis?

A. Insomnia disorder.
B. Circadian rhythm sleep-wake disorder.
C. Situational/acute insomnia.
D. Normal sleep variations (no sleep-wake disorder diagnosis).

12.4   Which of the following symptoms is most likely to indicate the presence of hypersomnolence disorder?

A. Sleep inertia.
B. Nonrestorative sleep.

C. Chronic sleepiness.

D. Multiple sleep latency test with mean sleep latency <10 minutes.

12.5 An obese 52-year-old man complains of daytime sleepiness, and his partner confirms snoring, snorting, and gasping during nighttime sleep. What polysomnographic finding is needed to confirm the diagnosis of obstructive sleep apnea hypopnea?

A. No polysomnography is necessary.

B. Apnea hypopnea index greater than 30.

C. Evidence by polysomnography of at least 5 obstructive apneas or hypopneas per hour of sleep.

D. Evidence by polysomnography of 15 or more obstructive apneas and/or hypopneas per hour of sleep.

12.6 Diagnostic Criterion B for narcolepsy requires the presence of cataplexy, hypocretin deficiency, *or* characteristic abnormalities on sleep polysomnography or multiple sleep latency testing. Which of the following is a defining characteristic of cataplexy?

A. It is sudden.

B. It occurs unilaterally.

C. It persists for hours.

D. It is accompanied by hypertonia.

12.7 A 68-year-old female patient complains of excessive daytime sleepiness. Nocturnal polysomnography demonstrates 10 episodes of apneas and hypopneas during sleep caused by variability in respiratory effort. Periods of breathing cessation last longer than 10 seconds. There are no nocturnal breathing disturbances and no sustained periods of oxygen desaturation. What is the appropriate DSM-5-TR diagnosis for this individual?

A. Insomnia due to substance use.

B. Sleep-related hypoventilation.

C. Obstructive sleep apnea hypopnea.

D. Central sleep apnea.

12.8 Which of the following metabolic changes is the cardinal feature of sleep-related hypoventilation?

A. Hypocretin deficiency.

B. Hypoxemia.

C. Hypercapnia.

D. Diabetes.

12.9 A 51-year-old man presents with symptoms of chronic fatigue. On weekday nights, it takes him several hours to fall asleep, with subsequent difficulty getting up to go to work in the morning and sleepiness for the first few hours of awake time. On weekends, he awakens later in the morning and feels less fatigue and sleepiness. Which of the following is the correct diagnosis?

A. Circadian rhythm sleep-wake disorder, advanced sleep phase type.
B. Circadian rhythm sleep-wake disorder, irregular sleep-wake type.
C. Circadian rhythm sleep-wake disorder, non-24-hour sleep-wake type.
D. Circadian rhythm sleep-wake disorder, delayed sleep phase type.

12.10 A 67-year-old woman complains of insomnia. She does not have trouble falling asleep between 10 and 11 P.M., but after 1–2 hours she awakens for several hours in the middle of the night, sleeps again for 2–4 hours in the early morning, and then naps three or four times during the day for 1–3 hours at a time. She has a family history of dementia. On examination, she appears fatigued and exhibits deficits in short-term memory, calculation, and abstraction. What is the most likely diagnosis?

A. Major neurocognitive disorder.
B. Circadian rhythm sleep-wake disorder, irregular sleep-wake type.
C. Insomnia disorder.
D. Major depressive disorder.

12.11 Following a traumatic brain injury resulting in blindness, a 50-year-old man develops waxing and waning daytime sleepiness interfering with daytime activity. Serial actigraphy (a method of measuring human activity/rest cycles) demonstrates that the time of onset of the major sleep period occurs progressively later day after day, with a normal duration of the major sleep period. What is the most likely diagnosis?

A. Major depressive disorder.
B. Circadian rhythm sleep-wake disorder, delayed sleep phase type.
C. Circadian rhythm sleep-wake disorder, non-24-hour sleep-wake type.
D. Neurodegenerative disorder.

12.12 A 50-year-old emergency department nurse complains of sleepiness at work interfering with her ability to function. History is notable for a recent switch from the 7 A.M. to 4 P.M. day shift to the 11 P.M. to 8 A.M. night shift. Symptoms include finding it difficult to sleep in the mornings at home, having little energy for recreational activities or household chores in the afternoon, and feeling exhausted by the middle of the overnight shift. What is the most likely diagnosis?

A. Normal variation in sleep with shift work.
B. Circadian rhythm sleep-wake disorder, shift work type.
C. Insomnia disorder.
D. Narcolepsy.

12.13 A 14-year-old adolescent wakes in the morning with clear recollection of very frightening dreams. Once awake, she is normally alert and oriented, but the dreams are a persistent source of distress. Her parents report occasional murmurs or groans but no talking or moving during the period before waking. Other pertinent positives include a history of having been homeless in a series of temporary shelter accommodations for 1 year during childhood. What is the most likely diagnosis?

   A. Sleep terror disorder.
   B. Rapid eye movement (REM) sleep behavior disorder.
   C. Nightmare disorder.
   D. Posttraumatic stress disorder (PTSD).

12.14 Which of the following is a type of rapid eye movement (REM) sleep arousal disorder?

   A. Sleepwalking.
   B. Sleep terrors.
   C. Nightmare disorder.
   D. Confusional arousals.

12.15 Which of the following is a specific subtype of non–rapid eye movement sleep arousal disorder, sleepwalking type?

   A. Sleep terrors.
   B. Sleep-related sexual behavior (sexsomnia).
   C. Parasomnia overlap syndrome.
   D. Night eating syndrome.

12.16 What is the key abnormality in sleep physiology in rapid eye movement (REM) sleep behavior disorder?

   A. Infrequent periodic extremity electromyography active during non-REM (NREM) sleep.
   B. Increased muscle activity uniformly across all muscle groups.
   C. Sleep paralysis.
   D. REM sleep without atonia.

12.17 Which of the following conditions is commonly associated with rapid eye movement (REM) sleep behavior disorder?

   A. Narcolepsy.
   B. Synucleinopathies.
   C. Seizure disorder.
   D. Dissociative disorders.

12.18 Which of the following classes of psychotropic drugs may result in rapid eye movement (REM) sleep without atonia and REM sleep behavior disorder?

A. Selective serotonin reuptake inhibitors (SSRIs).
B. Opioids.
C. Benzodiazepines.
D. Stimulants.

12.19 A 10-year-old boy is referred for evaluation of difficulty sitting still in school, which is interfering with his academic performance. He complains of an unpleasant "creepy-crawly" sensation in his legs for the past 3 months and an urge to move his legs when sitting still that is relieved by movement. This symptom is present most of the day but less so when he is playing sports after school or watching television in the evening, and it generally does not occur in bed at night. What aspect of this clinical presentation rules out a diagnosis of restless legs syndrome (RLS)?

A. The urge to move the legs is partially or totally relieved by movement.
B. The urge to move the legs begins or worsens during periods of rest or inactivity.
C. The symptoms have persisted for only 3 months.
D. The urge to move the legs is worse during the day than at night.

12.20 A 28-year-old pregnant patient reports restlessness and difficulty falling asleep at the onset of the sleep period, as well as daytime fatigue. There have been no changes in her sleep-work schedule. What sleep disorder is suggested by the onset of these symptoms in the third trimester of pregnancy?

A. Nocturnal leg cramps.
B. Narcolepsy.
C. Restless legs syndrome (RLS).
D. Obstructive sleep apnea.

12.21 Which of the following sleep disturbances is associated with *chronic* opioid use?

A. Increase in sleepiness.
B. Insomnia.
C. Increased total sleep time.
D. Increased rapid eye movement (REM) and slow-wave sleep.

12.22 Which of the following substances is associated with parasomnias?

A. Amphetamines.
B. Zolpidem.
C. Cannabis.
D. Caffeine.

12.23 A 56-year-old college professor complains of having difficulty sleeping for more than 5 hours per night over the past few weeks, with associated daytime sleepiness. Awakening occurs an hour or two before her intended waking time in the morning, with associated restless sleep with frequent awakenings until it is time to get up. There is no initial insomnia or depressed mood. She attributes the sleep trouble to intrusive thoughts that arise, after an initially momentary awakening, about the need to complete an overdue academic project. What is the most appropriate diagnosis?

A. Unspecified insomnia disorder.
B. Other specified insomnia disorder (restricted to nonrestorative sleep).
C. Insomnia disorder.
D. Other specified insomnia disorder (short-term insomnia disorder).

CHAPTER 13

Sexual Dysfunctions

13.1   Which of the following is required for a diagnosis of female sexual interest/
         arousal disorder?

A. The disturbance has been present since the individual became sexually active.
B. At least three manifestations of lack of, or significantly reduced, sexual interest/arousal.
C. The symptoms are not limited to certain types of stimulation, situations, or partners.
D. The symptoms have persisted for a minimum duration of approximately 6 weeks.

13.2   Which of the following is a subtype of sexual dysfunction in DSM-5-TR?

A. Lifelong.
B. Secondary to a medical condition.
C. Due to partner violence.
D. Due to an anxiety disorder.

13.3   A 65-year-old man presents with difficulty in obtaining an erection due to diabetes and severe vascular disease (previously diagnosed in DSM-IV as sexual dysfunction due to…[indicate the general medical condition] [coded as *607.84 male erectile disorder due to diabetes mellitus*]). What is the correct DSM-5-TR diagnosis for this presentation?

A. Sexual dysfunction due to a general medical condition.
B. Erectile disorder.
C. Erectile dysfunction.
D. No psychiatric diagnosis.

13.4   A 35-year-old man with new-onset diabetes presents with a 6-month history of inability to maintain an erection. The erectile dysfunction began suddenly 1 month after he was fired from his job. Serum glucose is well controlled with oral hypoglycemic medication. What is the appropriate DSM-5-TR diagnosis?

A. No psychiatric diagnosis.
B. Erectile disorder.

C. Substance/medication-induced sexual dysfunction.

D. Major depressive disorder.

13.5 Which of the following factors should be considered during assessment and diagnosis of a sexual dysfunction?

A. Biological factors only.

B. Factors related to the patient only and not their partner.

C. Cultural or religious factors.

D. The individual's specific sex assigned at birth.

13.6 A 30-year-old woman comes to your office and reports that she is there only because her mother pleaded with her to see you. She tells you that although she has a good social network with friends of both sexes, she has never had any feelings of sexual arousal in response to men or women, does not have any erotic fantasies, and has little interest in sexual activity. She has found other like-minded individuals, and she and her friends accept themselves as asexual. What is the appropriate diagnosis, if any?

A. Female sexual interest/arousal disorder.

B. Other specified sexual dysfunction.

C. No diagnosis because she does not have the minimum number of symptoms required for female sexual interest/arousal disorder.

D. No diagnosis because she does not have clinically significant distress or impairment.

13.7 Which of the following symptoms or conditions would rule out a diagnosis of erectile disorder?

A. Presence of diabetes mellitus.

B. Marked decrease in erectile rigidity.

C. Presence of alcohol use disorder.

D. Presence of symptoms for less than 3 months.

13.8 Which of the following is a distinctive feature of premature (early) ejaculation versus delayed ejaculation?

A. Symptoms have been present for at least 6 months.

B. Symptoms must be experienced during partnered sexual activity.

C. Symptoms cause clinically significant distress in the individual.

D. Severity is based on the level of distress experienced by the individual.

13.9 Which of the following medications is most likely to cause sexual dysfunction?

A. Bupropion.

B. Lamotrigine.

C. Citalopram.

D. Nefazodone.

13.10 Which of the following conditions would be appropriately diagnosed as *other specified sexual dysfunction*?

A. Substance/medication-induced sexual dysfunction.

B. Sexual aversion.

C. Delayed ejaculation.

D. Female sexual interest/arousal disorder.

CHAPTER 14

Gender Dysphoria

14.1   In order for a child to meet criteria for a diagnosis of gender dysphoria, which of the following *must* be present?

A. A co-occurring disorder of sex development.
B. A strong desire to be of the other gender or an insistence that one *is* the other gender (or some alternative gender different from one's assigned gender).
C. A strong dislike of one's sexual anatomy.
D. A strong desire for the primary and/or secondary sex characteristics that match one's experienced gender.

14.2   Which of the following statements about the diagnosis of gender dysphoria in adolescents and adults is *true*?

A. The *posttransition* specifier is used to indicate that the individual has undergone (or is preparing to have) at least one gender-affirming medical procedure or treatment regimen.
B. To qualify for the diagnosis, the individual must be pursuing some kind of sex reassignment treatment.
C. To qualify for the diagnosis, the individual must have a strong desire to be of a different gender or must insist that they *are* the other gender.
D. To qualify for the diagnosis, the individual must have an associated disorder of sex development.

14.3   Match each of the following terms (A–D) to its correct definition (i–iv).

A. Transgender.
B. Gender.
C. Sex.
D. Transsexual.

i.   The biological indicators of male or female.
ii. An individual's public, sociocultural (and usually legally recognized) lived role as boy or girl, man or woman.
iii. An individual whose gender identity is different from their birth-assigned gender.
iv. A term historically denoting an individual who seeks, or has undergone, a social transition from male to female or female to male.

14.4   How is a person's gender determined?

   A. Biological factors contribute, in interaction with social and psychological factors, to gender development.
   B. Gender is determined at birth.
   C. Gender is determined officially (and sometimes legally) when an individual changes gender.
   D. Gender is determined by medical procedures that align an individual's physical characteristics with their experienced gender.

14.5   What DSM-5-TR diagnosis has replaced the former DSM-IV diagnosis of gender identity disorder?

   A. Gender atypical.
   B. Transvestic disorder.
   C. Gender dysphoria.
   D. Nonconformity to gender roles.

CHAPTER 15

Disruptive, Impulse-Control, and Conduct Disorders

15.1   A 7-year-old boy has shown extreme stubbornness and defiance for the past year. This behavior is seen primarily at home and does not typically involve significant mood instability or anger, although he occasionally can be spiteful and vindictive. These symptoms have affected his sibling relationships in an extremely negative fashion, and more recently this behavior has been seen with peers and has begun to affect his friendships. His parents demonstrate a somewhat hostile parenting style. Which of the following statements about the diagnosis of oppositional defiant disorder (ODD) for this patient is correct?

A. The child does not qualify for a diagnosis of ODD because his symptoms lack a significant mood component.
B. The child may qualify for a diagnosis of ODD, despite lacking a persistently negative mood, if he meets the other symptom criteria.
C. The child does not qualify for a diagnosis of ODD because his symptoms are confined primarily to the home setting.
D. The child does not qualify for a diagnosis of ODD because his symptoms have not been present for a sufficient period of time.

15.2   A 3-year-old boy has had severe temper tantrums occurring approximately weekly for a 6-month period. The tantrums are characterized by anger and defiant behavior, with the boy arguing back against his parents' instructions. The tantrums are usually preceded by a change in routine, fatigue, or hunger and rarely include any aggression or property destruction. The boy is generally well behaved in nursery school and during periods between his tantrums. Which of the following is the most appropriate diagnosis?

A. Oppositional defiant disorder (ODD).
B. Intermittent explosive disorder (IED).
C. Disruptive mood dysregulation disorder (DMDD).
D. None of the above.

15.3 The diagnostic criteria for oppositional defiant disorder (ODD) include specifiers for indicating severity of the disorder as manifested by pervasiveness of symptoms across settings and relationships. Which of the following specifiers would be appropriate for an 11-year-old child who meets Criterion A symptoms at home and at school?

A. Mild.
B. Moderate.
C. Severe.
D. Insufficient information.

15.4 A previously well-behaved 13-year-old begins to display extremely defiant and oppositional behavior, with vindictiveness, for the past 8 months. They are angry and argumentative and refuse to accept responsibility for their behavior, which is significantly affecting their life at home and in school. Which aspect of this presentation fits poorly with a diagnosis of oppositional defiant disorder (ODD)?

A. Lack of remorse.
B. Duration of symptoms.
C. Age at onset.
D. Symptoms in multiple settings.

15.5 What is an associated risk factor with oppositional defiant disorder (ODD)?

A. Heightened cortisol reactivity.
B. Being bullied.
C. Permissive parenting.
D. Low emotional reactivity.

15.6 A 16-year-old boy with a long history of defiant behavior toward authority figures also has a history of aggression toward peers (gets into fights at school), his parents, and objects (punching holes in walls, breaking doors). He lies frequently. Recently, he began to steal merchandise from local stores and money and jewelry from his parents. He does not seem pervasively irritable or depressed, has no sleep disturbance, and denies any history of psychotic symptoms. What is the most likely diagnosis?

A. Oppositional defiant disorder (ODD).
B. Conduct disorder.
C. Attention-deficit/hyperactivity disorder (ADHD).
D. Disruptive mood dysregulation disorder (DMDD).

15.7 A 15-year-old boy has a history of episodic violent behavior that is out of proportion to the precipitant. During a typical episode, which escalates rapidly, he becomes extremely angry, punching holes in walls or destroying furniture in the home. There seems to be no specific purpose or gain associated with the outbursts, and within 30 minutes he is calm and "back to normal," a state that is not associated with any predominant mood disturbance. What diagnosis best fits this clinical picture?

A. Bipolar disorder.
B. Disruptive mood dysregulation disorder (DMDD).
C. Intermittent explosive disorder (IED).
D. Attention-deficit/hyperactivity disorder (ADHD).

15.8   Which of the following is *not* a risk factor for intermittent explosive disorder (IED)?

A. First-degree relatives with IED.
B. Separation from family members in refugee populations.
C. Schizotypal personality disorder.
D. Borderline personality disorder.

15.9   Which of the following biological markers is associated with intermittent explosive disorder (IED)?

A. Serotonergic abnormalities in the limbic system and orbitofrontal cortex.
B. Reduced amygdala responses to anger stimuli during functional MRI (fMRI) scanning.
C. Abnormalities in adrenal function.
D. Increased urinary catecholamines.

15.10 Which of the following statements about the differential diagnosis of intermittent explosive disorder (IED) is *false*?

A. In children, the diagnosis of IED can be made in the context of an adjustment disorder.
B. In contrast to IED, disruptive mood dysregulation disorder is characterized by a persistently negative mood state (i.e., irritability, anger) most of the day, nearly every day, between impulsive aggressive outbursts.
C. The level of impulsive aggression in individuals with antisocial personality disorder or borderline personality disorder is lower than that in individuals with IED.
D. Aggression in oppositional defiant disorder is typically characterized by temper tantrums and verbal arguments with authority figures, whereas impulsive aggressive outbursts in IED are in response to a broader array of provocation and include physical assault.

15.11 A 17-year-old adolescent with a history of bullying and initiating fights using bats and knives has also stolen from others, set fires, destroyed property, broken into homes, and "conned" others. Which conduct disorder Criterion A category is not met in this vignette?

A. Aggression to people and animals.
B. Destruction of property.

C. Deceitfulness or theft.

D. Serious violations of rules.

15.12 A 15-year-old adolescent with a history of cruelty to animals, stealing, school truancy, and running away from home shows no remorse when caught or when confronted with how these behaviors affect her family. She disregards the feelings of others and seems to not care that her conduct is compromising her school performance. The behavior has been present for more than a year and in multiple relationships and settings. Which of the following components of the *with limited prosocial emotions* specifier is absent in this clinical picture?

A. Lack of remorse or guilt.

B. Callous—lack of empathy.

C. Unconcerned about performance.

D. Shallow or deficient affect.

15.13 Which of the following does *not* qualify as aggressive behavior under Criterion A definitions for the diagnosis of conduct disorder?

A. Cyberbullying.

B. Forcing someone into sexual activity.

C. Stealing while confronting a victim.

D. Aggression in the context of a mood disorder.

15.14 A 16-year-old adolescent who has started to miss school at least three times a week this year is argumentative with her teachers and parents. Her parents recall many tantrums due to not getting her way when she was preschool age. Recently, she has been breaking curfew and returning home intoxicated around 2 A.M. There was a time last year where she was missing for 2 weeks. Which of this patient's symptoms is a symptom of conduct disorder?

A. School truancy.

B. Tantrums during preschool age.

C. Running away for a lengthy period.

D. Breaking curfew.

15.15 Compared with individuals with childhood-onset conduct disorder, what are patients with adolescent-onset conduct disorder more likely to have?

A. Oppositional defiant disorder (ODD).

B. Attention-deficit/hyperactivity disorder (ADHD).

C. Persistent symptoms into adulthood.

D. Normative peer relationships.

15.16 What is more common in individuals who qualify for the *with limited prosocial emotions* specifier for conduct disorder?

A. Personality features such as risk avoidance, fearfulness, and extreme sensitivity to punishment.
B. Engaging in aggression that is impulsive.
C. A *mild severity* specifier rating.
D. Childhood-onset subtype of conduct disorder.

15.17 When comparing populations, which population is associated with a higher prevalence of conduct disorder?

A. United States compared with other Western countries.
B. Socially oppressed adolescents compared with socially advantaged adolescents.
C. Females compared with males.
D. Children compared with adolescents.

15.18 Which of the following statements about the onset and developmental course of conduct disorder is *true*?

A. Onset may occur as early as the preschool years.
B. Age at onset has no bearing on the developmental course of the disorder.
C. Oppositional defiant disorder is generally not a precursor to the childhood-onset type of conduct disorder.
D. Onset is common after age 16.

15.19 Which of the following is a risk factor for the development of conduct disorder?

A. Higher-than-average verbal IQ.
B. Small family size.
C. Refugee status.
D. Parental history of attention-deficit/hyperactivity disorder (ADHD).

15.20 What is *not* a risk or prognostic factor associated with conduct disorder?

A. Biological sibling with conduct disorder.
B. Low skin conductance.
C. Adoptive parent with conduct disorder.
D. Increased autonomic fear conditioning

15.21 Which of the following helps distinguish conduct disorder from oppositional defiant disorder (ODD)?10

A. Conduct disorder is more likely to involve aggression toward other people.
B. ODD is more likely to involve conflict with parents.
C. Conduct disorder is more likely to involve an angry or irritable mood.
D. A diagnosis of conduct disorder supersedes and precludes the diagnosis of ODD.

15.22 Which of the following comorbid disorders is *not* associated with pyromania?

    A. Antisocial personality disorder.
    B. Substance use disorders.
    C. Obsessive-compulsive disorder
    D. Gambling disorder.

15.23 A 15-year-old student in private school, without known psychiatric history, has been caught stealing other students' laptops and cell phones, even though he comes from a wealthy family and his parents continue to purchase the newest electronics for him in an effort to deter him from stealing. Which of the following would raise your clinical suspicion that the patient may have kleptomania?

    A. He demonstrates recurrent failure to resist impulses to steal objects that are not needed for personal use or for their monetary value.
    B. He demonstrates recurrent failure to resist impulses to steal objects during periods of detachment or boredom.
    C. He experiences increased tension before committing the theft but does not experience relief, pleasure, or gratification while committing the theft.
    D. He has a strong family history for antisocial personality disorder and conduct disorder.

15.24 Which of the following statements about kleptomania is *false*?

    A. The prevalence of kleptomania in the general population is generally very low, and the disorder is more frequent among females.
    B. First-degree relatives of individuals with kleptomania may have higher rates of obsessive-compulsive disorder and/or substance use disorders than the general population.
    C. Kleptomania can occur in a manic episode as a response to a delusion or hallucination.
    D. Individuals with kleptomania generally do not preplan their thefts.

15.25 Which diagnosis is associated with higher risk for suicidal ideation and behavior?

    A. Intermittent explosive disorder (IED).
    B. Kleptomania.
    C. Oppositional defiant disorder (ODD).
    D. All of the above.

15.26 A 12-year-old boy with a history of verbal arguments with his parents and teachers was physically cruel to the family's pet hamster 3 months ago. Last month he stole his mother's credit card to purchase video games and clothes. He is brought to the emergency department after the police pick him up for setting a fire in one of the alleys near his parents' apartment building. What piece of information would indicate this could be due to pyromania rather than conduct disorder?

A. He burned the clothes he had stolen to avoid getting caught.
B. He is intoxicated and voices were commanding him to set the fire.
C. He practiced setting smaller fires at school and home and saved the ashes.
D. He set the fire on purpose.

CHAPTER 16

Substance-Related and Addictive Disorders

16.1 The diagnostic criteria for substance abuse, substance dependence, substance intoxication, and substance withdrawal were not equally applicable to all substances in DSM-IV and were changed in DSM-5. This remains the case in DSM-5-TR, with *substance use disorder* replacing the DSM-IV diagnoses of *substance abuse* and *substance dependence.* For which of the following substance classes is there adequate evidence to support diagnostic criteria in DSM-5 for the three major categories of *use disorder, intoxication,* and *withdrawal?*

A. Caffeine.
B. Cannabis.
C. Tobacco.
D. Hallucinogen.

16.2 Which of the following pairs of drugs falls into a single class in DSM-5-TR?

A. Cocaine and phencyclidine (PCP).
B. Cocaine and methylphenidate.
C. 3,4-Methylenedioxymethamphetamine (MDMA [ecstasy]) and methamphetamine.
D. Lorazepam and alcohol.

16.3 Which of the following statements about tolerance and withdrawal in the DSM-5-TR diagnosis of substance use disorder is *true?*

A. Tolerance and withdrawal are no longer considered to be valid diagnostic symptoms of substance use disorder.
B. The definitions of tolerance and withdrawal have been updated because the previous definitions had poor interrater reliability.
C. The presence of either tolerance or withdrawal is now required to make a substance use disorder diagnosis for some but not all classes of substances.
D. Tolerance and withdrawal are still listed as criteria, but if they occur during appropriate medically supervised treatment, they are not counted toward the diagnosis of a substance use disorder.

16.4   Which of the following differentiates alcohol use disorder from the other alcohol-related disorders?

A. Alcohol use disorder involves impaired control over alcohol use.
B. Alcohol use disorder requires a high quantity of alcohol to be consumed.
C. Alcohol use disorder is an intractable condition.
D. The majority of people who use heavy doses of alcohol develop the disorder.

16.5   Which of the following is *not* a recognized alcohol-related disorder in DSM-5-TR?

A. Alcohol dependence.
B. Alcohol use disorder.
C. Alcohol intoxication.
D. Alcohol withdrawal.

16.6   Which of the following statements is correct about the diagnosis of a caffeine-related disorder?

A. The individual must be aware of consuming caffeine.
B. In order to diagnose caffeine intoxication, the amount consumed must exceed 200 mg.
C. The diagnosis of caffeine withdrawal requires the preceding use of caffeine on a daily basis.
D. Caffeine withdrawal may be diagnosed even in the absence of clinically significant distress or impairment in social, occupational, or other important areas of functioning.

16.7   Which of the following symptoms is more common in women than men as a consequence of the abrupt termination of daily or near-daily cannabis use?

A. Less severe withdrawal symptoms.
B. Suicide.
C. Hunger.
D. Irritability.

16.8   Which of the following is *not* a recognized symptom associated with hallucinogen use?

A. Withdrawal.
B. Tolerance.
C. A persistent desire or unsuccessful efforts to cut down or control use of the substance.
D. Recurrent use of the substance in situations in which it is physically hazardous.

16.9   To meet proposed criteria for *neurobehavioral disorder associated with prenatal alcohol exposure,* an individual's prenatal alcohol exposure must have been "more than minimal." How is "more than minimal" exposure defined, in terms of how much alcohol was used by the mother during gestation?

A. Any exposure to alcohol during the pregnancy.
B. Fewer than 10 drinks per month and no more than 1 drink per drinking occasion.
C. Fewer than 7 drinks per month and no more than 3 drinks per drinking occasion.
D. Fewer than 13 drinks per month and no more than 2 drinks per drinking occasion.

16.10 Which of the following is the only non-substance-related disorder to be included in the DSM-5-TR chapter "Substance-Related and Addictive Disorders"?

A. Gambling disorder.
B. Internet gaming disorder.
C. Electronic communication addiction disorder.
D. Compulsive computer use disorder.

16.11 In most substance/medication-induced mental disorders (with the exception of substance/medication-induced major or mild neurocognitive disorder and hallucinogen persisting perception disorder), if the person abstains from substance use, the disorder will eventually disappear or no longer be clinically relevant even without formal treatment. In what time frame is this likely to happen?

A. One hour.
B. One month.
C. Three months.
D. One year.

16.12 Because opioid withdrawal and sedative, hypnotic, or anxiolytic withdrawal can involve very similar symptoms, distinguishing between the two can be difficult. Which of the following presenting symptoms would aid in differentiating opioid withdrawal from sedative, hypnotic, or anxiolytic withdrawal?

A. Nausea or vomiting.
B. Anxiety.
C. Yawning.
D. Restlessness or agitation.

16.13 In DSM-5-TR, the sedative, hypnotic, or anxiolytic class contains all prescription sleeping medications and almost all prescription antianxiety medications. What is the reason that nonbenzodiazepine antianxiety agents (e.g., buspirone, gepirone) are *not* included in this class?

A. They are not generally available in nonparenteral (intravenous or intramuscular) formulations.

B. They do not appear to be associated with significant misuse.

C. They are not associated with illicit manufacturing or diversion (e.g., Schedule I–V drugs in the United States, list of psychotropic substances recognized by the International Narcotics Control Board and the United Nations).

D. They are not respiratory depressants.

16.14 Which of the following criteria was *not* one of the criteria for either substance abuse or substance dependence in DSM-IV but was included in DSM-5 and has been continued in DSM-5-TR?

A. Important social, occupational, or recreational activities are given up or reduced because of substance use.

B. The substance is often taken in larger amounts or over a longer period than was intended.

C. Craving, or a strong desire or urge to use the substance, is present.

D. Recurrent substance use results in a failure to fulfill major role obligations at work, school, or home.

16.15 A 27-year-old woman presents for psychiatric evaluation after almost hitting someone with her car while driving under the influence of marijuana. She reports that her husband pushed her to seek treatment. He has told her that her ongoing marijuana use is a serious stress in the marriage. Nevertheless, she continues to smoke two joints daily and drive while under the influence of marijuana. What is the appropriate diagnosis?

A. Cannabis abuse.

B. Cannabis dependence.

C. Cannabis intoxication.

D. Cannabis use disorder.

16.16 A 35-year-old man with a long-standing history of heavy alcohol use is referred for psychiatric evaluation after his recent admission to the hospital for acute hepatitis. The patient reports that he drank 2–3 drinks daily in college. Over the past 10 years, he has gradually increased his nightly alcohol intake from a single 6-pack to two 12-packs of beer. He frequently oversleeps and does not get to work. He has tried to moderate his alcohol use on numerous occasions with little success, particularly after developing complications associated with alcoholic cirrhosis. The patient admits that he becomes anxious and gets hand tremors when he doesn't drink. This patient meets the criteria for which of the following diagnoses?

A. Alcohol abuse.

B. Alcohol dependence.

C. Alcohol use disorder, severe.

D. Alcohol use disorder, moderate.

16.17 Which of the following is the most accurate statement about predicting alcohol withdrawal or its consequences?

A. Fewer than 10% of individuals undergoing alcohol withdrawal experience dramatic symptoms such as severe autonomic hyperactivity, tremors, or alcohol withdrawal delirium.
B. All of the symptoms of alcohol withdrawal cease after 7 days.
C. Alcohol withdrawal varies widely across U.S. ethnoracial groups.
D. Tonic-clonic seizures occur in approximately 25% of individuals who meet criteria for alcohol withdrawal.

16.18 How many remission specifiers are included in the DSM-5-TR diagnostic criteria for alcohol use disorder?

A. One.
B. Two.
C. Three.
D. Four.

16.19 In which of the following situations would the specifier for a patient in remission be considered to be in a controlled environment?

A. Enlisted in the U.S. armed services.
B. Working on a cargo ship out at sea.
C. Imprisoned in a city jail.
D. Inpatient on a locked hospital unit.

16.20 Which of the following substances is most likely to be associated with poly-drug use?

A. Alcohol.
B. Tobacco.
C. 3,4-Methylenedioxymethamphetamine (MDMA [ecstasy]).
D. Methamphetamine.

16.21 For which of the following substances might laboratory testing be unreliable?

A. Lysergic acid diethylamide (LSD).
B. Cocaine.
C. Alcohol.
D. Opioids.

16.22 Alcohol intoxication, phencyclidine intoxication, cannabis intoxication, and inhalant intoxication have which Criterion C sign in common?

A. Depressed reflexes.
B. Generalized muscle weakness.
C. Nystagmus.
D. Impairment in attention or memory.

16.23 A 25-year-old medical student presents to the student health service at 7 A.M. complaining of having a "panic attack" and vomiting twice. He reports that he stayed up all night studying for his final exam in gross anatomy. The exam starts in an hour, but he feels too anxious to attend. The patient is restless and appears flushed, with visible muscle twitching. He is urinating excessively and has tachycardia, and his electrocardiogram shows premature ventricular complexes. His thoughts and speech appear to be rambling in nature. His urine toxicology screen is negative. What is the most likely diagnosis?

A. Panic disorder.
B. Amphetamine intoxication, amphetamine-like substance.
C. Caffeine intoxication.
D. Cocaine intoxication.

16.24 The use of which illicit psychoactive substance is the most prevalent in the United States?

A. 3,4-Methylenedioxymethamphetamine (MDMA [ecstasy]).
B. Phencyclidine.
C. Cannabis.
D. Lysergic acid diethylamide (LSD).

16.25 Which of the following laboratory tests can be used in combination with γ-glutamyltransferase (GGT) to monitor abstinence from alcohol?

A. Alanine aminotransferase (ALT).
B. Alkaline phosphatase.
C. Carbohydrate-deficient transferrin (CDT).
D. Mean corpuscular volume (MCV).

16.26 A patient presents to the student health clinic after a week of drinking several cans of cola eight times a day for a week to complete a bet he lost. The last soda was consumed yesterday. The patient is complaining of the sudden onset of extreme fatigue. With which of the following symptoms is he most likely to present?

A. Vomiting.
B. Drowsiness.
C. Flu-like symptoms.
D. Headache.

16.27 How much does cannabis use disorder increase the risk of an adult having any other substance disorder?

A. One time.
B. Five times.
C. Nine times.
D. Twenty times.

16.28　A patient presents to the emergency department complaining of vomiting that "comes and goes." Which drug is the patient likely using regularly?

A. Tobacco.
B. Alcohol.
C. Cannabis.
D. Cocaine.

16.29　Which adult ethnoracial group has the highest prevalence of cannabis use disorder?

A. Asians and Pacific Islanders.
B. American Indians/Alaska Natives.
C. African Americans.
D. Whites.

16.30　Which of the following drugs that can have hallucinogenic effects is not considered in the DSM-5-TR chemical classes of hallucinogens?

A. Mescaline.
B. 3,4-Methylenedioxymethamphetamine (MDMA [ecstasy]).
C. Cannabis.
D. Psilocybin.

16.31　Use of which of the following drugs is most likely to result in the development of a hallucinogen use disorder?

A. Lysergic acid diethylamide (LSD).
B. Psilocybin.
C. Dimethyltryptamine .
D. 3,4-Methylenedioxymethamphetamine (MDMA [ecstasy]).

16.32　For which of the following hallucinogens is there evidence of a withdrawal syndrome?

A. Lysergic acid diethylamide (LSD).
B. 3,4-Methylenedioxymethamphetamine (MDMA [ecstasy]).
C. Psilocybin.
D. Phencylidine.

16.33　What distinguishes substance/medication-induced mental disorders from substance use disorders?

A. They occur only during periods of intoxication.
B. Symptoms continue in spite of cessation of use of the substance.
C. Cognitive and behavioral symptoms contribute to the continued use.
D. They occur only if the medication is taken at higher than suggested doses.

16.34 Which two groups of inhalant agents are *not* among the recognized substances qualifying for the DSM-5-TR inhalant use disorder diagnosis?

A. Butane lighters and toluene.
B. Xylene and butane.
C. Trichloroethane and hexane.
D. Nitrous oxide and nitrite gases.

16.35 A 22-year-old university student presents to his primary care physician complaining of progressive worsening of numbness, tingling, and weakness in both of his legs over the past several weeks. His gait is unsteady, and he has difficulty grasping objects in his hands. He did not use any substances on the day of presentation but admits that over the past 3 months he has been consistently using one particular substance on a daily basis. Which substance use disorder most likely accounts for this patient's symptoms?

A. Other (or unknown) substance use disorder.
B. Other hallucinogen use disorder.
C. Inhalant use disorder.
D. Opioid use disorder.

16.36 Which organ system or anatomical function is most commonly affected by chronic use of 3,4-methylenedioxymethamphetamine (MDMA [ecstasy])?

A. Neurological.
B. Respiratory.
C. Cardiopulmonary.
D. Oral cavity.

16.37 What percentage of individuals who undergo untreated sedative, hypnotic, or anxiolytic withdrawal experience a grand mal seizure?

A. 5%–10%.
B. 10%–20%.
C. 20%–30%.
D. 30%–40%.

16.38 Which route of stimulant use is most prevalent among individuals who are in treatment for a stimulant use disorder?

A. Oral.
B. Intranasal.
C. Smoking.
D. Intravenous.

16.39 What is the most common co-occurring psychiatric diagnosis among individuals with a history of significant prenatal alcohol exposure?

A. Major depressive disorder.
B. Generalized anxiety disorder.
C. Attention-deficit/hyperactivity disorder (ADHD).
D. Oppositional defiant disorder.

16.40 Which of the following has been included in DSM-5-TR as a potential diagnosis?

A. Sex addiction.
B. Exercise addiction.
C. Shopping addiction.
D. Gaming addiction.

16.41 Which of the following is one of the most common medical consequences of drinking in people with alcohol use disorder?

A. Cirrhosis.
B. Cardiomyopathy.
C. Hypertension.
D. Pancreatitis.

CHAPTER 17

Neurocognitive Disorders

17.1 The essential feature of the DSM-5-TR diagnosis of delirium is a disturbance in attention/awareness and in cognition that develops over a short period of time, represents a change from baseline, and tends to fluctuate in severity during the course of a day. Which of the following additional conditions must apply?

   A. There must be laboratory evidence of an evolving dementia.
   B. The disturbance must be associated with a disruption of the sleep-wake cycle.
   C. The disturbance must not occur in the context of a severely reduced level of arousal, such as coma.
   D. The disturbance must not be superimposed on a preexisting neurocognitive disorder.

17.2 Both major and mild neurocognitive disorders can increase the risk of delirium and complicate its course. Delirium is distinguished from dementia on the basis of the key features of acute onset, impairment in attention, and which of the following?

   A. Fluctuating course.
   B. Steady course.
   C. Presence of depression.
   D. Cogwheeling movements.

17.3 A 79-year-old woman with a history of depression is being evaluated at a nursing home for a suspected urinary tract infection. She is easily distracted, perseverates on answers to questions, asks the same question repeatedly, is unable to focus, and cannot answer questions regarding orientation. The mental status changes evolved over a single day. Her family reports that they thought she "wasn't herself" when they saw her the previous evening, but the nursing report this morning indicates that the patient was cordial and appropriate. What is the most likely diagnosis?

   A. Major depressive disorder, recurrent episode.
   B. Depressive disorder due to another medical condition.
   C. Delirium.
   D. Major depressive disorder, with anxious distress.

17.4 The diagnostic criteria for major or mild neurocognitive disorder with Lewy bodies (NCDLB) include fulfillment of criteria for major or mild neurocognitive disorder and presence of a combination of core diagnostic features and suggested diagnostic features for either probable or possible neurocognitive disorder with Lewy bodies. Another feature necessary for the diagnosis is that the disturbance is not better explained by cerebrovascular disease, another neurodegenerative disease, the effects of a substance, or another mental, neurological, or systemic disorder. Which of the following completes the list of features necessary for the diagnosis?

A. An acute onset and rapid progression.
B. An insidious onset and gradual progression.
C. An insidious onset and rapid progression.
D. A waxing and waning presentation.

17.5 Which of the following is *not* a diagnostic criterion, feature, or marker of major or mild neurocognitive disorder with Lewy bodies (NCDLB)?

A. Concurrent symptoms of rapid eye movement (REM) sleep behavior disorder.
B. High striatal dopamine transporter uptake in basal ganglia demonstrated by single-photon emission computed tomography (SPECT) or positron emission tomography (PET) imaging.
C. Low striatal dopamine transporter uptake in basal ganglia demonstrated by SPECT or PET imaging.
D. Severe neuroleptic sensitivity.

17.6 A 72-year-old man with no history of alcohol or other substance use disorders and no psychiatric history is brought to the emergency department (ED) because of transient episodes of unexplained loss of consciousness. His wife reports that he has experienced repeated falls and syncope over the past year, as well as auditory and visual hallucinations. A thorough workup for cardiac disease has found no evidence of structural heart disease or arrhythmias. In the ED, he is found to have severe autonomic dysfunction, including orthostatic hypotension and urinary incontinence. What is the best provisional diagnosis for this patient?

A. New-onset schizophrenia.
B. Possible major or mild neurocognitive disorder with Lewy bodies (NCDLB).
C. Possible major or mild neurocognitive disorder due to Alzheimer's disease.
D. New-onset seizure disorder.

17.7 The diagnostic criteria for neurocognitive disorder (NCD) due to HIV infection include fulfillment of criteria for major or mild NCD and documented infection with HIV (as confirmed by established laboratory methods). Which of the following is a prominent feature of NCD due to HIV infection?

A. Impairment in executive functioning.
B. Significant delusions and hallucinations at onset of the disorder.

C. Marked difficulty with recall of learned information.

D. Rapid progression to profound neurocognitive impairment.

17.8 In addition to documented infection with HIV and fulfillment of criteria for major or mild neurocognitive disorder (NCD), what other requirement must be met to qualify for a diagnosis of major or mild NCD due to HIV infection?

A. Presence of HIV in the cerebrospinal fluid.

B. A pattern of cognitive impairment characterized by early predominance of aphasia and impaired memory for previously learned information.

C. Inability to attribute the NCD to non-HIV conditions (including secondary brain diseases), another medical condition, or a mental disorder.

D. Presence of Kayser-Fleischer rings.

17.9 Which of the following features characterizes alcohol-induced major or mild neurocognitive disorder, amnestic-confabulatory type?

A. Amnesia for new information and confabulation.

B. Seizures.

C. Amnesia for previously learned information and downward gaze paralysis.

D. Anosognosia and apraxia.

17.10 Which of the following statements about the diagnosis of neurocognitive disorder due to Huntington's disease (NCDHD) is *true*?

A. NCDHD is a laboratory-based diagnosis/disorder.

B. NCDHD is a disorder that requires positive neuroimaging for diagnosis.

C. NCDHD is a clinical diagnosis based on abnormal physical findings and family history/genetic findings.

D. NCDHD is a diagnosis that is best defined as patients who have a pill-rolling tremor.

17.11 Depression, irritability, anxiety, obsessive-compulsive symptoms, and apathy are frequently associated with Huntington's disease and often precede the onset of motor symptoms. Psychosis more rarely precedes the onset of motor symptoms. Which of the following is a core feature of major or mild neurocognitive disorder due to Huntington's disease?

A. Progressive cognitive impairment with early changes in executive function.

B. Prominent early memory impairment, mostly affecting short-term memory.

C. Psychosis in the early stages, with marked olfactory hallucinations.

D. Voluntary jerking movements.

17.12 Genetic testing is the primary laboratory test for the determination of Huntington's disease. Which of the following best characterizes the genetic nature of Huntington's disease?

A. X-linked recessive inheritance with incomplete penetrance.
B. Autosomal recessive inheritance with complete penetrance.
C. Autosomal dominant inheritance with complete penetrance.
D. X-linked dominant inheritance.

17.13 Major or mild neurocognitive disorder (NCD) due to prion disease encompasses NCDs associated with a group of subacute spongiform encephalopathies caused by transmissible agents known as *prions.* What is the most common prion disease?

A. Creutzfeldt-Jakob disease.
B. Bovine spongiform encephalopathy.
C. Huntington's disease.
D. Neurosyphilis.

17.14 Prion disease has been reported to occur in individuals of all ages, from the teenage years to late life. Which of the following best characterizes the time frame of disease progression?

A. Over a few months.
B. Over several days.
C. Over several weeks.
D. Over 5 years.

17.15 Major and mild neurocognitive disorders (NCDs) exist on a spectrum of cognitive and functional impairment. Which of the following constitutes an important threshold differentiating the two diagnoses?

A. Whether the individual is concerned about the decline in cognitive function.
B. Whether there is impairment in cognitive performance as measured by standardized testing or clinical assessment.
C. Whether the cognitive impairment is sufficient to interfere with independent completion of activities of daily living.
D. Whether the cognitive deficits occur exclusively in the context of a delirium.

17.16 Expressed as a percentile, what is the typical performance on neuropsychological testing of individuals with major neurocognitive disorder (NCD)?

A. Sixtieth percentile or below.
B. Fiftieth percentile or below.
C. Sixteenth percentile or below.
D. Third percentile or below.

17.17 A 68-year-old semiretired cardiologist with responsibility for electrocardiogram (ECG) interpretation at his community hospital is referred by the hospital's Employee Assistance Program for clinical evaluation because of concerns expressed by other clinicians that he has been making many mistakes in his

ECG interpretations over the past few months. The patient discloses symptoms of persistent sadness since the death of his wife 6 months prior to the evaluation, with frequent thoughts of death, trouble sleeping, and escalating usage of sedative-hypnotics and alcohol. He has some trouble concentrating, but he has been able to maintain his household, pay his bills, shop, and prepare meals by himself without difficulty. He scores 28/30 on the Mini-Mental State Examination (MMSE). Which of the following would be the primary consideration in the differential diagnosis?

A. Mild neurocognitive disorder (NCD).
B. Adjustment disorder.
C. Major depressive disorder.
D. No diagnosis.

17.18 A 69-year-old semiretired radiologist with responsibility for chest X-ray interpretation at his academic medical center has been referred by the hospital's Employee Assistance Program for clinical evaluation because of concerns expressed by other clinicians that he has been making many mistakes in his X-ray interpretations over the past few months. Evaluation discloses a remote history of alcohol dependence with sobriety for the past 20 years and a depressive episode following the death of his wife 9 years before the current problem, treated with cognitive-behavioral therapy with full resolution of symptoms after 6 months and no recurrence. He acknowledges some trouble concentrating but no other symptoms, and he minimizes the alleged X-ray interpretation problems. He cannot state the correct date or day of the week and cannot recall the previous day's news events, but he can describe highlights of his long career in medicine in great detail. Collateral history from his children reveals that on several occasions in the past year, neighbors in his apartment building had complained that he forgot to turn off his stove while cooking, resulting in a smoke-filled apartment. He scores 21/30 on the Mini-Mental State Examination. What diagnosis best fits this clinical picture?

A. Major neurocognitive disorder (NCD).
B. Mild NCD.
C. Major depressive disorder.
D. No diagnosis.

17.19 In a patient with *mild* neurocognitive disorder (NCD), which of the following would distinguish *probable* from *possible* Alzheimer's disease?

A. Evidence of a causative Alzheimer's disease genetic mutation from either genetic testing or family history.
B. Clear evidence of decline in memory and learning.
C. No evidence of mixed etiology.
D. Onset after age 80.

17.20 In major or mild frontotemporal neurocognitive disorder, which of the following is a diagnostic feature of the language variant?

A. Severe semantic memory impairment.

B. Severe deficits in perceptual-motor function.

C. Grammar, word-finding, or word-generation difficulty.

D. Hyperorality.

17.21 Which of the following neurocognitive disorders (NCDs) is especially characterized by deficits in domains such as speech production, word finding, object naming, or word comprehension, whereas episodic memory, perceptual-motor abilities, and executive function are relatively preserved?

A. Major or mild NCD due to Alzheimer's disease.

B. Major or mild NCD with Lewy bodies.

C. Behavioral-variant major or mild frontotemporal NCD.

D. Language-variant major or mild frontotemporal NCD.

17.22 Which of the following is a core feature of major or mild neurocognitive disorder with Lewy bodies?

A. Fluctuating cognition with pronounced variations in attention and alertness.

B. Recurrent auditory hallucinations.

C. Fulfillment of criteria for rapid eye movement (REM) sleep behavior disorder.

D. Evidence of low striatal dopamine transporter uptake in basal ganglia as demonstrated by single photon emission computed tomography (SPECT) or positron emission tomography (PET) imaging.

17.23 A previously healthy 67-year-old man is brought to the emergency department by his family. He is experiencing an acute change in mental status. There is no evidence in the initial history, physical examination, and laboratory studies to indicate substance intoxication or withdrawal or to suggest another medical problem as the cause of his altered mental state. Over the course of 1 hour of observation, his level of alertness varies from alert but distractible, with apparent auditory and visual hallucinations, to somnolent; he has difficulty sustaining attention to an examiner, and he cannot perform simple tasks such as serial subtractions or spelling words backward. What is the most appropriate diagnosis?

A. Delirium.

B. Delirium due to another medical condition.

C. Delirium due to substance intoxication.

D. Unspecified delirium.

17.24 A 35-year-old man brings his 60-year-old father for evaluation of cognitive and functional decline, stating that he thinks his father has dementia; the son is also worried about the possibility of a hereditary illness. The physician notes to herself that the patient has substantial cognitive impairment and features suggestive of the diagnosis of major neurocognitive disorder due to Huntington's disease, but she is not sure about the cause of the neurocognitive disorder. She also notes that the patient's son appears extremely anxious. She has a tight schedule and cannot provide a counseling session for the patient's son until the next day. What is the most appropriate diagnosis to record on the insurance claim form that the patient's son will submit on his father's behalf?

A. Unspecified central nervous system (CNS) disorder.
B. Unspecified neurocognitive disorder.
C. Unspecified mild neurocognitive disorder.
D. Huntington's disease.

CHAPTER 18

Personality Disorders

18.1 Which of the following DSM-IV personality disorder diagnoses is no longer present in DSM-5-TR?

A. Antisocial personality disorder.
B. Avoidant personality disorder.
C. Borderline personality disorder.
D. Personality disorder not otherwise specified (NOS).

18.2 While collaborating on a presentation to their customers, the members of a sales team become increasingly frustrated with their team leader. He insists that the members of the team adhere to strict rules for developing the project. This involves approaching the task in sequential manner such that no new task can be begun until the prior one is perfected. When other members suggest alternative approaches, the leader becomes frustrated and insists that the team stick to his approach. Although the results are inarguably of high quality, the team is convinced that they will not finish in time for the scheduled presentation. Which of the following disorders would best explain the behavior of this team leader?

A. Narcissistic personality disorder.
B. Obsessive-compulsive disorder (OCD).
C. Schizoid personality disorder.
D. Obsessive-compulsive personality disorder (OCPD).

18.3 Individuals with obsessive-compulsive personality disorder (OCPD) are primarily motivated by a need for which of the following?

A. Efficiency.
B. Admiration.
C. Control.
D. Intimacy.

18.4 Which of the following findings would rule out the diagnosis of obsessive-compulsive personality disorder (OCPD)?

A. A concurrent diagnosis of obsessive-compulsive disorder (OCD).
B. A concurrent diagnosis of hoarding disorder.

C. A concurrent diagnosis of narcissistic personality disorder.

D. Evidence that the behavioral patterns reflect culturally sanctioned interpersonal styles.

18.5 Despite working for a company for many years, a 36-year-old employee has not advanced beyond an entry level position. She gets good reviews and works long hours but has not asked for a promotion because she feels she is not as good as other employees and thus unworthy of promotion. She explains her long hours by saying that she is not very smart and needs to check over all her work because she is afraid that people will ridicule any mistakes. Which of the following personality disorders would best explain this woman's lack of job advancement?

A. Dependent personality disorder.

B. Avoidant personality disorder.

C. Paranoid disorder.

D. Schizoid personality disorder.

18.6 A cardiologist requests a psychiatric consultation for her patient, a 46-year-old man, because of concern that he "seems crazy." On evaluation, the patient makes poor eye contact, tends to ramble, and makes unusual word choices. He is modestly disheveled and wears clothes with mismatched colors. He expresses odd beliefs about supernatural phenomena, but these beliefs do not seem to be of delusional intensity. Collateral information from a sibling elicits the observation that the patient "has always been like this—weird, a loner, and likes it that way." Which of the following conditions best explains this patient's odd behaviors and beliefs?

A. Schizoid personality disorder.

B. Schizotypal personality disorder.

C. Delusional disorder.

D. Schizophrenia.

18.7 Which of the following statements most accurately describes the development, course, and prognosis of borderline personality disorder (BPD)?

A. Suicide attempts increase with age.

B. A childhood history of neglect, rather than abuse, is unusual.

C. Prospective follow-up studies have found that stable remissions of up to 8 years are very common.

D. Affective symptoms remit more rapidly than impulsive symptoms.

18.8 Which of the following is a characteristic of narcissistic personality disorder (NPD)?

A. A requirement for much attention of any kind.

B. Impulsive aggressivity and deceitfulness.

C. Immersion in perfectionism related to order and rigidity.

D. A pervasive pattern of grandiosity.

18.9   Which of the following cognitive or perceptual disturbances are most characteristic of borderline personality disorder (BPD)?

A. Overly concrete or overly abstract responses.

B. Ideas of reference.

C. Superstitiousness or preoccupation with paranormal phenomena.

D. Transient paranoid ideation during periods of stress.

18.10   A 43-year-old warehouse security guard comes to your office complaining of vague feelings of depression for the past few months, with no particular sense of fear or anxiety. He feels little desire for relationships but notes that his co-workers seem happier, and they have many relationships. He has never felt comfortable with other people, not even with family. He has lived alone since early adulthood and is self-sufficient. He almost always works night shifts to avoid interactions with others. He tries to remain low-key and undistinguished to discourage others from striking up conversations. Mental status examination is notable for significantly constricted, bland affect. No cognitive or perceptual disturbances are present. Which personality disorder would best fit with this presentation?

A. Paranoid.

B. Schizoid.

C. Schizotypal.

D. Avoidant.

18.11   Which of the following behaviors or states would be least likely to occur in an individual with schizoid personality disorder?

A. An angry outburst at a colleague who criticizes their work.

B. Turning down an invitation to a party.

C. Lacking desire for sexual experiences.

D. Drifting with regard to life goals.

18.12   What is the relationship between a history of conduct disorder before age 15 and the diagnosis of antisocial personality after age 18?

A. A history of some conduct disorder symptoms before age 15 is one of the required criteria for a diagnosis of antisocial personality disorder in adulthood.

B. Childhood onset of conduct disorder has no relationship to the likelihood of developing antisocial personality disorder in adult life.

C. Both antisocial personality disorder and conduct disorder can be diagnosed before age 18 years.

D. Both antisocial personality disorder and conduct disorder can be diagnosed in individuals older than 18 years.

18.13 A 25-year-old patient has a childhood history of repeated instances of torturing animals, setting fires, stealing, running away from home, and school truancy, beginning at age 9 years. As an adult, he repeatedly lies to others; engages in petty thefts, con games, and frequent fights (including episodes involving the use of objects at hand—pipe wrenches, chairs, steak knives—to injure others); and uses aliases to avoid paying child support. There is no history of manic, depressive, or psychotic symptoms. The patient is dressed in expensive clothing and displays an expensive wristwatch for which he demands admiration. He expresses feelings of specialness and entitlement and endorses a sense of deserving exemption from ordinary rules, as well as feelings of anger that his special talents have not been adequately recognized by others. He shows devaluation of, contempt for, and lack of empathy for others and lack of remorse for his behavior. There is no sign of psychosis. What is the appropriate DSM-5-TR diagnosis?

A. Antisocial personality disorder.
B. Narcissistic personality disorder.
C. Antisocial personality disorder and narcissistic personality disorder.
D. Other specified personality disorder (mixed personality features).

18.14 Which of the following is one of the general criteria for a personality disorder in DSM-5-TR?

A. The pattern of inner experience deviates markedly from the expectations of the individual's culture.
B. The pattern of inner experience is flexible and confined to a single personal or social situation.
C. The pattern of inner experience is fluctuating and of short duration.
D. The pattern of inner experience is ego-syntonic and does not lead to distress.

18.15 Which of the following presentations is characteristic of histrionic personality disorder?

A. A pervasive and excessive need to be taken care of that leads to submissive and clinging behavior and fears of separation.
B. A pervasive pattern of instability in interpersonal relationships, self-image, and affects and marked impulsivity.
C. A pervasive pattern of grandiosity, need for admiration, and lack of empathy.
D. A pervasive pattern of excessive emotionality and attention seeking.

18.16 Which of the following presentations is characteristic of borderline personality disorder?

A. A pervasive and excessive need to be taken care of that leads to submissive and clinging behavior and fears of separation.
B. A pervasive pattern of instability in interpersonal relationships, self-image, and affects and marked impulsivity.

C. A pervasive pattern of grandiosity, need for admiration, and lack of empathy.

D. Pervasive and excessive emotionality and attention seeking.

18.17 Which of the following presentations is characteristic of dependent personality disorder?

A. A pervasive and excessive need to be taken care of that leads to submissive and clinging behavior and fears of separation.

B. A pervasive pattern of instability in interpersonal relationships, self-image, and affects and marked impulsivity.

C. A pervasive pattern of grandiosity, need for admiration, and lack of empathy.

D. A pervasive pattern of social inhibition, feelings of inadequacy, and hypersensitivity to negative evaluation.

18.18 Which of the following presentations is characteristic of avoidant personality disorder?

A. A pervasive pattern of social inhibition, feelings of inadequacy, and hypersensitivity to negative evaluation.

B. A pervasive pattern of social and interpersonal deficits marked by acute discomfort with, and reduced capacity for, close relationships as well as by cognitive or perceptual distortions, and eccentricities of behavior.

C. A pervasive and excessive need to be taken care of that leads to submissive and clinging behavior and fears of separation.

D. A pervasive pattern of instability in interpersonal relationships, self-image, and affects and marked impulsivity.

18.19 Which of the following presentations is characteristic of schizotypal personality disorder?

A. A pervasive pattern of social inhibition, feelings of inadequacy, and hypersensitivity to negative evaluation.

B. A pervasive pattern of social and interpersonal deficits marked by acute discomfort with, and reduced capacity for, close relationships as well as by cognitive or perceptual distortions, and eccentricities of behavior.

C. A pervasive and excessive need to be taken care of that leads to submissive and clinging behavior and fears of separation.

D. A pervasive pattern of instability in interpersonal relationships, self-image, and affects and marked impulsivity.

18.20 Which of the following presentations is characteristic of paranoid personality disorder?

A. A pervasive pattern of social inhibition, feelings of inadequacy, and hypersensitivity to negative evaluation.

B. A pattern of pervasive distrust and suspiciousness of others such that their motives are interpreted as malevolent.

C. A pervasive and excessive need to be taken care of that leads to submissive and clinging behavior and fears of separation.

D. A pervasive pattern of instability in interpersonal relationships, self-image, and affects, and marked impulsivity.

18.21 Which of the following presentations is characteristic of narcissistic personality disorder?

A. A pervasive pattern of social inhibition, feelings of inadequacy, and hypersensitivity to negative evaluation.

B. A pervasive and excessive need to be taken care of that leads to submissive and clinging behavior and fears of separation.

C. A pervasive pattern of instability in interpersonal relationships, self-image, and affects and marked impulsivity.

D. A pervasive pattern of grandiosity, need for admiration, and lack of empathy.

18.22 Which of the following presentations is characteristic of schizoid personality disorder?

A. A pervasive pattern of social inhibition, feelings of inadequacy, and hypersensitivity to negative evaluation.

B. A pervasive pattern of social and interpersonal deficits marked by acute discomfort with, and reduced capacity for, close relationships, as well as by cognitive or perceptual distortions, and eccentricities of behavior.

C. A pervasive pattern of detachment from social relationships and a restricted range of expression of emotions in interpersonal settings.

D. A pervasive pattern of instability in interpersonal relationships, self-image, and affects and marked impulsivity.

18.23 Which of the following presentations is characteristic of antisocial personality disorder?

A. Preoccupation with orderliness, perfectionism, and mental and interpersonal control, at the expense of flexibility, openness, and efficiency.

B. A pervasive pattern of detachment from social relationships and a restricted range of expression of emotions in interpersonal settings.

C. A pattern of pervasive distrust and suspiciousness of others such that their motives are interpreted as malevolent.

D. A pervasive pattern of disregard for, and violation of, the rights of others.

18.24 Which of the following presentations is characteristic of obsessive-compulsive personality disorder?

A. A pervasive pattern of social inhibition, feelings of inadequacy, and hypersensitivity to negative evaluation.

B. A pervasive pattern of social and interpersonal deficits marked by acute discomfort with, and reduced capacity for, close relationships, as well as by cognitive or perceptual distortions, and eccentricities of behavior.

C. Preoccupation with orderliness, perfectionism, and mental and interpersonal control, at the expense of flexibility, openness, and efficiency.

D. A pervasive pattern of detachment from social relationships and a restricted range of expression of emotions in interpersonal settings.

CHAPTER 19

Paraphilic Disorders

19.1 Which of the following is not a classification scheme of paraphilic disorders in DSM-5-TR?

    A. Anomalous activity preferences.
    B. Courtship disorders.
    C. Algolagnic disorders.
    D. Asynchronous disorders.

19.2 Which of the following is *not* a true statement about paraphilias?

    A. The presence of a paraphilia does not always justify clinical intervention.
    B. Most paraphilias can be divided into those that involve an unusual activity and those that involve an unusual target.
    C. Paraphilias may coexist with normophilic sexual interests.
    D. It is rare for an individual to manifest more than one paraphilia.

19.3 Which of the following is *not* a paraphilic disorder?

    A. Sexual masochism disorder.
    B. Transvestic disorder.
    C. Transsexual disorder.
    D. Voyeuristic disorder.

19.4 Which of the following statements about a person with pedophilic disorder is *true*?

    A. Pedophilic disorder is found in 10%–12% of the male population.
    B. There is no evidence that neurodevelopmental perturbation in utero increases the probability of development of a pedophilic orientation.
    C. Adult males with pedophilia always report that they were sexually abused as children.
    D. The individual is at least age 16 years and at least 5 years older than the child or children.

19.5 Which of the following statements about pedophilic disorder is *true*?

A. The extensive use of pornography depicting prepubescent or early pubescent children is not a useful diagnostic indicator of pedophilic disorder.

B. Pedophilic disorder is stable over the course of a lifetime.

C. There is an association between pedophilic disorder and antisocial personality disorder.

D. Although normophilic sexual interest declines with age, pedophilic sexual interest remains constant.

19.6   A 35-year-old woman tells her therapist that she has recently become intensely aroused while watching movies in which people are tortured and that she regularly fantasizes about torturing people while masturbating. She is not distressed by these thoughts and denies ever having acted on these new fantasies; however, she fantasizes about these activities several times a day. Which of the following best summarizes the diagnostic implications of this patient's presentation?

A. She meets all of the criteria for sexual sadism disorder.

B. She does not meet the criteria for sexual sadism disorder because the fantasies are not sexual in nature.

C. She does not meet the criteria for sexual sadism disorder because she has never acted on the fantasies.

D. She does not meet the criteria for sexual sadism disorder because the interest and arousal began after age 35.

19.7   While intoxicated at a Mardi Gras celebration, a 19-year-old woman lifts her blouse and bra as a float goes by to get beads. The event appears on a cable news program watched by friends of her parents, who inform her parents. They insist that she get a psychiatric evaluation 2 months after the vacation. She denies any other similar events in her life but admits that the experience was "sort of sexy." She is currently extremely anxious and distressed about her parents' anger at her and their refusal to allow her to attend parties or go away on vacation until she has an evaluation. She reports that she is unable to attend classes or to focus on her work at college. What is the most appropriate diagnosis?

A. Exhibitionistic disorder.

B. Frotteuristic disorder.

C. Voyeuristic disorder.

D. Adjustment disorder.

19.8   A 16-year-old male tells his therapist that he can see into the bedroom of a woman across the street from his apartment house. He has been watching her since she moved into the apartment 6 months ago. He can see the woman dressing and undressing, which he finds sexually arousing. He has fantasies about the woman compelling him to have sex with her. He expresses no guilt about this because the woman has no shade on the window. The therapist requests a psychiatric consultation to evaluate the patient for a paraphilia. Which of the following is the correct diagnosis?

A. Voyeuristic disorder.
B. Unspecified paraphilic disorder.
C. Other specified paraphilic disorder.
D. Normal adolescent sexual behavior.

19.9 During an emergency department visit for asthma, a man has indications of being whipped. When asked about the welts, he reports that he self-flagellated during a religious ceremony. A psychiatric consultation is requested, and the man admits that he often fantasizes about being beaten and watches pornography of people being beaten, which is sexually arousing for him. He asks his partner to beat him and cannot achieve an erection if he is not beaten or humiliated. Which of the following describes the situation most accurately?

A. Sexual sadism disorder.
B. Sexual masochism disorder.
C. Voyeuristic disorder.
D. Masochistic personality disorder.

19.10 Following a syncopal episode, a man is examined in the emergency department and is found to be wearing women's undergarments. He is unable to give a history, and his wife is contacted. When asked about her husband's clothing, she reports that he has worn women's underwear on and off for years, which she finds distressing. She notes that they cannot have sex if he does not cross-dress. Except for wearing the clothing occasionally out of the house, and prior to sex, she states that he is otherwise a "regular guy." Which of the following diagnoses would be most appropriate?

A. Fetishistic disorder.
B. Gender dysphoria.
C. Transvestism.
D. Transvestic disorder.

.

CHAPTER 20

Medication-Induced Movement Disorders and Other Adverse Effects of Medication

20.1. Which of the following is *not* known to be a consistent risk factor in the development of medication-induced parkinsonism (MIP)?

A. Male sex.
B. Older age.
C. HIV disease.
D. Family history of Parkinson's disease,

20.2. Neuroleptic malignant syndrome is a potentially fatal syndrome with an incidence rate of 0.01%–0.02% among individuals treated with neuroleptics. Which of the following is not a sign or symptom of neuroleptic malignant syndrome?

A. Hyperthermia.
B. Generalized rigidity.
C. Elevated creatine kinase.
D. Unchanged mental status.

20.3. A 22-year-old patient with schizophrenia and no comorbid medical issues is admitted to an inpatient unit for treatment of a first episode of psychosis. Risperidone 1 mg is started for paranoia and derogatory auditory hallucinations. Within 24 hours the patient begins experiencing an oculogyric crisis. The muscle contractions are relieved by an injection of diphenhydramine 50 mg IM. Which of the following is the best explanation for what happened to this patient?

A. Neuroleptic malignant syndrome.
B. Medication-induced acute dystonia.
C. Medication-induced acute akathisia.
D. Tardive dystonia.

20.4. A 55-year-old patient with schizoaffective disorder presents to the emergency department in severe distress. His history includes feeling anxious and edgy for the past week and an inability to unwind at the end of the day. He is unable to sit still and has developed insomnia. The patient is observed to be shifting on the examination table and shaking both legs throughout the examination. His medication history includes risperidone 2 mg PO bid, which was increased from 2 mg daily a week earlier. Which of the following best explains what is happening to the patient?

A. Tobacco withdrawal.
B. Histrionic personality disorder.
C. Medication-induced acute akathisia.
D. Serotonin syndrome.

20.5. Which of the following is a true statement about tardive dyskinesias?

A. Tardive dyskinesias do not include movements that develop within 1 month after stopping an oral antipsychotic medication.
B. The overall prevalence of tardive dyskinesia in individuals who have been treated with long-term antipsychotic medications is between 10% and 20%.
C. Men are more likely to develop tardive dyskinesia than women.
D. Tardive dyskinesia includes several different types of movements.

20.6. A 41-year-old patient with recurrent depression and anxiety has been taking medication for a year. She has been experiencing "brain zaps," nausea, terrible headaches, and anxiety for the past 3 days. The psychiatrist assesses for any other symptoms and asks about medication adherence, learning that the patient stopped taking her antidepressant "cold turkey" a few days ago. Which of the following medications did the patient likely stop taking?

A. Venlafaxine.
B. Fluoxetine.
C. Thyroid hormone.
D. Lithium.

20.7. Which of the following factors does *not* increase the risk of lithium tremor?

A. Anxiety.
B. High serum lithium levels.
C. Personal or family history of tremor.
D. Young age.

20.8. Which of the following is *not* true about medication-induced postural tremor?

A. The essential feature is a fine tremor occurring during attempts to maintain a posture and developing in association with the use of medication.

B. The tremor is a regular, rhythmic oscillation of the limbs, head, mouth, or tongue with a frequency between 3 and 6 Hz.

C. Medication-induced postural tremor is not diagnosed if the tremor is better accounted for by medication-induced parkinsonism.

D. The tremor can be an early feature of serotonin syndrome.

CHAPTER 21

Assessment Measures (DSM-5-TR Section III)

21.1 Which of the following factors about traditional categorical diagnosis supports the incorporation of dimensional concepts?

A. Specific treatment guidance.
B. Stable, definitive diagnoses.
C. Low rates of comorbidity.
D. Frequent use of *other* or *unspecified* diagnoses.

21.2 Which of the following statements accurately describes the World Health Organization Disability Assessment Schedule, Version 2.0 (WHODAS 2.0)?

A. It focuses only on disabilities due to psychiatric illness.
B. It assesses a patient's ability to perform activities in six functional areas.
C. It may not be completed on behalf of a patient with impaired capacity.
D. It primarily measures physical disability.

21.3 What is the function of the DSM-5 Level 1 Cross-Cutting Symptom Measure?

A. It assesses a patient's ability to perform activities in six areas of daily life functioning.
B. It assesses the presence and frequency of symptoms in 13 psychiatric domains.
C. It clarifies symptoms present *at the time of the interview* only.
D. It is intended primarily as a research tool.

21.4 In clinician review of item scores on the DSM-5 Level 1 Cross-Cutting Symptom Measure for an adult patient, a rating of "slight" would call for further inquiry if found for any item in which of the following domains?

A. Depression.
B. Mania.
C. Anger.
D. Suicidal ideation.

21.5   If a parent answers "I don't know" to the question "In the past TWO (2) WEEKS, has your child had an alcoholic beverage (beer, wine, liquor, etc.)?" in the parent/guardian-rated version of the DSM-5 Level 1 Cross-Cutting Symptom Measure, what is the appropriate clinician response?

A. Ask the child questions from the substance use domain of the child-rated Level 2 Cross-Cutting Symptom Measure.
B. Rely on other questions from the substance use domain and do not incorporate this answer into the final score.
C. Ask the parent to ask the child, and schedule a follow-up visit to readminister the questionnaire.
D. Consider reporting the parent to child protective services.

21.6   Which of the following is *not* assessed by the Clinician-Rated Dimensions of Psychosis Symptom Severity measure?

A. Social function.
B. Cognitive function.
C. Depression.
D. Mania.

21.7   When reviewing a patient's responses to items on the World Health Organization Disability Assessment Schedule 2.0 (WHODAS 2.0), the clinician notes that in response to the question "How much time did you spend on your health condition or its consequences?" the patient answered, "Hardly any." The clinician, who has treated the patient for several years, is surprised to see this because she is quite certain that the patient spends most of the day dealing with health concerns. What is the appropriate action for this clinician?

A. Leave the patient's response as is and score accordingly.
B. Indicate on the form that the clinician is making a correction and revise the score.
C. Attempt to obtain additional information from family members in order to clarify the discrepancy.
D. Take the average of the patient's and clinician's differing scores and use that for the final score.

21.8   The cross-cutting symptom measures in DSM-5 are modeled on which of the following?

A. The International Classification of Functioning, Disability, and Health.
B. The general medical review of systems.
C. The Brief Psychiatric Rating Scale.
D. The Clinical Global Impression Scale.

21.9   Which of the following is an intended use of severity measures in DSM-5-TR?

    A. To evaluate transdiagnostic symptom severity.
    B. To quantify treatment-associated side effects.
    C. To establish any psychiatric diagnosis.
    D. To estimate severity in patients who do not meet full diagnostic criteria for
       a particular disorder.

CHAPTER 22

Culture and Psychiatric Diagnosis (DSM-5-TR Section III)

22.1 Updated in DSM-5-TR, the expanded Outline for Cultural Formulation assesses which of the following items?

A. Cultural preferences in leisure and entertainment choices.
B. Risk factors for specific psychiatric diagnoses.
C. Cultural features of vulnerability and resilience.
D. Definitions of cultural groups and their unified belief structures.

22.2 *Cultural identity of the individual* is one of several categories in the DSM-5-TR Outline for Cultural Formulation. Which of the following is a feature of cultural identity of the individual?

A. How cultural constructs influence the individual's experiences of symptoms or psychological problems.
B. Religious affiliation and spirituality.
C. Social determinants of mental health.
D. Prior experiences of racism and discrimination in mental health care.

22.3 In what type of clinical setting is the Cultural Formulation Interview (CFI) meant to be used?

A. Any setting.
B. Outpatient clinic.
C. Emergency department.
D. Inpatient hospital.

22.4 In which of the following clinical situations is the Cultural Formulation Interview (CFI) meant to be helpful?

A. The clinician and patient have a shared belief system regarding the nature of the problem and the appropriate therapeutic approach.

B. The patient presents with a symptom complex that is distressing but does not fit any DSM-5-TR diagnosis.

C. The clinician and the patient speak different languages.

D. The clinician is finding it difficult to identify the correct code for the patient's primary clinical diagnosis.

22.5   Which of the following accurately distinguishes the concept of race from that of ethnicity?

A. Race is based on superficial physical attributes, whereas ethnicity is based on culturally constructed group identity.

B. Race is a biological construct, whereas ethnicity is socially constructed.

C. Race is generally region-specific, whereas ethnicity is a construct generally carried across societies.

D. Race tends to be self-assigned by the identified group, whereas ethnicity is attributed by outsiders.

22.6   In DSM-5-TR, which of the following is included in *cultural concepts of distress*?

A. Culturally specific alternative names for DSM-5-TR psychiatric disorders.

B. Culturally specific subtypes of psychiatric disorders.

C. Culturally influenced explanations of symptoms.

D. A unifying explanation of variable symptom expression in psychiatric disorders.

22.7   Which of the following best defines *cultural idioms of distress*?

A. Idiosyncratic clusters of symptoms restricted to specific geographic regions.

B. Collective, shared ways of experiencing and discussing concerns.

C. Perceived causes or explanatory models regarding distress.

D. Culturally specific terms that correspond to specific DSM-5-TR diagnoses.

22.8   Which of the following accurately characterizes *ataque de nervios*?

A. Intense emotional upset, including acute anxiety, anger, and grief, and crying or screaming and shouting uncontrollably.

B. Intense anxiety about and avoidance of interpersonal situations for fear of inadequacy or offensiveness.

C. A frightening event perceived to cause the soul to leave the body, resulting in illness or sadness.

D. A general state of vulnerability to stressful life events.

22.9   What is the term for a cultural concept of distress, coined in South Asia, involving an individual's fear that various symptoms may be attributed to semen loss?

A. *Kufungisisa.*
B. *Dhat syndrome.*
C. *Maladi dyab.*
D. *Shenjing shuairuo.*

22.10 Which of the following does the term *kufungisisa* represent?

A. Idiom of distress.
B. Cultural explanation.
C. Both.
D. Neither.

22.11 Which of the following psychiatric disorders is associated with *hikikomori*?

A. Obsessive-compulsive disorder.
B. Alcohol use disorder.
C. Schizophrenia.
D. Attention-deficit/hyperactivity disorder.

22.12 Which of the following accurately describes *Khyâl cap*?

A. Social withdrawal involving the complete cessation of in-person interaction with others.
B. Physical or mental illness, distress, or dysfunction caused by another's ill will toward the sufferer.
C. A general vulnerability to stressful life events and difficult experiences.
D. A sudden onset of dizziness, palpitations, shortness of breath, anxiety, or autonomic arousal.

22.13 How do cultural concepts of distress relate to DSM-5-TR nosology?

A. One-to-one correspondence.
B. Providing specific diagnostic criteria.
C. Static correspondence across time and geography.
D. May apply to multiple disorders.

CHAPTER 23

Alternative DSM-5 Model for Personality Disorders (DSM-5-TR Section III)

23.1 Which of the following terms best describes the diagnostic approach proposed in the Alternative DSM-5 Model for Personality Disorders?

A. Categorical.
B. Dimensional.
C. Hybrid.
D. Developmental.

23.2 In the Alternative DSM-5 Model for Personality Disorders, personality disorders are characterized by pathological personality traits and which of the following?

A. Impairments in personality functioning.
B. Impairments in identity.
C. Impairments in self-direction.
D. Impairments in empathy.

23.3 Which of the following is a domain of the Alternative DSM-5 Model for Personality Disorders?

A. Emotional lability.
B. Intimacy avoidance.
C. Disinhibition.
D. Cognitive and perceptual dysregulation.

23.4 In addition to negative affectivity, which of the following maladaptive trait domains is most associated with avoidant personality disorder?

A. Detachment.
B. Antagonism.

C. Disinhibition.

D. Psychoticism.

23.5   Which of the following is included in the Section III personality trait system?

A. The Personality Psychopathology Five (PSY-5).

B. The Level of Personality Functioning Scale (LPFS).

C. The Five Factor Model of personality (FFM).

D. The Personality Inventory for DSM-5 (PID-5).

23.6   Disturbances in self and interpersonal functioning constitute the core of personality psychopathology, and in the alternative DSM-5-TR diagnostic model for personality disorders they are evaluated on a continuum. Which of the following is a characteristic of healthy self functioning?

A. Comprehension and appreciation of others' experiences and motivations.

B. Variability of self-esteem.

C. Fluctuating boundaries between self and others.

D. Experience of oneself as unique.

23.7   Which of the following is a general criterion for personality disorder in the Alternative DSM-5-TR Model for Personality Disorders?

A. The individual experiences mild impairment in personality (self/interpersonal) functioning.

B. The individual demonstrates two or more pathological personality traits.

C. The impairments in personality functioning and the individual's personality trait expression may fluctuate over time.

D. The impairments in personality functioning and the individual's personality trait expression are not better explained by another mental disorder.

23.8   In order to meet the proposed diagnostic criteria for antisocial personality disorder in the Alternative DSM-5 Model for Personality Disorders, an individual must have maladaptive personality traits in which of the following domains?

A. Negative affectivity.

B. Detachment.

C. Antagonism.

D. Psychoticism.

23.9   Which of the following statements best characterizes the relationship between severity of personality dysfunction—as rated on the Level of Personality Functioning Scale (LPFS)—and presence of a personality disorder?

A. A moderate level of impairment in personality functioning is required for the diagnosis of a personality disorder.

B. Impairment in personality functioning is unrelated to the presence of a personality disorder.

C. The severity of impairment in personality functioning is unrelated to the number of personality disorders.

D. The severity of impairment in personality functioning is unrelated to the severity of the personality disorder.

23.10 Which of the following statements about the Level of Personality Functioning Scale (LPFS) is most accurate?

A. A rating of moderate or greater impairment is necessary for the diagnosis of a personality disorder.

B. A rating of mild impairment is necessary for the diagnosis of a personality disorder.

C. The LPFS can be used only with specification of a personality disorder diagnosis.

D. To use the LPFS, the clinician selects the level that captures the person's lowest lifetime level of impairment.

PART II

Answer Guide

DSM-5-TR Introduction

I.1 Which of the following differentiates the vetting process of contributors to DSM-5 from previous editions of DSM?

A. Only clinicians were on the task force.
B. Only researchers were on the task force.
C. Disclosure of all income for members of the task force.
D. Only physicians were on the task force.

Correct Answer: C. Disclosure of all income for members of the task force.

Explanation: In 2006, the American Psychiatric Association (APA) named David J. Kupfer, M.D., as Chair and Darrel A. Regier, M.D., M.P.H., as Vice-Chair of the DSM-5 Task Force. They were charged with recommending chairs for the 13 diagnostic work groups and additional task force members with a multidisciplinary range of expertise who would oversee the development of DSM-5. An additional vetting process was initiated by the APA Board of Trustees to disclose sources of income and thus avoid conflicts of interest by task force and work group members. The full disclosure of all income and research grants from commercial sources, including the pharmaceutical industry, in the previous 3 years; the imposition of an income cap from all commercial sources; and the publication of disclosures on a website set a new standard for the field.

I.1—Introduction / DSM-5 Revision Process (p. 6)

I.2 Which of the following was not a principle guiding the DSM-5 draft revision process?

A. DSM-5 was primarily intended to be a manual to be used by clinicians, and revisions must be feasible for routine clinical practice.
B. Recommendations for revisions should be guided by research evidence.
C. There were no considerations for maintaining continuity with previous editions of DSM.
D. No a priori constraints should be placed on the degree of change between DSM-IV and DSM-5.

Correct Answer: C. There were no considerations for maintaining continuity with previous editions of DSM.

Explanation: Four principles guided the draft revisions: 1) DSM-5 is primarily intended to be a manual to be used by clinicians, and revisions must be feasible for routine clinical practice; 2) recommendations for revisions should be guided by research evidence; 3) where possible, continuity should be maintained with previous editions of DSM; and 4) no a priori constraints should be placed on the degree of change between DSM-IV and DSM-5.

I.2—Introduction / Proposals for Revision (p. 7)

I.3   Which of the following best describes the use of DSM-5-TR in forensic settings?

   A. Anyone involved in forensic cases can use DSM-5-TR to arrive at a psychiatric diagnosis.
   B. A person who meets criteria of a diagnosis will also meet the standard for having a mental illness as defined by law.
   C. There is a risk that the diagnoses will be misused or misunderstood.
   D. A diagnosis carries implications regarding the etiology of the person's mental disorder.

Correct Answer: C. There is a risk that the diagnoses will be misused or misunderstood

Explanation: The use of DSM-5-TR in forensic settings should be informed by an awareness of the risks and limitations of its use. When DSM-5-TR categories, criteria, and textual descriptions are employed for forensic purposes, there is a risk that diagnostic information will be misused or misunderstood. These dangers arise because of the imperfect fit between the questions of ultimate concern to the law and the information contained in a clinical diagnosis. In most situations, the clinical diagnosis of a DSM-5-TR mental disorder such as intellectual developmental disorder (intellectual disability), schizophrenia, major neurocognitive disorder, gambling disorder, or pedophilic disorder does not imply that an individual with such a condition meets legal criteria for the presence of a mental disorder or *mental illness* as defined in law or a specified legal standard (e.g., for competence, criminal responsibility, or disability). Use of DSM-5-TR to assess the presence of a mental disorder by nonclinical, nonmedical, or otherwise insufficiently trained individuals is not advised. Nonclinical decision-makers should also be cautioned that a diagnosis does not carry any necessary implications regarding the etiology or causes of the individual's mental disorder or the individual's degree of control over behaviors that may be associated with the disorder.

I.3—Cautionary Statement for Forensic Use of DSM-5 (p. 29)

C H A P T E R   1

Neurodevelopmental Disorders

1.1   Which of the following is *not* required for a DSM-5-TR diagnosis of intellectual developmental disorder (intellectual disability)?

A. Full-scale IQ below 70.
B. Deficits in intellectual functions confirmed by clinical assessment and individualized, standardized intelligence testing.
C. Deficits in adaptive functioning that result in failure to meet developmental and sociocultural standards for personal independence and social responsibility.
D. Symptom onset during the developmental period.

Correct Answer: A. Full-scale IQ below 70.

Explanation: The essential features of intellectual developmental disorder (intellectual disability) relate to both intellectual impairment and deficits in adaptive function. In contrast to DSM-IV, which specified "an IQ of approximately 70 or below" for the former diagnosis of mental retardation, DSM-5-TR has no specific requirement for IQ in the renamed diagnosis of intellectual disability. Intellectual developmental disorder (intellectual disability) is a disorder with onset during the developmental period. Intellectual functioning is typically measured with individually administered and psychometrically valid, comprehensive, and culturally appropriate tests of intelligence. Clinical training and judgment are required for interpreting test results and assessing intellectual performance. Deficits in adaptive functioning (Criterion B) refer to how well a person meets community standards of personal independence and social responsibility in comparison with others of similar age and sociocultural background.

1.1—Intellectual Developmental Disorder (Intellectual Disability) / diagnostic criteria (p. 37); Diagnostic Features (p. 38)

1.2   A 7-year-old boy in second grade displays significant delays in his ability to reason, solve problems, and learn from experiences. He has been slow to develop skills in reading, writing, and mathematics. These skills have lagged behind peers throughout the child's development, although he is making slow progress. The deficits significantly impair his ability to play in an age-appropriate manner with peers and to begin to acquire independent skills at home. He requires ongoing assistance with basic skills (dressing, feeding, bathing, and doing any type of schoolwork) on a daily basis. Which of the following diagnoses best fits this presentation?

A. Childhood-onset major neurocognitive disorder.
B. Intellectual developmental disorder (intellectual disability).
C. Communication disorder.
D. Autism spectrum disorder.

Correct Answer: B. Intellectual developmental disorder (intellectual disability).

Explanation: Intellectual developmental disorder is characterized by deficits in general mental abilities, which result in impairments of intellectual and adaptive functioning. In communication disorders, there is no general intellectual impairment. Autism spectrum disorder must include history suggesting "persistent deficits in social communication and social interaction across multiple contexts" (Criterion A) or "restricted, repetitive patterns of behavior, interests, or activities" (Criterion B). Intellectual developmental disorder is categorized as a neurodevelopmental disorder and is distinct from the neurocognitive disorders, which are characterized by a *loss* of cognitive functioning. There is no evidence for a neurocognitive disorder in this case, although major neurocognitive disorder may co-occur with intellectual developmental disorder (e.g., an individual with Down syndrome who develops Alzheimer's disease or an individual with intellectual developmental disorder who loses further cognitive capacity following a head injury). In such cases, the diagnoses of intellectual developmental disorder and neurocognitive disorder may both be given.

1.2—Intellectual Developmental Disorder (Intellectual Disability): Development and Course (p. 43) and Differential Diagnosis (p. 45)

1.3   A 7-year-old boy in second grade displays significant delays in his ability to reason, solve problems, and learn from his experiences. He has been slow to develop reading, writing, and mathematics skills in school. All through development, these skills lagged behind peers, although he is making slow progress. These deficits significantly impair his ability to play in an age-appropriate manner with peers and to begin to acquire independent skills at home. He requires ongoing assistance with basic skills (dressing, feeding, bathing, and doing any type of schoolwork) on a daily basis. What is the appropriate severity rating for this patient's current presentation?

A. Mild.
B. Moderate.

C. Severe.

D. Cannot be determined without an IQ score.

Correct Answer: B. Moderate.

Explanation: With respect to severity, the *moderate* qualifier reflects this patient's skills (which have chronically lagged behind those of peers) and his need for assistance in most activities of daily living; however, it also takes into account the fact that he is slowly developing these skills (which would peak at roughly the elementary school level, according to DSM-5-TR).

Although IQ testing would be informative in diagnosing intellectual developmental disorder (in previous DSM classifications, subtypes of mild, moderate, severe, and profound were categories based on IQ scores), DSM-5-TR specifies that "the various levels of severity are defined on the basis of adaptive functioning, and not IQ scores, because it is adaptive functioning that determines the level of supports required" (p. 388). Deficits in adaptive functioning refer to how well a person meets community standards of personal independence and social responsibility in comparison with others of similar age and sociocultural background. Adaptive functioning is assessed using both clinical evaluation and individualized, culturally appropriate, psychometrically sound measures.

Adaptive functioning involves adaptive reasoning in three domains: conceptual, social, and practical. The *conceptual (academic) domain* involves competence in memory, language, reading, writing, math reasoning, acquisition of practical knowledge, problem-solving, and judgment in novel situations, among others. The *social domain* involves awareness of others' thoughts, feelings, and experiences; empathy; interpersonal communication skills; friendship abilities; and social judgment, among others. The *practical domain* involves learning and self-management across life settings, including personal care, job responsibilities, money management, recreation, self-management of behavior, and school and work task organization. Intellectual capacity, education, motivation, socialization, personality features, vocational opportunity, cultural experience, and coexisting general medical conditions or mental disorders influence adaptive functioning. With mild severity, the individual may function age-appropriately in personal care. With severe severity, the individual generally has little understanding of written language or of concepts involving numbers, quantity, time, and money.

1.3—Intellectual Developmental Disorder (Intellectual Disability) / Specifiers (p. 38) and Diagnostic Features (pp. 38–42)

1.4   What can lead to an invalid assessment of overall mental abilities and adaptive functioning in individuals with intellectual developmental disorder?

A. Comparing the individual with age- and gender-matched peers from the same linguistic and sociocultural group.

B. A full-scale IQ score with highly discrepant subtest scores.
C. Using multiple IQ or other cognitive tests to create a profile.
D. Accounting for factors that may limit performance, such as sociocultural background, native language, associated communication/language disorder, and motor or sensory handicap.

Correct Answer: B. A full-scale IQ score with highly discrepant subtest scores.

Explanation: Invalid scores may result from the use of brief intelligence screening tests or group tests; highly discrepant individual subtest scores may make an overall IQ score invalid. Instruments must be normed for the individual's sociocultural background and native language. Co-occurring disorders that affect communication, language, and/or motor or sensory function may affect test scores. Individual cognitive profiles based on neuropsychological testing as well as cross-battery intellectual assessment (using multiple IQ or other cognitive tests to create a profile) are more useful than a single IQ score for understanding intellectual abilities.

1.4—Intellectual Developmental Disorder (Intellectual Disability) / Diagnostic Features (p. 38)

1.5   A 15-year-old patient is enrolled in the eighth grade in a special education setting. She has an IQ of 70 and has trouble keeping track of time, although she is able to read a digital watch. It has taken considerable time for her family to teach her how to do simple tasks in the kitchen, and she continues to need supervision with the stove. She is able to socialize with other peers in her class but is no longer friends with other kids of similar age in the neighborhood. She attends a social skills group, but her parents must keep track of the appointments. What is the specifier for her current severity of intellectual developmental disorder (intellectual disability)?

A. Normal variation.
B. Mild.
C. Moderate.
D. Severe

Correct Answer: C. Moderate

Explanation: Severity specifiers are included in the diagnostic criteria for intellectual developmental disorder (intellectual disability). The various levels of severity are defined on the basis of adaptive functioning, not IQ scores, because it is adaptive functioning that determines the level of supports required. In moderate severity, progress in reading, writing, mathematics, and understanding of time and money occurs slowly across the school years and is markedly limited compared with that of peers. Friendships with typically developing peers are often affected by communication or social limitations. Significant social and communicative support is needed in work settings for success. Participation in all household tasks can be achieved by adulthood, although an extended period of teaching is needed, and ongoing supports will typically occur for adult-level performance.

1.5—Intellectual Developmental Disorder (Intellectual Disability) / Table 1 [Severity levels for intellectual developmental disorder (intellectual disability)] (pp. 39–41)

1.6   Which of the following is *not* a diagnostic feature of intellectual developmental disorder (intellectual disability)?

   A. Repetitive, seemingly driven, and apparently purposeless motor behavior (e.g., hand shaking, body rocking).
   B. Inability to perform complex daily living tasks (e.g., money management, medical decision-making) without support.
   C. Gullibility, with naiveté in social situations and a tendency to be easily led by others.
   D. Lack of age-appropriate communication skills for social and interpersonal functioning.

Correct Answer: A. Repetitive, seemingly driven, and apparently purposeless motor behavior (e.g., hand shaking, body rocking).

Explanation: In general, individuals with intellectual disability may have difficulty with social judgment. Lack of communication skills may also predispose them to disruptive and aggressive behaviors. Communication, conversation, and language are more concrete or immature than expected for any given age. Furthermore, gullibility is an important feature of intellectual developmental disorder. It is especially important in forensic situations and may affect judgment. Repetitive, seemingly driven, and apparently purposeless motor behavior can be a part of autism spectrum disorder, stereotypic movement disorder, or obsessive-compulsive disorder.

1.6—Intellectual Developmental Disorder (Intellectual Disability) / Diagnostic Features and Associated Features (pp. 42–43)

1.7   How is adaptive functioning related to the diagnosis of intellectual developmental disorder (intellectual disability)?

   A. Adaptive functioning is based on an individual's IQ score.
   B. Impairment in at least two domains of adaptive functioning must be present to meet Criterion B for the diagnosis of intellectual developmental disorder.
   C. Adaptive functioning in intellectual developmental disorder tends to improve over time, although the threshold of cognitive capacities and associated developmental disorders can limit it.

D. Individuals diagnosed with intellectual developmental disorder in childhood will typically continue to meet criteria in adulthood even if their adaptive functioning improves.

Correct Answer: C. Adaptive functioning in intellectual developmental disorder tends to improve over time, although the threshold of cognitive capacities and associated developmental disorders can limit it.

Explanation: In the DSM-5-TR diagnosis of intellectual developmental disorder (intellectual disability), unlike the DSM-IV diagnosis of mental retardation, the various levels of severity are defined on the basis of adaptive functioning rather than IQ scores alone because it is adaptive functioning that determines the level of support required. Moreover, IQ measures are less valid in the lower end of the IQ range. Criterion B is met when at least one domain of adaptive functioning—conceptual, social, or practical—is sufficiently impaired that ongoing support is needed in order for the person to perform adequately across multiple environments, such as home, school, work, and community. Severity levels are meant to refer only to functioning at the time of the assessment, and they can change over time in a positive direction if the individual receives support and can develop compensatory strategies. Improvement in adaptive functioning can occur to a degree such that the individual no longer meets criteria for the diagnosis in adulthood.

1.7—Intellectual Developmental Disorder (Intellectual Disability) / Specifiers (p. 38); Diagnostic Features (p. 42); Development and Course (pp. 43–44)

1.8   In which of the following clinical scenarios could comorbid intellectual developmental disorder (intellectual disability) occur as an acquired disorder?

A. Lesch-Nyhan syndrome.
B. Prader-Willi syndrome.
C. Head trauma occurring during the developmental period.
D. Rett syndrome.

Correct Answer: C. Head trauma occurring during the developmental period.

Explanation: When intellectual developmental disorder is associated with a genetic syndrome, there may be a characteristic physical appearance (e.g., as in Down syndrome). Some syndromes have a behavioral phenotype, which refers to specific behaviors that are characteristic of a particular genetic disorder (e.g., Lesch-Nyhan syndrome). In acquired forms, the onset may be abrupt, following an illness such as meningitis or encephalitis or head trauma occurring during the developmental period. When intellectual developmental disorder results from a loss of previously acquired cognitive skills, as in severe traumatic brain injury, the diagnoses of both intellectual developmental disorder and a neurocognitive disorder may be assigned. Although intellectual developmental disorder is generally nonprogressive, in certain genetic disorders (e.g., Rett syndrome) there are periods of worsening, followed by stabilization, and in others (e.g., Sanfilippo syndrome, Down syndrome) there is progressive worsening of intellectual function in varying degrees.

1.8—Intellectual Developmental Disorder (Intellectual Disability) / Development and Course (p. 43)

1.9   Which of the following is a true statement about the developmental course of intellectual developmental disorder (intellectual disability)?

   A. Delayed motor, language, and social milestones are not identifiable until after the first 2 years of life.
   B. Intellectual disability caused by an illness (e.g., encephalitis) or by head trauma occurring during the developmental period would be diagnosed as a neurocognitive disorder, not as intellectual developmental disorder (intellectual disability).
   C. Major neurocognitive disorder may co-occur with intellectual developmental disorder.
   D. Even if early and ongoing interventions throughout childhood and adulthood lead to improved adaptive and intellectual functioning, the diagnosis of intellectual developmental disorder (intellectual disability) would continue to apply.

Correct Answer: C. Major neurocognitive disorder may co-occur with intellectual developmental disorder.

Explanation: intellectual developmental disorder (intellectual disability) is categorized as a neurodevelopmental disorder and is distinct from the neurocognitive disorders, which are characterized by a loss of cognitive functioning. Major neurocognitive disorder may co-occur with intellectual developmental disorder (e.g., an individual with Down syndrome who develops Alzheimer's disease or an individual with intellectual developmental disorder who loses further cognitive capacity following a head injury). In such cases, the diagnoses of both intellectual developmental disorder and neurocognitive disorder may be given.

   Delayed motor, language, and social milestones may be identifiable within the first 2 years of life among those with more severe intellectual developmental disorder. Head trauma with subsequent cognitive deficits would represent an acquired form of intellectual developmental disorders. Although intellectual developmental disorder is generally nonprogressive, in certain genetic disorders (e.g., Rett syndrome) there are periods of worsening, followed by stabilization, and in others (e.g., San Philippo syndrome) there is progressive worsening of intellectual function. After early childhood, the disorder is generally lifelong, although severity levels may change over time. If early and ongoing interventions improve adaptive functioning and significant improvement of intellectual functioning occurs, the diagnosis of intellectual developmental disorder may no longer be appropriate.

1.9—Intellectual Developmental Disorder (Intellectual Disability) / Development and Course (pp. 43–44); Differential Diagnosis (p. 45); Comorbidity (p. 45)

1.10   The DSM-5-TR diagnosis of intellectual developmental disorder (intellectual disability) includes severity specifiers—mild, moderate, severe, and profound—to indicate the level of support required in various domains of adaptive functioning. Which of the following features would be characteristic of an individual with a *mild* level of impairment?

A. The individual generally has little understanding of written language or of concepts involving numbers, quantity, time, and money.
B. The individual's spoken language is quite limited in terms of vocabulary and grammar.
C. The individual requires support for all activities of daily living, including meals, dressing, bathing, and toileting.
D. In adulthood, the individual may be able to sustain competitive employment in a job that does not emphasize conceptual skills.

Correct Answer: D. In adulthood, the individual may be able to sustain competitive employment in a job that does not emphasize conceptual skills.

Explanation: Competitive employment may be attainable by individuals with a *mild* level of impairment but would not be characteristic of those with a *severe* level of impairment. Intellectual developmental disorder (intellectual disability) is a disorder with onset during the developmental period that includes both intellectual and adaptive functioning deficits in conceptual, social, and practical domains (DSM-5-TR, Table 1, pp. 39–41). The *conceptual (academic) domain* involves competence in memory, language, reading, writing, math reasoning, acquisition of practical knowledge, problem-solving, and judgment in novel situations, among others. The *social domain* involves awareness of others' thoughts, feelings, and experiences; empathy; interpersonal communication skills; friendship abilities; and social judgment, among others. The *practical domain* involves learning and self-management across life settings, including personal care, job responsibilities, money management, recreation, self-management of behavior, and school and work task organization, among others. Individuals with a *severe* level of impairment would demonstrate the deficits in the conceptual, social, and practical domains mentioned in options A–C.

1.10—Intellectual Developmental Disorder (Intellectual Disability) / diagnostic criteria (pp. 37–38) / Table 1 [Severity levels for intellectual developmental disorder (intellectual disability)] (pp. 39–41); Diagnostic Features (p. 42)

1.11 A 10-year-old boy with a history of dyslexia, who is otherwise developmentally normal, is in a skateboarding accident in which he experiences severe traumatic brain injury. This results in significant global intellectual impairment (with a persistent reading deficit that is more pronounced than his other newly acquired but stable deficits, along with a full-scale IQ of 75). There is mild impairment in his adaptive functioning such that he requires support in some areas of functioning. He is also displaying anxious and depressive symptoms in response to the accident and hospitalization. What is the *least likely* diagnosis?

A. Intellectual developmental disorder (intellectual disability).
B. Traumatic brain injury.
C. Major neurocognitive disorder due to traumatic brain injury.
D. Adjustment disorder.

Correct Answer: C. Major neurocognitive disorder due to traumatic brain injury.

Explanation: There are no exclusion criteria for a diagnosis of intellectual developmental disorder in DSM-5-TR, which notes that both specific learning disorder and communication disorders can co-occur if the criteria are met. Although the patient's full-scale IQ is 75, the statistical model associated with his intellect would allow for his actual IQ to be ±5 points. His adaptive functioning would be the key factor in his receiving the diagnosis of intellectual developmental disorder, with a mild level of severity due to needing to receive only some support in most of his areas of functioning. His emotional symptoms in response to the accident would yield a potential diagnosis of an adjustment disorder. The boy's deficits are not severe enough to qualify for a diagnosis of major neurocognitive disorder. Criterion A for a major neurocognitive disorder is "evidence of significant cognitive decline from a previous level of performance in one or more cognitive domains (complex attention, executive function, learning and memory, language, perceptual-motor, or social cognition)."

1.11—Intellectual Developmental Disorder (Intellectual Disability) / Differential Diagnosis (p. 45)

1.12 In which of the following situations would a diagnosis of global developmental delay be *inappropriate*?

A. The patient is a child who is too young to fully manifest specific symptoms or to complete requisite assessments.
B. The patient, a 7-year-old child, has a full-scale IQ of 65 and severe impairment in adaptive functioning.
C. The patient's scores on psychometric tests suggest intellectual developmental disorder (intellectual disability), but there is insufficient information about the patient's adaptive functional skills.
D. The patient's impaired adaptive functioning suggests intellectual developmental disorder, but there is insufficient information about the level of cognitive impairment measured by standardized instruments.

Correct Answer: B. The patient, a 7-year-old child, has a full-scale IQ of 65 and severe impairment in adaptive functioning.

Explanation: Enough information is present to diagnose intellectual developmental disorder (intellectual disability) in this child. The diagnosis of global developmental delay is used when there is insufficient information to make the diagnosis of intellectual developmental disorder. The diagnosis of global developmental delay is reserved for individuals younger than age 5 years, when the clinical severity level cannot be reliably assessed during early childhood. Individuals do not meet expected developmental milestones in several areas of intellectual functioning. This category is diagnosed when an individual fails to meet expected developmental milestones in several areas of intellectual functioning and applies to individuals who are unable to undergo systematic assessments of intellectual functioning, including children who are too young to participate in standardized testing.

1.12—Global Developmental Delay (p. 46)

1.13 For whom should a clinician consider the diagnosis of global developmental delay?

A. Children younger than age 5 years.
B. Children who can undergo systematic assessments.
C. Children with a full-scale IQ <65.
D. Children with a diagnosis of intellectual developmental disorder (intellectual disability), severe.

Correct Answer: A. Children younger than age 5 years.

Explanation: The diagnosis of global developmental delay is reserved for individuals younger than age 5 years when the clinical severity level cannot be reliably assessed during early childhood. Individuals do not meet expected developmental milestones in several areas of intellectual functioning. The diagnosis is used for individuals who are unable to undergo systematic assessments of intellectual functioning, including children who are too young to participate in standardized testing. The diagnosis does not require an identified etiology and requires reassessment over time. The course of the condition can be variable and can be a precursor to more specific neurodevelopmental disorders that can be diagnosed with systematic testing, older age, and ability to participate in testing.

1.13—Global Developmental Delay (p. 46)

1.14 A 3½-year-old girl with a history of lead exposure and a seizure disorder demonstrates substantial delays across multiple domains of functioning, including communication, learning, attention, and motor development, which limit her ability to interact with same-age peers and require substantial support in all activities of daily living at home. Unfortunately, her parents are extremely poor historians, and the child has received no formal psychological or learning evaluation to date. She is about to be evaluated for readiness to attend preschool. What is the most appropriate diagnosis?

A. Major neurocognitive disorder.
B. Autism spectrum disorder.
C. Global developmental delay.
D. Specific learning disorder.

Correct Answer: C. Global developmental delay.

Explanation: Although this child's deficits may be suggestive of intellectual developmental disorder (intellectual disability), that diagnosis cannot be made in this case because information is lacking (e.g., about age at onset of her symptoms) and she is too young to participate in standardized testing. At this point, there is no information to suggest that this child has dementia (no evidence of a major neurocognitive disorder), an autism spectrum disorder (no evidence of symptoms in the core autism spectrum disorder categories), or a specific area of learning weakness (which generally would not be able to be diagnosed until the elementary school years).

1.14—Global Developmental Delay (p. 46)

1.15   A 5-year-old boy has difficulty making friends and has problems with initiating and sustaining back-and-forth conversation, reading social cues, and sharing his feelings with others. He makes good eye contact, has normal speech intonation, displays facial gestures, and has a range of affect that generally seems appropriate to the situation. He demonstrates an interest in trains that seems abnormal in intensity and focus, and he engages in little imaginative or symbolic play. Which of the following diagnostic requirements for autism spectrum disorder are *not* met in this case?

A. Deficits in social-emotional reciprocity.
B. Deficits in nonverbal communicative behaviors used for social interaction.
C. Deficits in developing and maintaining relationships.
D. Restricted, repetitive patterns of behavior, interests, or activities as manifested by symptoms in two of the specified four categories.

Correct Answer: B. Deficits in nonverbal communicative behaviors used for social interaction.

Explanation: DSM-5-TR Criterion A for autism spectrum disorder specifies that all three symptom clusters (summarized in options A, B, and C above) must be met. This child's nonverbal communication is reported to be unimpaired (although this should be confirmed with a standard instrument such as the Autism Diagnostic Observation Schedule). On the basis of the current history, he could not be diagnosed with autism spectrum disorder in DSM-5-TR. In order to meet Criterion B, at least two symptom clusters must be met. Although the child has "highly restricted, fixated interests that are abnormal in intensity or focus," he would need to have at least one other symptom from categories in Criterion B (which includes stereotyped or repetitive motor movements, use of objects, or speech; insistence on sameness, inflexible adherence to routines, or ritualized patterns of verbal or nonverbal behavior; or hyper- or hyporeactivity to sensory input or unusual interest in sensory aspects of the environment).

1.15—Autism Spectrum Disorder / diagnostic criteria (pp. 56–57)

1.16   Which of the following statements about the development and course of autism spectrum disorder is *false*?

A. Symptoms of autism spectrum disorder are usually not noticeable until ages 5–6 years or later.
B. First symptoms frequently involve delayed language development, often accompanied by lack of social interest or unusual social interactions.
C. Autism spectrum disorder is not a degenerative disorder, and it is typical for learning and compensation to continue throughout life.
D. Because many normally developing young children have strong preferences and enjoy repetition, distinguishing restricted and repetitive behaviors that are diagnostic of autism spectrum disorder can be difficult in preschoolers.

Correct Answer: A. Symptoms of autism spectrum disorder are usually not noticeable until ages 5–6 years or later.

Explanation: Details about the age at and pattern of onset are important and should be noted in the history. Symptoms of autism spectrum disorder are typically recognized during the second year of life (age 12–24 months) but may be seen earlier than 12 months if developmental delays are severe or may be noted later than 24 months if symptoms are more subtle. The pattern of onset description might include information about early developmental delays or any losses of social or language skills. In cases where skills have been lost, parents or caregivers may give a history of a gradual or relatively rapid deterioration in social behaviors or language skills. Typically, this would occur between ages 12 and 24 months and is distinguished from the rare instances of developmental regression occurring after at least 2 years of normal development (previously described as childhood disintegrative disorder).

Autism spectrum disorder is not a degenerative disorder, and it is typical for learning and compensation to continue throughout life. Symptoms are often most marked in early childhood and early school years, with developmental gains typical in later childhood in at least some areas. First symptoms of autism spectrum disorder frequently involve delayed language development, often accompanied by lack of social interest or unusual social interactions, odd play patterns, and unusual communication patterns. Because many typically developing young children have strong preferences and enjoy repetition, distinguishing restricted and repetitive behaviors that are diagnostic of autism spectrum disorder can be difficult in preschoolers. The clinical distinction is based on the type, frequency, and intensity of the behavior.

1.16—Autism Spectrum Disorder / Development and Course (pp. 63–64)

1.17   Which of the following was a criterion symptom for autistic disorder in DSM-IV that was eliminated from the diagnostic criteria for autism spectrum disorder in DSM-5-TR?

A. Stereotyped or restricted patterns of interest.
B. Stereotyped and repetitive motor mannerisms.
C. Inflexible adherence to routines.
D. Persistent preoccupation with parts of objects.

Correct Answer: D. Persistent preoccupation with parts of objects.

Explanation: In DSM-5-TR, the older requirement regarding objects was restated as follows: "Highly restricted, fixated interests that are abnormal in intensity or focus (e.g., strong attachment to or preoccupation with unusual objects, excessively circumscribed or perseverative interests)" in Criterion B3. In Criterion B4, hyper- or hyporeactivity to sensory input or unusual interest in sensory aspects of the environment, DSM-5-TR mentions "visual fascination with lights or movement." There is no mention of preoccupation with "parts of objects" in DSM-5-TR (Criterion A3d in DSM-IV autistic disorder).

1.17—Autism Spectrum Disorder / diagnostic criteria (pp. 56–57)

1.18   A 7-year-old girl presents with a history of normal language skills (vocabulary and grammar intact) but is unable to use language in a socially pragmatic manner to share ideas and feelings. She has never made good eye contact and has difficulty reading social cues. Consequently, she has had difficulty making friends, which is further complicated by her obsession with cartoon characters, which she repetitively scripts. She tends to excessively smell objects. Because she insists on wearing the same shirt and shorts every day, regardless of the season, getting dressed is a difficult activity. These symptoms date from early childhood and cause significant impairment in her functioning. What diagnosis best fits this child's presentation?

A. Asperger's disorder.
B. Autism spectrum disorder.
C. Social (pragmatic) communication disorder.
D. Rett syndrome.

Correct Answer: B. Autism spectrum disorder.

Explanation: This child might have met criteria for Asperger's disorder or pervasive developmental disorder not otherwise specified (NOS) in DSM-IV. Autism spectrum disorder in DSM-5-TR incorporated Asperger's disorder and pervasive developmental disorder NOS. Although the child has intact formal language skills, it is the use of language for social communication that is particularly affected in autism spectrum disorder. A specific language delay is not required. She meets all three components of Criterion A (deficits in social-emotional reciprocity; deficits in nonverbal communicative behaviors used for social interaction; and deficits in developing, maintaining, and understanding relationships) and two components of Criterion B (highly restricted, fixated interests that are abnormal in intensity or focus and hyper- or hyporeactivity to sensory input or unusual interest in sensory aspects of the environment). Disruption of social interaction may be observed during the regressive phase of Rett syndrome (typically between ages 1 and 4 years), and after this period, most individuals with Rett syndrome improve their social communication skills, and autistic features are no longer a major area of concern. Autism spectrum disorder can be differentiated from social (pragmatic) communication disorder by the presence in autism spectrum disorder of restricted/repetitive patterns of behavior, interests, or activities and their absence in social (pragmatic) communication disorder.

1.18—Autism Spectrum Disorder / diagnostic features (p. 60) and Differential Diagnosis (pp. 66–67)

1.19   A 15-year-old teenager has a long history of nonverbal communication deficits. As an infant, he was unable to shift his gaze in the direction someone else pointed. As a toddler, he was not interested in social events, discussing feelings, or playing games with others, including his own family. From school age into adolescence, his speech was odd in tonality and phrasing, and his body language was awkward. What do these symptoms represent?

A. Restricted range of interests.
B. Developmental regression.
C. Prodromal schizophreniform symptoms.
D. Deficits in nonverbal communicative behaviors.

Correct Answer: D. Deficits in nonverbal communicative behaviors.

Explanation: These symptoms are examples of deficits in nonverbal communicative behavior, as described in Criterion A2 for autism spectrum disorder criteria in DSM-5-TR:

A. Persistent deficits in social communication and social interaction across multiple contexts, as manifested by all of the following, currently or by history (examples are illustrative, not exhaustive; see text):

1. Deficits in social-emotional reciprocity, ranging, for example, from abnormal social approach and failure of normal back-and-forth conversation; to reduced sharing of interests, emotions, or affect; to failure to initiate or respond to social interactions.
2. Deficits in nonverbal communicative behaviors used for social interaction, ranging, for example, from poorly integrated verbal and nonverbal communication; to abnormalities in eye contact and body language or deficits in understanding and use of gestures; to a total lack of facial expressions and nonverbal communication.
3. Deficits in developing, maintaining, and understanding relationships, ranging, for example, from difficulties adjusting behavior to suit various social contexts; to difficulties in sharing imaginative play or in making friends; to absence of interest in peers.

1.19—Autism Spectrum Disorder / diagnostic criteria (p. 56) and Diagnostic Features (p. 60)

1.20 A 10-year-old boy demonstrates hand-flapping and finger flicking. He repetitively flips coins and lines up his trucks. He tends to "echo" the last several words of a question posed to him before answering, mixes up his pronouns (refers to himself in the second person), tends to repeat phrases in a perseverative fashion, and is quite fixated on routines related to dress, eating, travel, and play. He spends hours in the garage playing with his father's tools. What do these behaviors represent?

A. Restricted, repetitive patterns of behaviors, interests, or activities characteristic of autism spectrum disorder.
B. Symptoms of obsessive-compulsive disorder.
C. Prototypical manifestations of obsessive-compulsive personality.
D. Complex tics.

Correct Answer: A. Restricted, repetitive patterns of behaviors, interests, or activities characteristic of autism spectrum disorder.

Explanation: In DSM-5-TR, the symptoms in the category of "restrictive, repetitive patterns of behaviors, interests, or activities" (Criterion B) associated with autism spectrum disorder demonstrated by this patient include stereotyped or repetitive motor movements, use of objects, or speech; insistence on sameness, inflexible adherence to routines, or ritualized patterns of verbal or nonverbal behavior; and highly restricted, fixated interests that are abnormal in intensity or focus. Only two of the four symptoms in this category (along with meeting Criterion A) are needed to qualify for the autism spectrum disorder diagnosis. The fourth symptom in Criterion B (which this patient does not display) is hyper- or hyporeactivity to sensory input or unusual interest in sensory aspects of the environment. In obsessive-compulsive disorder, intrusive thoughts are often related to contamination, organization, or sexual or religious themes. Compulsions are performed in response to these intrusive thoughts in attempts to relieve anxiety. Motor stereotypies are among the diagnostic characteristics of autism spectrum disorder and can usually be differentiated from tics on the basis of the former's earlier age at onset (often younger than 3 years), prolonged duration (seconds to minutes), being repetitive and rhythmic in form and location, lacking a premonitory sensation or urge, and cessation with distraction.

1.20—Autism Spectrum Disorder / diagnostic features (p. 61) and Differential Diagnosis (p. 67)

1.21   A 25-year-old man presents with long-standing nonverbal communication deficits, inability to have a back-and-forth conversation or share interests in an appropriate fashion, and a complete lack of interest in having relationships with others. His speech reflects awkward phrasing and intonation and is mechanical in nature. He has a history of sequential fixations and obsessions with various games and objects throughout childhood; however, this is not currently a major issue for him. He is living in an assisted living residence and follows the same routine daily. He works at the register in the store in the residence because he enjoys math, and his wages are managed by a guardian. When the store is closed for holidays, he has a hard time adjusting to the change. What is the appropriate diagnosis?

A. Intellectual developmental disorder (intellectual disability), moderate.
B. Intellectual developmental disorder (intellectual disability), severe.
C. Autism spectrum disorder, level 1 ("requiring support").
D. Autism spectrum disorder, level 2 ("requiring substantial support").

Correct Answer: D. Autism spectrum disorder, level 2 ("requiring substantial support").

Explanation: This patient presents with all criteria for autism spectrum disorder, with deficits in social communication and social interaction across multiple contexts and restricted, repetitive patterns of behavior, interests, or activities both currently and by history, and symptoms were present in the early developmental period. He requires substantial support with his living situation and having a guardian. The deficits in independence and social relationships are due to nonverbal communication deficits, lack of interest, and need for repetition. In intellectual developmental disorder, regardless of severity, the desire for social connection and use of language to establish relationships is evident; individuals will initiate and respond to social interactions through gestural and emotional cues.

1.21—Autism Spectrum Disorder / Table 2 [Severity levels for autism spectrum disorder (examples of level of support needs)] (p. 58)

1.22   A 9-year-old girl presents with a history of intellectual impairment, a structural language impairment, nonverbal communication deficits, disinterest in peers, and inability to use language in a social manner. She has extreme food and tactile sensitivities. She is obsessed with one particular computer game that she plays for hours each day, scripting and imitating the characters. She is clumsy, has an odd gait, and walks on her tiptoes. In the past year, she developed a seizure disorder and has begun to bang her wrists against the wall repetitively, causing bruising. On the other hand, she plays several musical instruments in an extremely precocious manner. Which feature of this child's clinical presentation fulfills a criterion symptom for DSM-5-TR autism spectrum disorder?

A. Motor abnormalities.
B. Structural language impairment.
C. Intellectual impairment.
D. Nonverbal communicative deficits.

Correct Answer: D. Nonverbal communicative deficits.

Explanation: Criterion A2 of autism spectrum disorder lists nonverbal communicative deficits as one of the symptoms. The rest of the options represent associated features supporting diagnosis, which according to the DSM-5-TR text notes that "the gap between intellectual and adaptive functional skills is often large."

1.22—Autism Spectrum Disorder / diagnostic criteria (p. 56); Associated Features (p. 62)

1.23   An 11-year-old girl with autism spectrum disorder displays no spoken language and is minimally responsive to overtures from others. She can be somewhat inflexible, which interferes with her ability to travel, do schoolwork, and be managed in the home. She has difficulty planning, organizing, and transitioning activities. These problems can usually be managed with incentives and reinforcers. What severity levels should be specified in the DSM-5-TR diagnosis?

A. Level 3 (requiring very substantial support) for social communication and level 1 (requiring support) for restricted, repetitive behaviors.
B. Level 1 (requiring support) for social communication and level 3 (requiring very substantial support) for restricted, repetitive behaviors.
C. Level 1 (requiring support) for social communication and level 1 (requiring support) for restricted, repetitive behaviors.
D. Level 2 (requiring substantial support) for social communication and level 1 (requiring support) for restricted, repetitive behaviors.

Correct Answer: A. Level 3 (requiring very substantial support) for social communication and level 1 (requiring support) for restricted, repetitive behaviors.

Explanation: In DSM-5-TR, severity is noted separately for social communication impairments and for restricted, repetitive patterns of behavior. In this case, the social communication deficits are quite severe, warranting a classification of level 3, but the restricted, repetitive behaviors are milder, reflecting the lowest classification of level 1. Level 2 is an intermediate category reflecting the need for "substantial support."

1.23—Autism Spectrum Disorder / Table 2 [Severity levels for autism spectrum disorder (examples of level of support needs)] (p. 58)

1.24 Which of the following is *not* a specifier included in the diagnostic criteria for autism spectrum disorder?

A. With or without accompanying intellectual impairment.
B. With or without associated dementia.
C. Associated with a known medical or genetic condition or environmental factor.
D. Associated with another neurodevelopmental, mental, or behavioral disorder.

Correct Answer: B. With or without associated dementia.

Explanation: The specifier *with or without associated dementia* is not included in the diagnostic criteria for autism spectrum disorder.

1.24—Autism Spectrum Disorder / diagnostic criteria (p. 57)

1.25 Which of the following is *not* typical for the developmental course of children diagnosed with autism spectrum disorder?

A. Developmental gains in later childhood.
B. Early, prominent lack of interest in social interaction.
C. Regression across multiple domains occurring after age 2–3 years.
D. First symptoms that often include delayed language development.

Correct Answer: C. Regression across multiple domains occurring after age 2–3 years.

Explanation: Regression across multiple domains after age 2–3 years may occur, but it is not typical of the developmental course in autism spectrum disorder. As noted in DSM-5-TR, some children with autism spectrum disorder experience developmental plateaus or regression, with a gradual or relatively rapid deterioration in social behaviors or use of language, often during the first 2 years of life. Such losses are rare in other disorders and may be a useful "red flag" for autism spectrum disorder. Much more unusual and warranting more extensive medical investigation are losses of skills beyond social communication (e.g., loss of self-care, toileting, or motor skills) or those occurring after the second birthday. The first symptoms of autism spectrum disorder frequently involve delayed language development, which is often accompanied by lack of social interest or unusual social interactions (e.g., pulling individuals by the hand without any attempt to look at them), odd play patterns (e.g., carrying toys around but never playing with them), and unusual communication patterns (e.g., knowing the alphabet but not responding to own name).

1.25—Autism Spectrum Disorder / Development and Course (p. 63)

1.26   A 4-year-old girl has some food aversions. She enjoys having the same book read to her at night but does not become terribly upset if her mother asks her to choose a different book. She spins around repeatedly when her favorite show is on television. She generally likes her toys neatly arranged in bins and complains when her sister leaves them on the floor. With which of the following diagnoses are these behaviors consistent?

   A. Obsessive-compulsive disorder.
   B. Autism spectrum disorder.
   C. Attention-deficit/hyperactivity disorder.
   D. Typical development.

Correct Answer: D. Typical development.

Explanation: The child described in the question meets none of the criteria for autism spectrum disorder. Because many typically developing young children have strong preferences and enjoy repetition (e.g., eating the same foods, watching the same video multiple times), distinguishing restricted and repetitive behaviors that are diagnostic of autism spectrum disorder can be difficult in preschoolers. The clinical distinction is based on the type, frequency, and intensity of the behavior (e.g., a child who daily lines up objects for hours and is very distressed if any item is moved). In obsessive-compulsive disorder, intrusive thoughts are often related to organization, and compulsions are performed in response to these intrusive thoughts in attempts to relieve anxiety. In attention-deficit/hyperactivity disorder, *hyperactivity* refers to excessive motor activity (such as a child running about) when it is not appropriate or excessive fidgeting, tapping, or talkativeness.

1.26—Autism Spectrum Disorder / Development and Course (p. 63)

1.27   Which of the following is typical for the developmental course for autism spectrum disorder?

   A. Lack of degenerative course.
   B. Behavioral deterioration during adolescence.
   C. Reduction in learning throughout life.
   D. Absence of symptoms in early childhood and early school years, with developmental losses in later childhood in areas such as social interaction.

Correct Answer: A. Lack of degenerative course.

Explanation: Most adolescents with autism spectrum disorder improve behaviorally; only a minority further deteriorates. Autism spectrum disorder is not a degenerative disorder, and it is typical for learning and compensation to continue throughout life. Symptoms are often most marked in early childhood and early school years, with developmental gains typical in later childhood in at least some areas. As more individuals are able to find a niche that matches their special interests and skills, they are productively employed. Access to vocational rehabilitation services significantly improves competitive employment outcomes for transition-age youth with autism spectrum disorder. In general, individuals with lower levels of impairment may be better able to function independently.

1.27—Autism Spectrum Disorder / Development and Course (pp. 63–64)

1.28   A 21-year-old patient, who was not previously diagnosed with a developmental disorder, presents for evaluation after taking a leave from college for psychological reasons. He makes little eye contact, does not appear to pick up on social cues, has become disinterested in friends, spends hours each day on the computer surfing the internet and playing games, and has become so sensitive to smells that he keeps multiple air fresheners in all locations of the home. He reports that he has had long-standing friendships dating from childhood and high school (corroborated by his parents). He reports making many friends in his social club at college. His parents report good social and communication skills in childhood, although he was quite shy and somewhat inflexible and ritualistic at home. What is the *least likely* diagnosis?

A. Depression.
B. Schizophreniform disorder or schizophrenia.
C. Autism spectrum disorder.
D. Social anxiety disorder (social phobia).

Correct Answer: C. Autism spectrum disorder.

Explanation: The history of good social and communication skills in childhood and long-standing friendships is not consistent with autism spectrum disorder. With respect to schizophrenia specifically, DSM-5-TR text notes that "schizophrenia with childhood onset usually develops after a period of normal, or near normal, development. A prodromal state has been described in which social impairment and atypical interests and beliefs occur, which could be confused with the social deficits seen in autism spectrum disorder. Hallucinations and delusions, which are defining features of schizophrenia, are not features of autism spectrum disorder."

1.28—Autism Spectrum Disorder / Differential Diagnosis (p. 67)

1.29 Which of the following characteristics is generally *not* associated with autism spectrum disorder?

   A. Anxiety, depression, and isolation as an adult.
   B. Catatonia.
   C. Insistence on routines and aversion to change.
   D. Successful adaptation in regular school settings.

   Correct Answer: D. Successful adaptation in regular school settings.

   Explanation: In young children with autism spectrum disorder, lack of social and communication abilities may hamper learning, especially learning through social interaction or in settings with peers. In the home, insistence on routines and aversion to change, as well as sensory sensitivities, may interfere with eating and sleeping and make routine care (e.g., haircuts, dental work) extremely difficult. Adaptive skills are typically below measured IQ. Extreme difficulties in planning, organization, and coping with change negatively impact academic achievement, even for students with above-average intelligence. During adulthood, these individuals may have difficulties establishing independence because of continued rigidity and difficulty with novelty. In general, individuals with lower levels of impairment may be better able to function independently. However, even these individuals may remain socially naive and vulnerable, may have difficulties organizing practical demands without aid, and are prone to anxiety and depression. Many adults report using compensation strategies and coping mechanisms to mask their difficulties in public but suffer from the stress and effort of maintaining a socially acceptable facade. It is possible for individuals with autism spectrum disorder to experience a marked deterioration in motor symptoms and display a full catatonic episode with symptoms such as mutism, posturing, grimacing, and waxy flexibility. The risk period for comorbid catatonia appears to be greatest in the adolescent years.

   1.29—Autism Spectrum Disorder / Functional Consequences of Autism Spectrum Disorder (pp. 65–66) and Comorbidity (p. 68)

1.30 Which of the following disorders is generally *not* comorbid with autism spectrum disorder?

   A. Attention-deficit/hyperactivity disorder (ADHD).
   B. Selective mutism.
   C. Intellectual developmental disorder (intellectual disability).
   D. Stereotypic movement disorder.

   Correct Answer: B. Selective mutism.

   Explanation: Children with selective mutism have appropriate communication skills in certain contexts and do not demonstrate severe impairments in social interaction and restricted patterns of behavior; in selective mutism, there are typically no abnormalities in early development and no restricted and repetitive behavior or interests. ADHD can be comorbid with autism spectrum disorder in DSM-5-TR (unlike in DSM-IV); such comorbidity would be coded with the specifier *associated with another neurodevelopmental, mental, or behavioral disorder*. Autism spectrum disorder can be comorbid with intellectual developmental disorder when all criteria for both disorders are met and "social communication and interaction are significantly impaired relative to the developmental level of the individual's nonverbal skills"; that is, there is a discrepancy between social-communicative skills and nonverbal skills. Autism spectrum disorder can be comorbid with stereotypic movement disorder if the repetitive movements cannot be accounted for as part of the autism spectrum disorder (e.g., hand flapping). In general, when criteria for another disorder are met along with meeting the criteria for autism spectrum disorder, both disorders are diagnosed. Comorbidity with additional diagnoses is common in autism spectrum disorder (about 70% of individuals with autism spectrum disorder have one comorbid mental disorder, and 40% have two or more comorbid mental disorders).

1.30—Autism Spectrum Disorder / Differential Diagnosis (pp. 66–67) and Comorbidity (pp. 67–68)

1.31   Which of the following is *not* a criterion for the DSM-5-TR diagnosis of attention-deficit/hyperactivity disorder (ADHD)?

A. Onset of several inattentive or hyperactive-impulsive symptoms prior to age 12 years.
B. Manifestation of several inattentive or hyperactive-impulsive symptoms in two or more settings (e.g., at home, school, or work; with friends or relatives; in other activities).
C. Persistence of symptoms for at least 12 months.
D. Inability to explain symptoms as a manifestation of another mental disorder (e.g., mood disorder, anxiety disorder, dissociative disorder, personality disorder, substance intoxication or withdrawal).

Correct Answer: C. Persistence of symptoms for at least 12 months.

Explanation: The essential feature of ADHD is a pervasive pattern of *inattention* and/or *hyperactivity-impulsivity* that interferes with functioning or development, with persistence of symptoms for at least 6 months to a degree that is inconsistent with developmental level and that negatively impacts social and academic/occupational activities directly. ADHD begins in childhood. The requirement that several symptoms be present before age 12 years conveys the importance of a substantial clinical presentation during childhood. Manifestations of the disorder must be present in more than one setting (e.g., home and school, work). Confirmation of substantial symptoms across settings typically cannot be done accurately without consulting informants who have seen the individual in those settings.

1.31—Attention-Deficit/Hyperactivity Disorder / diagnostic criteria (pp. 68–69); Diagnostic Features (p. 70)

1.32   The parents of a 15-year-old tenth grader believe that she should be doing better in high school, given how bright she seems and the fact that she received mostly As through eighth grade. However, her papers are frequently handed in late, and she makes careless mistakes on examinations. On formal testing, her Wechsler Adult Intelligence Scale, 4th Edition (WAIS-IV) results are as follows: Verbal IQ, 125; Perceptual Reasoning Index, 122; Full-Scale IQ, 123; Working Memory Index, 55th percentile; Processing Speed Index, 50th percentile. Weaknesses in executive function are noted. During a psychiatric evaluation, the teenager reports a long history of failing to give close attention to details; difficulty sustaining attention while in class or doing homework; failing to finish chores and tasks; and significant difficulties with time management, planning, and organization. She is forgetful, often loses things, and is easily distracted. She has no history of restlessness or impulsivity and is well liked by peers. What is the most likely diagnosis?

A. Adjustment disorder with anxiety.
B. Specific learning disorder.
C. Attention-deficit/hyperactivity disorder, predominantly inattentive.
D. Major depressive disorder.

Correct Answer: C. Attention-deficit/hyperactivity disorder, predominantly inattentive.

Explanation: The patient has six symptoms in the inattention cluster of attention-deficit/hyperactivity disorder (ADHD) and meets criteria for this disorder. She has common associated features of ADHD, including weaknesses in working memory and processing speed and problems handing in her work (especially writing) on time. There is no evidence from the testing or history that her writing difficulty is secondary to a primary disorder involving writing or that she has any other specific learning disorder. She is not demonstrating sadness or irritability and/or anhedonia, which are required to diagnose a major depressive disorder. Poor concentration in mood disorders becomes prominent only during a depressive episode. Additionally, there is no mention of a triggering event leading to the onset of concentration difficulties, which would lead to considering an adjustment disorder.

1.32—Attention-Deficit/Hyperactivity Disorder / Differential Diagnosis (pp. 73–74)

1.33   A 7-year-old boy is having behavioral and social difficulties in his second-grade class. Although he seems to be able to pay attention and is doing "well" from an academic standpoint (although seemingly not up to his assumed capabilities), he is constantly interrupting, fidgeting, talking excessively, and getting out of his seat. He has friends but sometimes annoys his peers because of difficulty sharing and taking turns and frequently talking over others. Although he seeks out play dates, he exhausts his friends by wanting to play sports nonstop. At home, he can barely stay in his seat for a meal and is unable to play quietly. Although he shows remorse when the consequences of his behavior are pointed out to him, he can become angry in response and nevertheless is unable to inhibit himself. What is the most likely diagnosis?

A. Autism spectrum disorder.
B. Generalized anxiety disorder.
C. Attention-deficit/hyperactivity disorder, predominantly hyperactive/impulsive.
D. Specific learning disorder.

Correct Answer: C. Attention-deficit/hyperactivity disorder, predominantly hyperactive/impulsive.

Explanation: This child has all the cardinal features in the hyperactivity/impulsivity cluster of attention-deficit/hyperactivity disorder (ADHD). Although he is not currently displaying inattention or impairment in his academic functioning, it is quite likely that this will become more of an issue as schoolwork becomes more complex and tedious and academic demands increase. His behaviors are somewhat alienating to peers, as is common in ADHD. There is no evidence that he has comorbid autism spectrum disorder, especially because he seeks out friendships. He meets Criterion C in that "several inattentive or hyperactive-impulsive symptoms are present in two or more settings (e.g., at home, school, or work; with friends or relatives; in other activities)" and Criterion D in that "there is clear evidence that the symptoms interfere with, or reduce the quality of, social, academic, or occupational functioning." He is not demonstrating any evidence of worry or rumination, which would be seen in anxiety disorder and would lead to disruption in attention. Children with specific learning disorder alone may appear inattentive because of frustration, lack of interest, or limited ability in neurocognitive processes, including working memory and processing speed, whereas their inattention is much reduced when performing a skill that does not require the impaired cognitive process.

1.33—Attention-Deficit/Hyperactivity Disorder / Differential Diagnosis (pp. 73–74)

1.34   A 37-year-old stock trader schedules a visit after his 8-year-old son is diagnosed with attention-deficit/hyperactivity disorder (ADHD), combined inattentive and hyperactive. Although the patient does not currently note motor restlessness like his son, he recalls being that way as a child, along with being quite inattentive, being impulsive, talking excessively, interrupting, and having problems waiting his turn. He was an underachiever in high school and college, when he did his work inconsistently and had difficulty following rules. Nevertheless, he never failed any classes and was never evaluated by a psychologist or psychiatrist. Currently, he works about 60–80 hours a week and often gets insufficient sleep. He tends to make impulsive business decisions, can be impatient and short-tempered, and notes that his mind tends to wander both in one-on-one interactions with associates and his wife and during business meetings, for which he is often late; he is forgetful and disorganized. Overall, he tends to perform fairly well and is quite successful, but he frequently feels overwhelmed and demoralized. What is the most likely diagnosis?

A. Major depressive disorder.
B. Generalized anxiety disorder.
C. Specific learning disorder.
D. ADHD, in partial remission.

Correct Answer: D. ADHD, in partial remission.

Explanation: This is a not uncommon story of a parent who presents to treatment after a son or daughter is diagnosed with ADHD and the parent recognizes similarities from their own childhood. This patient presents with a possible history of ADHD during childhood, along with a possible *prior* history of oppositional defiant disorder. Currently, there is no evidence that he has difficulty with rules, and the fact that he is no longer restless is common for the developmental course of ADHD. Currently, his ADHD symptoms include three symptoms in the inattention cluster (difficulty sustaining attention, difficulty organizing tasks and activities, forgetfulness), and only one clear symptom of impulsivity (impatience); because he has retained only some of the symptoms, a diagnosis of ADHD, *in partial remission*, is appropriate and is provided for in DSM-5-TR. It is unclear to what degree his work schedule and insufficient sleep are also contributing to his distress.

1.34—Attention-Deficit/Hyperactivity Disorder / Differential Diagnosis (pp. 73–74)

1.35   A hyperactive, impulsive, and inattentive 5-year-old boy presents with hypertelorism, highly arched palate, and low-set ears. He is uncoordinated and clumsy, has no sense of time, and constantly leaves toys and clothes strewn all over the house. He recently developed what appears to be a motor tic involving blinking. He enjoys playing with peers, who tend to like him, although he seems to willfully defy all requests from parents and teachers, which does not seem to be due simply to inattention. He is delayed in beginning to learn how to read. What is the *least likely* diagnosis?

A. Autism spectrum disorder.
B. Developmental coordination disorder.

C. Oppositional defiant disorder (ODD).

D. Attention-deficit/hyperactivity disorder (ADHD).

Correct Answer: A. Autism spectrum disorder.

Explanation: There is no evidence that this child has a disorder of relatedness, especially because he enjoys playing with peers, who like him. He has signs and symptoms of ADHD, along with some soft neurological signs and minor physical anomalies that can be associated with ADHD (although genetic and neurological evaluations seem warranted). He may have a comorbid diagnosis of ODD because his oppositional behavior is not simply due to inattention.

1.35—Attention-Deficit/Hyperactivity Disorder / Differential Diagnosis (pp. 73–74)

1.36   What is the prevalence of attention-deficit/hyperactivity disorder (ADHD) in children?

A. 2%.

B. 7%.

C. 10%.

D. 12%.

Correct Answer: B. 7%.

Explanation: Population surveys suggest that ADHD occurs worldwide in about 7.2% of children; however, cross-national prevalence ranges widely, from 0.1% to 10.2% of children and adolescents. Prevalence is higher in special populations such as foster children or correctional settings. Differences in ADHD prevalence rates across regions appear to be attributable mainly to different diagnostic and methodological practices. However, there also may be cultural variation in attitudes toward or interpretations of children's behaviors. Clinical identification rates in the United States for African American and Latinx populations tend to be lower than for non-Latinx white populations. Underdetection may result from mislabeling of ADHD symptoms as oppositional or disruptive in socially oppressed ethnic or racialized groups because of explicit or implicit clinician bias, leading to overdiagnosis of disruptive disorders. Higher prevalence in non-Latinx white youth may also be influenced by greater parental demand for diagnosis of behaviors seen as ADHD related.

1.36—Attention-Deficit/Hyperactivity Disorder / Prevalence (p. 71); Culture-Related Diagnostic Issues (p. 72)

1.37   What is the prevalence of attention-deficit/hyperactivity disorder (ADHD) in adults?

A. 0.5%.
B. 2.5%.
C. 5%.
D. 8%.

Correct Answer: B. 2.5%.

Explanation: Population surveys suggest that ADHD occurs in most cultures in about 2.5% of adults and about 7% of children.

1.37—Attention-Deficit/Hyperactivity Disorder / Prevalence (p. 71)

1.38   What is the gender ratio of attention-deficit/hyperactivity disorder (ADHD) in children?

A. Male:female ratio of 2:1.
B. Male:female ratio of 3:2.
C. Male:female ratio of 5:1.
D. Male:female ratio of 1:2.

Correct Answer: A. Male:female ratio of 2:1.

Explanation: ADHD is more prevalent in males than in females in the general population, with a gender ratio of approximately 2:1 in children and 1.6:1 in adults. Females are more likely than males to present primarily with inattentive features.

1.38—Attention-Deficit/Hyperactivity Disorder / Sex- and Gender-Related Diagnostic Issues (p. 72)

1.39   A child is born with very low birth weight and had prenatal exposure to smoking. He is currently being treated for encephalitis. Which neurodevelopmental disorder should the parents consider as a possibility for their child?

A. Attention deficit/hyperactivity disorder (ADHD).
B. Specific learning disorder.
C. Stereotypic movement disorder.
D. Childhood-onset fluency disorder.

Correct Answer: A. Attention deficit/hyperactivity disorder (ADHD).

Explanation: Very low birth weight and degree of prematurity convey a greater risk for ADHD; the more extreme the low weight, the greater the risk. Prenatal exposure to smoking is associated with ADHD even after controlling for parental psychiatric history and socioeconomic status. Neurotoxin exposure (e.g., lead), infections (e.g., encephalitis), and alcohol exposure in utero have been correlated with subsequent ADHD, but it is not known whether these associations are causal.

1.39—Attention-Deficit/Hyperactivity Disorder / Risk and Prognostic Factors (p. 71)

1.40   Which of the following is *not* associated with attention-deficit/hyperactivity disorder (ADHD)?

A. Reduced school performance.
B. Higher probability of unemployment.
C. Elevated interpersonal conflict.
D. Reduced risk of substance use disorders.

Correct Answer: D. Reduced risk of substance use disorders.

Explanation: Children with ADHD are significantly more likely than their peers without ADHD to develop conduct disorder in adolescence and antisocial personality disorder in adulthood, consequently increasing the likelihood for substance use disorders and incarceration. The risk of subsequent substance use disorders is elevated, especially when conduct disorder or antisocial personality disorder develops. ADHD is associated with reduced school performance and academic attainment. Adults with ADHD show higher probability of unemployment, as well as elevated interpersonal conflict. On average, individuals with ADHD obtain less schooling, have poorer vocational achievement, and have reduced intellectual scores than their peers, although there is great variability.

1.40—Attention-Deficit/Hyperactivity Disorder / Functional Consequences of Attention-Deficit/Hyperactivity Disorder (pp. 72–73)

1.41   Which of the following is *not* associated with attention-deficit/hyperactivity disorder (ADHD)?

A. Social rejection.
B. Increased risk of developing conduct disorder in childhood and antisocial personality disorder in adulthood.
C. Increased risk of Alzheimer's disease.
D. Increased risk of accidental injury.

Correct Answer: C. Increased risk of Alzheimer's disease.

Explanation: The risk of Alzheimer's disease is not elevated in individuals with ADHD. Peer relationships in individuals with ADHD are often disrupted by peer rejection, neglect, or teasing. Children with ADHD are significantly more likely than their peers without ADHD to develop conduct disorder in adolescence and antisocial personality disorder in adulthood, consequently increasing the likelihood for substance use disorders and incarceration. Individuals with ADHD are more likely than peers to be injured.

1.41—Attention-Deficit/Hyperactivity Disorder / Functional Consequences of Attention-Deficit/Hyperactivity Disorder (pp. 72–73)

1.42   A 15-year-old has developed concentration problems in school that have been associated with a significant decline in grades. When interviewed, he explains that his mind is occupied with worrying about his mother, who has a serious autoimmune disease. As his grades falter, he becomes increasingly demoralized and sad and notices that his energy levels drop, further compromising his ability to pay attention in school. At the same time, he complains of feeling restless and unable to sleep. What is the most likely diagnosis?

A. Specific learning disorder.
B. Attention-deficit/hyperactivity disorder (ADHD).
C. Adjustment disorder with mixed anxiety and depressed mood.
D. Separation anxiety disorder.

Correct Answer: C. Adjustment disorder with mixed anxiety and depressed mood.

Explanation: The inattention seen in this teenager relates to anxiety and depressive symptoms that are reactions to his mother's illness and his own subsequent decline in grades. Inattention related to ADHD is not associated with worry and rumination, as would be the case in anxiety disorders. Children with specific learning disorder alone may appear inattentive because of frustration, lack of interest, or limited ability in neurocognitive processes. When separated from major attachment figures, children and adults with separation anxiety disorder may exhibit social withdrawal, apathy, sadness, or difficulty concentrating on work or play. In this vignette, the patient is not expressing a developmentally inappropriate and excessive fear or anxiety concerning separation from his mother.

1.42—Attention-Deficit/Hyperactivity Disorder / Differential Diagnosis (pp. 73–75)

1.43   A 5-year-old boy is consistently moody, irritable, and intolerant of frustration. In addition, he is pervasively and chronically restless, impulsive, and inattentive. Which diagnosis best fits the clinical picture?

A. Attention-deficit/hyperactivity disorder (ADHD).
B. ADHD and disruptive mood dysregulation disorder (DMDD).
C. Bipolar disorder.
D. Oppositional defiant disorder (ODD).

Correct Answer: B. ADHD and DMDD.

Explanation: The child's mood symptoms cannot be accounted for by ADHD alone, and they are characteristic of DMDD; ADHD is not associated with this level of affective symptoms on its own. Individuals with bipolar disorder may have increased activity, poor concentration, and increased impulsivity, but these features are episodic, unlike ADHD, in which the symptoms are persistent. Moreover, in bipolar disorder, increased impulsivity or inattention is accompanied by elevated mood, grandiosity, and other specific bipolar features. Children with ADHD may show significant changes in mood within the same day; such lability is distinct from a manic or hypomanic episode, which must last 4 or more days to be a clinical indicator of bipolar disorder, even in children. Individuals with ODD may resist work or school tasks that require self-application because they resist conforming to others' demands. Their behavior is characterized by negativity, hostility, and defiance. These symptoms must be differentiated from aversion to school or mentally demanding tasks because of difficulty in sustaining mental effort, forgetting instructions, and impulsivity in individuals with ADHD.

1.43—Attention-Deficit/Hyperactivity Disorder / Differential Diagnosis (pp. 73–75)

1.44 Which comorbidity is found in a minority of children with attention-deficit/hyperactivity disorder (ADHD)?

    A. Oppositional defiant disorder (ODD).
    B. Disruptive mood dysregulation disorder (DMDD).
    C. Intermittent explosive disorder.
    D. Specific learning disorder.

Correct Answer: C. Intermittent explosive disorder.

Explanation: Although ADHD is more common in males, females with ADHD have higher rates of a number of comorbid disorders, particularly ODD, autism spectrum disorder, and personality and substance use disorders. ODD co-occurs with ADHD. Most children and adolescents with DMDD have symptoms that also meet criteria for ADHD; a smaller percentage of children with ADHD have symptoms that meet criteria for DMDD. Anxiety disorders, major depressive disorder, obsessive-compulsive disorder, and intermittent explosive disorder occur in a minority of individuals with ADHD but more often than in the general population. Specific learning disorder commonly co-occurs with ADHD.

1.44—Attention-Deficit/Hyperactivity Disorder / Comorbidity (p. 75)

1.45 What are the characteristics of specific learning disorder?

A. It is part of a more general learning impairment as manifested in intellectual developmental disorder (intellectual disability).
B. It usually can be attributed to a sensory, physical, or neurological disorder.
C. It involves pervasive and wide-ranging deficits across multiple domains of information processing.
D. It consists of persistent difficulties learning keystone academic skills with onset during the years of formal schooling.

Correct Answer: D. It consists of persistent difficulties learning keystone academic skills with onset during the years of formal schooling.

Explanation: The DSM-5-TR diagnosis of specific learning disorder combines the DSM-IV diagnoses of reading disorder, mathematics disorder, disorder of written expression, and learning disorder not otherwise specified. The difficulties seen in specific learning disorder are considered *specific* for four reasons. First, they are not attributable to intellectual disabilities (intellectual developmental disorder [intellectual disability]), global developmental delay, hearing or vision disorders, or neurological or motor disorders (Criterion D). Second, the learning difficulty cannot be attributed to more general external factors, such as economic or environmental disadvantage, chronic absenteeism, or lack of education as typically provided in the individual's community context. Third, the learning difficulty cannot be attributed to a neurological disorder (e.g., pediatric stroke) or motor disorder or to vision or hearing disorders, which are often associated with problems learning academic skills but are distinguishable by the presence of neurological signs. Finally, the learning difficulty may be restricted to one academic skill or domain (e.g., reading single words, retrieving or calculating number facts).

1.45—Specific Learning Disorder / diagnostic criteria (pp. 76–78) and Diagnostic Features (pp. 78–80)

1.46 DSM-5-TR classifies all learning disorders under the diagnosis of specific learning disorder, along with the requirement to "specify all academic domains and subskills that are impaired" at the time of assessment. What is *not* characteristic of specific learning disorder?

A. The persistent learning difficulties manifest as restricted progress in learning for at least 6 months despite the provision of extra help at home or school.
B. Current skills in one or more of these academic areas are well below the average range for the individual's age, gender, cultural group, and level of education.
C. There usually is a discrepancy of more than 3 standard deviations (SDs) between achievement and IQ.
D. The learning difficulties significantly interfere with academic achievement, occupational performance, or activities of daily living that require these academic skills.

Correct Answer: C. There usually is a discrepancy of more than 3 standard deviations (SDs) between achievement and IQ.

Explanation: One robust clinical indicator of difficulties learning academic skills is low academic achievement for the individual's age or average achievement that is sustainable only by extraordinarily high levels of effort or support. The learning difficulties are persistent, not transitory. In children and adolescents, persistence is defined as restricted progress in learning (i.e., no evidence that the individual is catching up with classmates) for at least 6 months despite the provision of extra help at home or school. In children, the low academic skills cause significant interference in school performance. Another clinical indicator, particularly in adults, is avoidance of activities that require the academic skills. Also in adulthood, low academic skills interfere with occupational performance or everyday activities requiring those skills. Academic skills are distributed along a continuum, so there is no natural cut point that can be used to differentiate individuals with and without specific learning disorder. Thus, any threshold used to specify what constitutes significantly low academic achievement is to a large extent arbitrary. Low achievement scores on one or more standardized tests or subtests within an academic domain (i.e., at least 1.5 SDs below the population mean for age, which translates to a standard score of 78 or less, which is below the 7th percentile) are needed for the greatest diagnostic certainty. However, precise scores will vary according to the particular standardized tests that are used. On the basis of clinical judgment, a more lenient threshold may be used (e.g., 1.0 SD below the population mean for age) when learning difficulties are supported by converging evidence from clinical assessment, academic history, school reports, or test scores. Moreover, because standardized tests are not available in all languages, the diagnosis may then be based in part on clinical judgment of scores on available test measures.

1.46—Specific Learning Disorder / Diagnostic Features (pp. 78–80)

1.47   What is associated with the diagnosis of specific learning disorder?

    A. A neurodegenerative cognitive disorder.
    B. An uneven profile of abilities.
    C. Lack of educational opportunity.
    D. There are four formal subtypes of specific learning disorder.

Correct Answer: B. An uneven profile of abilities.

Explanation: An uneven profile of abilities is common, such as a combination of above-average visuospatial abilities and slow, effortful, and inaccurate reading and poor reading comprehension and written expression. Specific learning disorder is distinguished from learning problems associated with neurodegenerative cognitive disorders. In specific learning disorder, the clinical expression of specific learning difficulties occurs during the developmental period, and the difficulties do not manifest as a marked decline from a former state. Specific learning disorder is distinguished from normal variations in academic attainment attributable to external factors (e.g., lack of educational opportunity, consistently poor instruction, learning in a second language) because the learning difficulties persist in the presence of adequate educational opportunity, exposure to the same instruction as the peer group, and competency in the language of instruction, even when it is different from one's primary spoken language. In DSM-5-TR, there are no formal subtypes of specific learning disorder. Learning deficits in the areas of reading, written expression, and mathematics are coded as separate specifiers.

1.47—Specific Learning Disorder / Differential Diagnosis (pp. 84–85)

1.48   What is associated with prevalence rates for specific learning disorder?

    A. Prevalence rates range from 1% to 5% among school-age children across languages and cultures.
    B. Specific learning disorder is equally common among males and females.
    C. Prevalence rates vary according to the range of ages in the sample, selection criteria, severity of specific learning disorder, and academic domains investigated.
    D. Gender ratios can be attributed to factors such as ascertainment bias, definitional or measurement variation, language, race, or socioeconomic status.

Correct Answer: C. Prevalence rates vary according to the range of ages in the sample, selection criteria, severity of specific learning disorder, and academic domains investigated.

Explanation: Specific learning disorder is more common in males than in females (ratios range from about 2:1 to 3:1, and gender ratios cannot be attributed to factors such as ascertainment bias, definitional or measurement variation, language, race, or socioeconomic status). The prevalence of specific learning disorder across the academic domains of reading, writing, and mathematics is approximately 5%–15% among school-age children across different languages and cultures.

1.48—Specific Learning Disorder / Prevalence (p. 81); Sex- and Gender-Related Diagnostic Issues (p. 84)

1.49   What disorder(s) is/are typically comorbid with specific learning disorders?

    A. Attention-deficit/hyperactivity disorder (ADHD).
    B. Speech sound disorder.
    C. Developmental coordination disorder.
    D. All of the above.

Correct Answer: D. All of the above.

Explanation: Specific learning disorder commonly co-occurs with neurodevelopmental disorders (e.g., ADHD, communication disorders, developmental coordination disorder, autistic spectrum disorder) or other mental disorders (e.g., anxiety disorders, depressive and bipolar disorders). These comorbidities do not necessarily exclude the diagnosis of specific learning disorder but may make testing and differential diagnosis more difficult because each of the co-occurring disorders independently interferes with the execution of activities of daily living, including learning. Thus, clinical judgment is required to attribute such impairment to learning difficulties.

1.49—Specific Learning Disorder / Comorbidity (p. 85)

1.50 Which of the following is *not* associated with developmental coordination disorder (DCD)?

A. Additional (usually suppressed) motor activity, such as choreiform movements of unsupported limbs or mirror movements.
B. Improvement in learning new tasks involving complex/automatic motor skills, including driving and using tools.
C. Prenatal exposure to alcohol.
D. Impairments in underlying neurodevelopmental processes affecting visuomotor skills.

Correct Answer: B. Improvement in learning new tasks involving complex/automatic motor skills, including driving and using tools.

Explanation: Regarding the choreiform or mirror movements seen in DCD, DSM-5-TR states, "these 'overflow' movements are referred to as *neurodevelopmental immaturities* or *neurological soft signs* rather than neurological abnormalities. In both current literature and clinical practice, their role in diagnosis is still unclear, requiring further evaluation." In adulthood, there are often ongoing problems with learning new tasks involving complex/automatic motor skills. DCD is more common following prenatal exposure to alcohol and in preterm and low–birth weight children. In DCD, deficits have been identified in both visuomotor perception and spatial mentalizing; these deficits affect the ability to make rapid motoric adjustments as the complexity of the required movements increases.

1.50—Developmental Coordination Disorder / Associated Features; Prevalence; Risk and Prognostic Factors (p. 87)

1.51 Which of the following statements about developmental coordination disorder (DCD) is *true*?

A. Symptoms have usually improved significantly at 1-year follow-up.
B. In most cases, symptoms are no longer evident by adolescence.
C. DCD has no clear relationship with prenatal alcohol exposure, preterm birth, or low birth weight.
D. Cerebellar dysfunction is hypothesized to play a role in DCD.

Correct Answer: D. Cerebellar dysfunction is hypothesized to play a role in DCD.

Explanation: DCD is usually not diagnosed before age 5 years, and the course has been demonstrated to be stable up to 1-year follow-up. In about 50%–70% of cases, symptoms continue into adolescence. Prenatal alcohol exposure, prematurity, and low birth weight may be risk factors.

1.51—Developmental Coordination Disorder / Development and Course (p. 87)

1.52   Which of the following is *not* a criterion for the DSM-5-TR diagnosis of stereotypic movement disorder?

A. Repetitive, seemingly driven, and apparently purposeless movements are present.
B. Onset occurs during the early developmental period.
C. Behaviors result in self-inflicted bodily injury.
D. Behaviors are not attributable to the effects of a substance or neurological condition.

Correct Answer: C. Behaviors result in self-inflicted bodily injury.

Explanation: Although the repetitive behaviors *may* result in self-injury, that is not a criterion for the diagnosis. All of the other options represent criteria for the diagnosis of stereotypic movement disorder.

1.52—Stereotypic Movement Disorder / diagnostic criteria (p. 89)

1.53   Which of the following is *not* consistent with stereotypic movement disorder?

A. The presence of stereotypic movements may indicate an undetected neurodevelopmental problem, especially in children ages 1–3 years.
B. Among typically developing children, the repetitive movements may be stopped when attention is directed to them or when the child is distracted from performing them.
C. In some children, the stereotypic movements would result in self-injury if protective measures were not used.
D. Stereotypic movements typically begin within the first year of life.

Correct Answer: D. Stereotypic movements typically begin within the first year of life.

Explanation: The movements typically begin within the first 3 years of life. Simple stereotypic movements are common in infancy and may be involved in acquisition of motor mastery. In children who develop complex motor stereotypies, approximately 80% exhibit symptoms before age 24 months, 12% between 24 and 35 months, and 8% at 36 months or older.

1.53—Stereotypic Movement Disorder / Development and Course (pp. 90–91)

1.54   Which of the following is a DSM-5-TR diagnostic criterion for Tourette's disorder?

A. Tics occur throughout a period of more than 1 year without a tic-free period of more than 3 consecutive months.
B. Onset is before age 5 years.
C. Tics may wax and wane in frequency but have persisted for more than 1 year since first tic onset.
D. Motor tics must precede vocal tics.

Correct Answer: C. Tics may wax and wane in frequency but have persisted for more than 1 year since first tic onset.

Explanation: Only option C is a criterion for the DSM-5-TR diagnosis of Tourette's disorder. In DSM-IV, Criterion B specified that tics must have been present for "a period of more than 1 year, and during this period there was never a tic-free period of more than 3 consecutive months." In DSM-5-TR, this criterion was simplified to the requirement that tics must have persisted for more than 1 year since first tic onset.

1.54—Tic Disorders / diagnostic criteria (p. 93)

1.55   At an 8-year-old boy's third office visit, his mother describes a 6-month history of excessive eye blinking and intermittent chirping, noting that these characteristics have also been accompanied by grunting sounds since the recent start of a new school term. What is the most likely diagnosis?

A. Tourette's disorder.
B. Provisional tic disorder.
C. Persistent (chronic) vocal tic disorder.
D. Transient tic disorder, recurrent.

Correct Answer: B. Provisional tic disorder.

Explanation: The presence of single or multiple motor and/or vocal tics for *less* than 1 year meets Criteria A and B for provisional tic disorder. This is in contrast to Tourette's disorder, in which tics must be present for *more* than 1 year.

Thus, option A is incorrect. Persistent (chronic) vocal tic disorder (option C) is incorrect because in this vignette the boy has *both* motor and vocal tics, and they have been present for less than 1 year. Transient tic disorder, recurrent (option D), would have been correct if the question were asking for a DSM-IV diagnosis; however, transient tic disorder was revised and renamed provisional tic disorder in DSM-5.

1.55—Tic Disorders / diagnostic criteria (p. 93)

1.56   A 5-year-old girl is referred to your care with a DSM-IV diagnosis of chronic motor or vocal tic disorder. She has had motor tics only since a year ago, and there were 2 months when there were no tics. Which diagnosis is consistent under DSM-5-TR criteria?

A. Tourette's disorder.
B. Provisional tic disorder.
C. Persistent (chronic) motor tic disorder.
D. Other specified tic disorder.

Correct Answer: C. Persistent (chronic) motor tic disorder.

Explanation: Under DSM-5-TR criteria for persistent (chronic) motor or vocal tic disorder, tics may wax and wane but need to be present for more than 1 year since tic onset. There is no requirement for a tic-free period. Tourette's disorder incorporates having both motor and vocal tics. In provisional tic disorder, symptoms have been present for less than 6 months. The category other specified tic disorder applies to presentations in which symptoms characteristic of a tic disorder that cause clinically significant distress or impairment in social, occupational, or other important areas of functioning predominate but do not meet the full criteria for a tic disorder or any of the disorders in the neurodevelopmental disorders diagnostic class.

1.56—Tic Disorders / diagnostic criteria (pp. 93 and 98)

1.57   A highly functional 20-year-old college student with a history of anxiety symptoms and attention-deficit/hyperactivity disorder, for which she is prescribed lisdexamfetamine (Vyvanse), tells her psychiatrist that she has been researching the side effects of her medication for one of her class projects. In addition, she says that for the past week she has been feeling stressed by her schoolwork, and her friends have been asking her why she intermittently bobs her head up and down multiple times a day. What is the most likely diagnosis?

A. Provisional tic disorder.
B. Unspecified tic disorder.
C. Unspecified stimulant use disorder.
D. Unspecified stimulant-induced disorder.

Correct Answer: B. Unspecified tic disorder.

Explanation: Given the data provided by the vignette, unspecified tic disorder (option B) is the best answer. Included in this category are presentations in which there is uncertainty about whether the tic is primary versus attributable to medication. By definition, onset must be before age 18 years for provisional, persistent motor, and persistent vocal tic disorders and Tourette's disorder. Tic onset after age 18 years would be diagnosed as unspecified tic disorder. Option C is incorrect given that the student is highly functioning, lacks significant functional impairment (on the basis of the limited details provided in the vignette), and takes lisdexamfetamine, which may have less abuse potential because it is a prodrug.

1.57—Tic Disorders / Differential Diagnosis (p. 97)

1.58   Which of the following is *not* a DSM-5-TR diagnostic criterion for language disorder?

  A. Persistent difficulties in the acquisition and use of language across modalities due to deficits in comprehension or production.
  B. Language abilities that are substantially and quantifiably below those expected for age.
  C. Inability to attribute difficulties to hearing or other sensory impairment, motor dysfunction, or another medical or neurological condition.
  D. Failure to meet criteria for mixed receptive-expressive language disorder or a pervasive developmental disorder.

Correct Answer: D. Failure to meet criteria for mixed receptive-expressive language disorder or a pervasive developmental disorder.

Explanation: Options A through C constitute the DSM-5-TR diagnostic criteria for language disorder. This diagnosis replaced the DSM-IV diagnoses expressive language disorder and mixed receptive-expressive language disorder. In contrast to DSM-IV, in DSM-5-TR, meeting criteria for autism disorder does not preclude one from being diagnosed with language disorder. Language disorder may be associated with other neurodevelopmental disorders in terms of specific learning disorder (literacy and numeracy), intellectual developmental disorder, attention-deficit/hyperactivity disorder, autism spectrum disorder, and developmental coordination disorder.

1.58—Language Disorder / diagnostic criteria (p. 47)

1.59   Which of the following statements about speech sound disorder is *true*?

  A. Speech sound production must be present by age 2 years.
  B. "Failure to use developmentally expected speech sounds" is assessed by comparison of a child with their peers of the same age and dialect.

C. The difficulties in speech sound production need not result in functional impairment to meet diagnostic criteria.

D. Symptom onset is in the early developmental period.

Correct Answer: D. Symptom onset is in the early developmental period.

Explanation: The diagnosis of speech sound disorder in DSM-5-TR replaces the diagnosis of phonological disorder in DSM-IV. According to DSM-IV, Criterion A in the classification of phonological disorder is the "failure to use developmentally expected speech sounds that are appropriate for age and dialect." This has been revised in DSM-5-TR such that presence of "persistent difficulty with speech sound production that interferes with speech intelligibility or prevents verbal communication" suffices for Criterion A. Thus, option B is incorrect. Option C is a false statement because Criterion B of speech sound disorder *does* require that difficulties from speech sound production interfere with one's function in social, academic, and occupational performance. There is also no specific age at onset for symptoms in speech sound disorder, but Criterion D specifies that symptom onset must be in the early developmental period. Thus, option A is incorrect, and D is the correct answer.

1.59—Speech Sound Disorder / diagnostic criteria (p. 50)

1.60   A parent brings a 4-year-old child to you for an evaluation with concerns that he has struggled with speech articulation since early development. He has not sustained any head injuries, is otherwise healthy, and has a normal IQ. His preschool teacher reports that it is difficult to understand what the boy is saying and that other children tease him by calling him a "baby" because of his difficulty with communication. He does not have trouble relating to other people or understanding nonverbal social cues. What is the most likely diagnosis?

A. Selective mutism.

B. Global developmental delay.

C. Speech sound disorder.

D. Unspecified anxiety disorder.

Correct Answer: C. Speech sound disorder.

Explanation: In this vignette, the child exhibits "persistent difficulty with speech sound production that interferes with speech intelligibility" leading to functional limitations in effective communication that interfere with social participation. Additionally, his symptoms are not attributable to a congenital or acquired medical condition, and his symptom onset is in the early developmental period. These are the criteria for speech sound disorder. The child's difficulty in communication is in sound production rather than lack of communication during specific situations, which is seen in selective mutism. Option B is also incorrect because apart from difficulty with speech sound production, the child relates well to other people and understands nonverbal cues. Finally, although the child may have some anxiety symptoms from the teasing, this is difficult to assess without additional information about worries, fears, or avoidant behaviors, making option D incorrect.

1.60—Speech Sound Disorder / diagnostic criteria (p. 50)

1.61 A 6-year-old boy is failing school and continues to struggle significantly with grammar, sentence construction, and vocabulary. He also interjects "and" in between all words when speaking. He is generally quiet and does not cause trouble otherwise. He is playful with peers and enjoys playing soccer at recess. He switches between music class and lunch easily. Which of the following diagnoses would be on your differential?

    A. Language disorder.
    B. Expressive language disorder.
    C. Childhood-onset fluency disorder.
    D. Autism spectrum disorder.

Correct Answer: A. Language disorder.

Explanation: This question asks for DSM-5-TR *diagnoses*, so option B is incorrect because expressive and mixed receptive-expressive language disorders are from DSM-IV. They are now consolidated into *language disorder* in DSM-5-TR. Option A, language disorder, would be an important consideration in the differential diagnosis because the child has persistent difficulties with both the production and possibly comprehension of language. The child may need additional repetition to understand commands and may not interact with peers as readily because of communication difficulty and thus appears quiet. Option C is incorrect because word interjections (e.g., "and") are no longer considered a type of speech disturbance in DSM-5-TR. Autism spectrum disorder manifests with delayed language development. However, autism spectrum disorder is often accompanied by behaviors not present in language disorder, such as lack of social interest, odd play patterns, and rigid adherence to routines and repetitive behaviors. No such items are present, ruling out option D.

1.61—Language Disorder / Comorbidity (p. 49)

1.62 Which of the following types of disturbance in speech is *not* included in the DSM-5-TR criteria for childhood-onset fluency disorder (stuttering)?

    A. Sound prolongation.
    B. Reduced vocabulary.
    C. Circumlocutions.
    D. Sound and syllable repetitions.

Correct Answer: B. Reduced vocabulary.

Explanation: Criterion A for childhood-onset fluency disorder in DSM-5-TR requires the presence of one or more of seven types of disturbances, including sound prolongation, circumlocutions, and sound and syllable repetitions. The other speech disturbances are words produced with an excess of physical tension, broken words, audible or silent blocking, and monosyllabic whole-word repetitions. Reduced vocabulary is a DSM-5-TR criteria in language disorder.

1.62—Language Disorder and Childhood-Onset Fluency Disorder (Stuttering) / diagnostic criteria (pp. 47 and 51–52)

1.63 A 14-year-old in regular education tells you that he believes a classmate likes him. His mother is surprised to hear this because, since a young age, he has often struggled with making inferences or understanding nuances from what other people say. His teacher has also noticed that he sometimes misses nonverbal cues. He tends to get along better with adults, perhaps because they are not as likely to be put off by a stilted speech pattern. When he makes jokes, his peers do not always find the humor appropriate. Although he enjoys spending time with his best friend engaging in a wide range of activities, he can be talkative and struggles with taking turns in conversation. What is the most likely diagnosis?

A. Social (pragmatic) communication disorder.
B. Autism spectrum disorder.
C. Social anxiety disorder.
D. Language disorder.

Correct Answer: A. Social (pragmatic) communication disorder.

Explanation: Social (pragmatic) communication disorder is a new DSM-5-TR diagnosis, first introduced in DSM-5, characterized by "persistent difficulties in the social use of verbal and nonverbal communication as manifested by all of the following: 1) deficits in using communication for social purposes…in a manner that is appropriate for the social context, 2) impairment in the ability to change communication to match context or needs of the listener…, 3) difficulties following rules for conversation and storytelling…and knowing how to use verbal and nonverbal signals to regulate interaction, [and] 4) difficulties understanding what is not explicitly stated." These deficits manifest in the early development period and result in functional limitations. Autism spectrum disorder can be differentiated by the presence of restricted/repetitive patterns of behavior, interests, or activities or history of this and their absence in social (pragmatic) communication disorder. Social anxiety disorder would not affect one's ability to understand nuances in verbal and nonverbal communication. Language disorder is incorrect because the boy does not have difficulty with the production or comprehension of language, but rather has difficulty with the nuances and social appropriateness of language content.

1.63—Social (Pragmatic) Communication Disorder / Differential Diagnosis (pp. 55–56)

1.64   A 15-year-old with a prior diagnosis of Tourette's disorder is referred to your care. His mother tells you that during middle school, he was teased for having vocal and motor tics. Since he started ninth grade, his tics have become less frequent. Currently, only mild motor tics remain. What is the appropriate DSM-5-TR diagnosis?

A. Tourette's disorder.
B. Persistent (chronic) motor tic disorder.
C. Provisional tic disorder.
D. Unspecified tic disorder.

Correct Answer: A. Tourette's disorder.

Explanation: There are four tic disorder diagnostic categories, and they follow a hierarchical order: 1) Tourette's disorder, 2) persistent (chronic) motor or vocal tic disorder, 3) provisional tic disorder, and 4) unspecified tic disorder. According to Criterion E for tic disorders in DSM-5-TR, once someone is diagnosed with a tic disorder at one level of the hierarchy, a diagnosis that is lower in the hierarchy cannot be made. In this case, option A is the correct answer because the teenager has already been previously diagnosed with Tourette's disorder, which is at the top of the tic disorder hierarchy. Thus, at this point, he can no longer be diagnosed with persistent (chronic) motor tic disorder (option B) and does not qualify for provisional tic disorder. The unspecified tic disorder category is used in situations in which the clinician chooses *not* to specify the reason that the criteria are not met for a tic disorder.

1.64—Tic Disorders / diagnostic criteria (p. 93)

1.65   The onset of tics typically occurs for the first time during which developmental stage?

A. Prepuberty.
B. Latency.
C. Adolescence.
D. Adulthood.

Correct Answer: A. Prepuberty.

Explanation: Although it is not uncommon for adolescents and adults to present for an initial diagnostic assessment for tics, the initial onset of tics generally occurs during the prepubertal stage (ages 4–6 years). Tics then reach peak severity around ages 10–12 years, followed by a decline during adolescence. The incidence of new tic disorders decreases during the teen years and even more so during adulthood. Clinicians should be wary of new-onset abnormal movements suggestive of tics outside the usual age range.

1.65—Tic Disorders / Development and Course (p. 95)

1.66   A 7-year-old boy with a history of speech delay presents with long-standing repetitive hand waving, arm flapping, and finger wiggling. His mother reports that these symptoms first appeared when he was a toddler and wonders whether they could represent tics. She reports that he tends to flap more when he is engrossed in activities, such as while watching a favorite television program, but will stop when called or distracted. On the basis of the mother's report, which of the following conditions would be highest on your list of possible diagnoses?

A. Persistent (chronic) motor or vocal tic disorder.
B. Chorea.
C. Dystonia.
D. Motor stereotypies.

Correct Answer: D. Motor stereotypies.

Explanation: The child's movements are not tics, but stereotypies. *Motor stereotypies* are defined as involuntary rhythmic, repetitive, predictable movements that appear purposeful but serve no obvious adaptive function or purpose and stop with distraction. Motor stereotypies can be differentiated from tics on the basis of the former's earlier age at onset (younger than 3 years), prolonged duration (seconds to minutes), constant repetitive fixed form and location, exacerbation when the individual is engrossed in activities, lack of a premonitory urge, and cessation with distraction (e.g., name called or touched). Clinical history is crucial for differentiation.

Chorea represents rapid, random, continual, abrupt, irregular, unpredictable, nonstereotyped actions that are usually bilateral and affect all parts of the body (i.e., face, trunk, and limbs). The timing, direction, and distribution of movements vary from moment to moment, and movements usually worsen during attempted voluntary action. *Dystonia* is the simultaneous sustained contracture of both agonist and antagonist muscles, resulting in a distorted posture or movement of parts of the body. Dystonic postures are often triggered by attempts at voluntary movements and are not seen during sleep. The child's movements do not fit these categories.

1.66—Stereotypic Movement Disorder / Differential Diagnosis (pp. 91–92)

1.67   Assessment of co-occurring conditions is important for understanding the overall functional consequence of tics on an individual. Which of the following conditions has been associated with tic disorders?

A. Attention-deficit/hyperactivity disorder (ADHD).
B. Obsessive-compulsive and related disorders.
C. Depressive disorders.
D. All of the above.

Correct Answer: D. All of the above.

Explanation: Many medical and psychiatric conditions have been described as co-occurring with tic disorders, with ADHD and obsessive-compulsive and related disorders being particularly common. Children with ADHD may demonstrate disruptive behavior, social immaturity, and learning difficulties that may interfere with academic progress and interpersonal relationships and lead to greater impairment than that caused by a tic disorder. Individuals with tic disorders can also have other movement disorders and other mental disorders, such as depressive, bipolar, or substance use disorders.

1.67—Tic Disorders / Comorbidity (pp. 97–98)

1.68   By what age should most children have acquired adequate speech and language ability to understand and follow social rules of verbal and nonverbal communication, follow rules for conversation and storytelling, and change language according to the needs of the listener or situation?

A. Age 3–4 years.
B. Age 4–5 years.
C. Age 5–6 years.
D. Age 6–7 years.

Correct Answer: B. Age 4–5 years.

Explanation: Because social (pragmatic) communication depends on adequate developmental progress in speech and language, diagnosis of social (pragmatic) communication disorder is rare among children younger than 4 years. By age 4 or 5 years, most children should possess adequate speech and language abilities to permit identification of specific deficits in social communication. Milder forms of the disorder may not become apparent until early adolescence, when language and social interactions become more complex.

1.68—Social (Pragmatic) Communication Disorder / Development and Course (p. 55)

1.69   Having a family history of which of the following psychiatric disorders increases an individual's risk of social (pragmatic) communication disorder?

A. Social anxiety disorder (social phobia).
B. Autism spectrum disorder.
C. Attention-deficit/hyperactivity disorder (ADHD).
D. Intellectual developmental disorder (intellectual disability)

Correct Answer: B. Autism spectrum disorder.

Explanation: A family history of autism spectrum disorder, communication disorders, or specific learning disorder appears to increase the risk of social (pragmatic) communication disorder. Although deficits stemming from

ADHD, intellectual developmental disorder, and social anxiety disorder may overlap with symptoms of social communication disorder and may represent important considerations in the differential diagnosis, their presence in an individual's family history is not currently known to increase that person's risk of social (pragmatic) communication disorder.

1.69—Social (Pragmatic) Communication Disorder / Development and Course (p. 55)

1.70 A 6-year-old boy with a history of mild language delay is brought to your office by his mother, who is concerned that the boy is being teased in school because he misinterprets nonverbal cues and speaks in overly formal language with his peers. She tells you that her son was in an early intervention program, but his written and spoken language is now at grade level. The boy does not have a history of repetitive movements, sensory issues, or ritualized behaviors. Although he prefers constancy, he adapts fairly well to new situations. Additionally, he has a long-standing interest in trains and cars and is able to recite for you all the car models he memorized from a book on the history of transportation. Which of the following disorders would be a primary consideration in the differential diagnosis?

A. Social (pragmatic) communication disorder.
B. Autism spectrum disorder.
C. Global developmental delay.
D. Language disorder.

Correct Answer: A. Social (pragmatic) communication disorder.

Explanation: The presence of restricted interests and repetitive behaviors, interests, and activities beginning from early development is the primary diagnostic difference between autism spectrum disorder and social (pragmatic) communication disorder. In this vignette, the child does not meet Criterion B for autism spectrum disorder, which requires evidence of at least two restricted, repetitive patterns of behavior, interests, or activities. Furthermore, although the child has an interest in cars and trains, these are not necessarily atypical interests for children his age. According to DSM-5-TR, an individual who shows impairment in social communication and social interactions but does not show restricted and repetitive behavior or interests may meet criteria for social communication disorder instead of autism spectrum disorder. "The diagnosis of autism spectrum disorder supersedes that of social (pragmatic) communication disorder whenever the criteria for autism spectrum disorder are met, and care should be taken to inquire carefully regarding past or current restricted/repetitive behavior." Option D is incorrect because, from the limited data in the case, the mother suggests that the boy's language is no longer a problem. Similarly, although option C would also be a consideration in the differential diagnosis, it is not the best answer given the data.

1.70—Social (Pragmatic) Communication Disorder / Differential Diagnosis (pp. 55–56)

1.71 Below what age is it difficult to distinguish a language disorder from normal developmental variations?

A. <3 years.
B. <4 years.
C. <5 years.
D. <6 years.

Correct Answer: B. <4 years.

Explanation: During the early developmental period, there is significant variation in early language acquisition, and it may be difficult to distinguish normal variations from impairments. By the time a child is 4 years old, language ability becomes more stable.

1.71—Language Disorder / Differential Diagnosis (p. 49)

1.72 Which of the following psychiatric diagnoses is strongly associated with language disorder?

A. Attention-deficit/hyperactivity disorder (ADHD).
B. Diurnal enuresis.
C. Generalized anxiety disorder.
D. Disruptive mood dysregulation disorder.

Correct Answer: A. Attention-deficit/hyperactivity disorder (ADHD).

Explanation: Language disorder is strongly associated with other neurodevelopmental disorders in terms of specific learning disorder (literacy and numeracy), ADHD, autism spectrum disorder, and developmental coordination disorder. It is also associated with social (pragmatic) communication disorder. A positive family history of speech or language disorders is often present.

1.72—Language Disorder / Comorbidity (p. 49)

1.73 Which of the following statements about the development of speech as it applies to speech sound disorder is *false*?

A. Most children with speech sound disorder respond well to treatment.
B. Speech sound production should be mostly intelligible by age 3 years.
C. Most speech sounds should be pronounced clearly and accurately according to age and community norms before age 10 years.
D. It is abnormal for children to shorten words when they are learning to talk.

Correct Answer: D. It is abnormal for children to shorten words when they are learning to talk.

Explanation: Speech sound production requires both phonological knowledge and the ability to coordinate movements of the jaw, tongue, lips, and breath. A speech sound disorder is diagnosed when the speech sound production is not what is expected on the basis of the child's age and developmental stage. Developmentally, children often shorten words and syllables when they are learning to talk, but by age 3–4 years, most of their speech should be intelligible. By age 7, most speech sounds should be articulated clearly according to age and community norms. Lisping is common in speech sound disorder and may be associated with an abnormal tongue-thrust swallowing pattern.

1.73—Speech Sound Disorder / Development and Course (p. 50)

1.74 Which of the following would likely *not* be an important condition to rule out in the differential diagnosis of speech sound disorder?

A. Normal variations in speech.
B. Hearing or other sensory impairment.
C. Dysarthria.
D. Depression.

Correct Answer: D. Depression.

Explanation: All of the options except option D are important considerations when making a diagnosis of speech sound disorder. Regional and cultural variations are important to consider, as well as abnormalities of speech due to hearing impairments. Dysarthria includes speech impairments due to a motor disorder and must also be considered, especially because this may be difficult to differentiate in young children.

1.74—Speech Sound Disorder / Differential Diagnosis (p. 51)

1.75 Which of the following statements about the development of childhood-onset fluency disorder (stuttering) is *true*?

A. Stuttering occurs by age 6 for 80%–90% of affected individuals.
B. Stuttering always begins abruptly and is noticeable to everyone.
C. Stress and anxiety do not exacerbate disfluency.
D. Motor movements are not associated with this disorder.

Correct Answer: A. Stuttering occurs by age 6 for 80%–90% of affected individuals.

Explanation: The key feature of childhood-onset fluency disorder is a disturbance in the normal fluency and time patterning of speech that is inappropriate for the individual's age. Age at onset ranges from 2 to 7 years and occurs by age 6 for 80%–90% of affected individuals. Disfluencies can be gradual or sudden and even subtle (thus, option B is incorrect). Emotional stress or anxiety can exacerbate stuttering, and motor movements may sometimes accompany this disorder (thus, options C and D are incorrect).

1.75—Childhood-Onset Fluency Disorder (Stuttering) / Development and Course (pp. 52–53)

1.76   An 18-year-old who moved from Mexico to the United States when he was 8 years old is now entering college. He has been able to arrange financial aid and a work study schedule. He wants academic support in college, and the Office of Academic Support has referred him to you. In the process of completing an evaluation, you contact the student's high school teachers, who share that he struggled with essay writing in all social studies and literature classes. In his last 6 months of high school, he used study hall and tutoring sessions to work on grammar and organization and needed extra time to complete written assignments. With these supports, he was able to pass these courses with a 75% average. What is the most likely diagnosis?

A. Expressive language disorder.
B. Specific learning disorder with impairment in written expression.
C. Social (pragmatic) communication disorder.
D. Intellectual developmental disorder (intellectual disability), mild.

Correct Answer: B. Specific learning disorder with impairment in written expression.

Explanation: In specific learning disorder, there are difficulties learning and using academic skills, as indicated by the presence of at least one of six symptom categories that have persisted for at least 6 months, despite the provision of interventions that target those difficulties: The reports from the teachers indicate that the student has difficulties with written expression (e.g., multiple grammatical or punctuation errors within sentences; poor paragraph organization; written expression of ideas that lacks clarity). Language disorder is incorrect because the student does not have difficulty with the production or comprehension of language. Social communication disorder involves nuances and social appropriateness of language content, which this vignette does not recount. Intellectual developmental disorder (intellectual disability) is a disorder of both intellectual and adaptive functioning deficits in conceptual, social, and practical domains; this vignette does not describe deficits in adaptive functioning.

1.76—Specific Learning Disorder / diagnostic criteria (pp. 77–78)

CHAPTER 2

Schizophrenia Spectrum and Other Psychotic Disorders

2.1   Criterion A for schizoaffective disorder requires an uninterrupted period of illness during which Criterion A for schizophrenia is met. Which of the following additional symptoms must be present to fulfill diagnostic criteria for schizoaffective disorder?

   A. An anxiety episode—either panic or general anxiety.
   B. Rapid eye movement (REM) sleep behavior disorder.
   C. A major depressive or manic episode.
   D. Cyclothymia.

Correct Answer: C. A major depressive or manic episode.

Explanation: The diagnosis of schizoaffective disorder is based on the presence of an uninterrupted period of illness during which Criterion A for schizophrenia is met. Criterion B (social dysfunction) and Criterion F (exclusion of autism spectrum disorder or other communication disorder of childhood onset) for schizophrenia do not have to be met. In addition to meeting Criterion A for schizophrenia, there must be a major mood episode (major depressive or manic) (Criterion A for schizoaffective disorder). Because loss of interest or pleasure is common in schizophrenia, to meet Criterion A for schizoaffective disorder, the major depressive episode must include pervasive depressed mood (i.e., the presence of markedly diminished interest or pleasure is not sufficient). The episodes of depression or mania must be present for the majority of the total duration of the illness (i.e., after Criterion A has been met) (Criterion C for schizoaffective disorder).

2.1—Schizoaffective Disorder / Diagnostic Features (pp. 122–123)

2.2   In order to differentiate schizoaffective disorder from depressive or bipolar disorder with psychotic features, which of the following symptoms must be present for at least 2 weeks in the absence of a major mood episode at some point during the lifetime duration of the illness?

A. Delusions or hallucinations.
B. Delusions or paranoia.
C. Regressed behavior.
D. Projective identification.

Correct Answer: A. Delusions or hallucinations.

Explanation: To separate schizoaffective disorder from a depressive or bipolar disorder with psychotic features, Criterion B for schizoaffective disorder specifies that delusions or hallucinations must be present for at least 2 weeks in the absence of a major mood episode (depressive or manic) at some point during the lifetime duration of the illness.

2.2—Schizoaffective Disorder / Diagnostic Features (pp. 122–123)

2.3   A 27-year-old unmarried truck driver has a 5-year history of active and residual symptoms of schizophrenia. He develops symptoms of depression, including depressed mood and anhedonia. These symptoms last 4 months and resolve with treatment but do not meet criteria for major depression. Which diagnosis best fits this clinical presentation?

A. Schizoaffective disorder.
B. Unspecified schizophrenia spectrum and other psychotic disorder.
C. Unspecified depressive disorder.
D. Schizophrenia and unspecified depressive disorder.

Correct Answer: D. Schizophrenia and unspecified depressive disorder.

Explanation: The depressive episode does not occupy more than 1 year during the 5-year history. Thus, the presentation does not meet Criterion C for schizoaffective disorder, and the diagnosis remains schizophrenia. The additional diagnosis of unspecified depressive disorder may be added to indicate the superimposed depressive episode.

2.3—Schizoaffective Disorder / Differential Diagnosis (p. 125)

2.4   How common is schizoaffective disorder relative to schizophrenia?

A. Twice as common.
B. Equally common.
C. One-half as common.
D. One-third as common.

Correct Answer: D. One-third as common.

Explanation: Schizoaffective disorder appears to be about one-third as common as schizophrenia, with a lifetime prevalence of 0.3%.

2.4—Schizoaffective Disorder / Prevalence (p. 123)

2.5   A 30-year-old single woman reports having experienced auditory and persecutory delusions for 2 months, followed by a full major depressive episode with sad mood, anhedonia, and suicidal ideation lasting 3 months. Although the depressive episode resolves with pharmacotherapy and psychotherapy, the psychotic symptoms persist for another month before resolving. What diagnosis best fits this clinical picture?

   A. Brief psychotic disorder.
   B. Schizoaffective disorder.
   C. Major depressive disorder.
   D. Major depressive disorder with psychotic features.

Correct Answer: B. Schizoaffective disorder.

Explanation: During this period of illness, the woman's symptoms concurrently met criteria for a major depressive episode and Criterion A for schizophrenia. Auditory hallucinations and delusions were present both before and after the depressive phase. The total period of illness lasted for about 6 months, with psychotic symptoms alone present during the initial 2 months, both depressive and psychotic symptoms present during the next 3 months, and psychotic symptoms alone present during the last month. The duration of the depressive episode was not brief relative to the total duration of the psychotic disturbance (Criterion C for schizoaffective disorder).

2.5—Schizoaffective Disorder / Diagnostic Features (pp. 122–123); Differential Diagnosis (p. 125)

2.6   Which of the following statements about the incidence of schizoaffective disorder is *true*?

   A. The incidence is equal in women and men.
   B. The incidence is higher in men.
   C. The incidence is higher in women.
   D. The incidence rates vary based on seasonality of birth.

Correct Answer: C. The incidence is higher in women.

Explanation: When DSM- IV diagnostic criteria are used, the incidence of schizoaffective disorder is higher in women than in men. This rate is expected to be lower with DSM-5-TR because of the more stringent requirement of Criterion C, which specifies that a major mood episode must be present for the majority of the total duration of the active and residual portion of the illness.

2.7   Substance/medication-induced psychotic disorder cannot be diagnosed if the disturbance is better explained by an independent psychotic disorder that is not induced by a substance or medication. Which of the following psychotic symptom presentations would *not* be evidence of an independent psychotic disorder?

   A. Psychotic symptoms that meet full criteria for a psychotic disorder and that persist for a substantial period after cessation of severe intoxication or acute withdrawal.
   B. Psychotic symptoms that are substantially in excess of what would be expected given the type or amount of the substance used or the duration of use.
   C. Psychotic symptoms that occur during a period of sustained substance abstinence.
   D. Psychotic symptoms that occur during a medical admission for substance withdrawal.

Correct Answer: D. Psychotic symptoms that occur during a medical admission for substance withdrawal.

Explanation: A substance/medication-induced psychotic disorder is distinguished from a primary psychotic disorder by considering the onset, course, and other factors. For drugs of abuse, there must be evidence from the history, physical examination, or laboratory findings of substance use, intoxication, or withdrawal. Substance/medication-induced psychotic disorders arise during or soon after exposure to a medication or after substance intoxication or withdrawal but can persist for weeks, whereas primary psychotic disorders may precede the onset of substance/medication use or may occur during times of sustained abstinence. Once initiated, the psychotic symptoms may continue as long as the substance/medication use continues. Another consideration is the presence of features that are atypical of a primary psychotic disorder (e.g., atypical age at onset or course). For example, the appearance of delusions de novo in a person older than 35 years without a known history of a primary psychotic disorder should suggest the possibility of a substance/medication-induced psychotic disorder. Even a prior history of a primary psychotic disorder does not rule out the possibility of a substance/medication-induced psychotic disorder. In contrast, factors that suggest that the psychotic symptoms are better accounted for by a primary psychotic disorder include a history of prior recurrent primary psychotic disorders or persistence of psychotic symptoms for a substantial period of time (i.e., a month or more) after the end of substance intoxication or acute substance withdrawal or after cessation of medication use. Other causes of psychotic symptoms must be considered even in an individual with substance intoxication or withdrawal because substance use problems are not uncommon among individuals with non-substance/medication-induced psychotic disorders.

2.7—Substance/Medication-Induced Psychotic Disorder / Diagnostic Features (p. 128)

2.8   A 55-year-old man with a known history of alcohol dependence and schizophrenia is brought to the emergency department because of frank delusions and visual hallucinations. Which of the following would *not* be a diagnostic possibility for inclusion in the differential diagnosis?

   A. Substance/medication-induced psychotic disorder.
   B. Alcohol dependence.
   C. Psychotic disorder due to another medical condition.
   D. Borderline personality disorder with psychotic features.

Correct Answer: D. Borderline personality disorder with psychotic features.

Explanation: No evidence is provided for a diagnosis of borderline personality disorder. A prior history of a primary psychotic disorder (schizophrenia) does not rule out the possibility of a substance/medication-induced psychotic disorder. The appearance of delusions de novo in a person older than 35 years without a known history of primary psychotic disorder should suggest the possibility of a substance/medication-induced psychotic disorder.

2.8—Substance/Medication-Induced Psychotic Disorder / Differential Diagnosis (pp. 130–131)

2.9   Which of the following sets of specifiers is included in the DSM-5-TR diagnostic criteria for substance/medication-induced psychotic disorder?

   A. *With onset before intoxication* and *with onset before withdrawal*.
   B. *With onset during intoxication* and *with onset during withdrawal*.
   C. *With good prognostic features* and *without good prognostic features*.
   D. *With catatonia* and *without catatonia*.

Correct Answer: B. *With onset during intoxication* and *with onset during withdrawal*.

Explanation: The specifier *with onset during intoxication* should be used if criteria for intoxication with the substance are met and the symptoms develop during intoxication. The specifier *with onset during withdrawal* should be used if criteria for withdrawal from the substance are met and the symptoms develop during, or shortly after, withdrawal.

2.9—Substance/Medication-Induced Psychotic Disorder / diagnostic criteria (pp. 126–127)

2.10   A 65-year-old man with systemic lupus erythematosus, who is being treated with corticosteroids, witnesses a serious motor vehicle accident. He begins to have disorganized speech, which lasts for several days before resolving. What diagnosis best fits this clinical picture?

A. Psychotic disorder associated with systemic lupus erythematosus.
B. Steroid-induced psychosis.
C. Brief psychotic disorder, with marked stressor.
D. Schizoaffective disorder.

Correct Answer: C. Brief psychotic disorder, with marked stressor.

Explanation: The essential features of psychotic disorder due to another medical condition are prominent delusions or hallucinations that are judged to be attributable to the physiological effects of another medical condition and are not better explained by another mental disorder (e.g., the symptoms are not a psychologically mediated response to a severe medical condition). In this vignette, the symptoms are better understood as being a psychologically mediated response to the trauma of witnessing the accident.

2.10—Psychotic Disorder Due to Another Medical Condition / Diagnostic Features (pp. 131–132)

2.11   Which of the following psychotic symptom presentations would *not* be appropriately diagnosed as *other specified schizophrenia spectrum and other psychotic disorder*?

A. Psychotic symptoms that have lasted for less than 1 month but have not yet remitted, so the criteria for brief psychotic disorder are not met.
B. Persistent auditory hallucinations occurring in the absence of any other features.
C. Postpartum psychosis that does not meet criteria for a depressive or bipolar disorder with psychotic features, brief psychotic disorder, psychotic disorder due to another medical condition, or substance/medication-induced psychotic disorder.
D. Psychotic symptoms that are temporally related to use of a substance.

Correct Answer: D. Psychotic symptoms that are temporally related to use of a substance.

Explanation: Psychotic symptoms that are temporally related to use of a substance would likely meet criteria for a DSM-5-TR substance/medication-induced psychotic disorder. The category *other specified schizophrenia spectrum and other psychotic disorder* applies to presentations in which symptoms characteristic of a schizophrenia spectrum and other psychotic disorder that cause clinically significant distress or impairment in social, occupational, or other important areas of functioning predominate but do not meet the full criteria for any of the disorders in the schizophrenia spectrum and other psychotic disorders diagnostic class. The other specified schizophrenia spectrum and other psychotic disorder category is used in situations in which the clinician chooses to communicate the specific reason that the presentation does not meet the criteria for any specific schizophrenia spectrum and other psychotic disorder. This is done by recording "other specified schizophrenia spectrum and other psychotic disorder" followed by the specific reason (e.g., "persistent auditory hallucinations").

2.11—Other Specified Schizophrenia Spectrum and Other Psychotic Disorder (p. 138)

2.12   Which of the following patient presentations would *not* be classified as psychotic for the purpose of diagnosing schizophrenia?

A. A patient is hearing a voice that tells him he is a special person.
B. A patient believes he is being followed by a secret police organization that is focused exclusively on him.
C. A patient has a flashback to a war experience that feels like it is happening again.
D. A patient cannot organize his thoughts and stops responding in the middle of an interview.

Correct Answer: C. A patient has a flashback to a war experience that feels like it is happening again.

Explanation: Schizophrenia spectrum and other psychotic disorders are defined by abnormalities in one or more of the following five domains, the first four of which are considered to be psychotic symptoms: delusions, hallucinations, disorganized thinking (speech), grossly disorganized or abnormal motor behavior (including catatonia), and negative symptoms. A flashback to a traumatic experience is an intense, emotionally laden memory but does not reach the level of a psychotic symptom.

2.12—chapter introduction / Key Features That Define the Psychotic Disorders (pp. 101–103)

2.13   Which of the following would rule out a diagnosis of brief psychotic disorder?

A. Continuation of symptoms for 6 weeks, followed by complete resolution.
B. Visions of a religious figure occurring in several individuals during a religious ceremony.
C. Severe impairment from the symptoms that requires nutritional support.
D. A suicide attempt.

Correct Answer: A. Continuation of symptoms for 6 weeks, followed by complete resolution.

Explanation: The essential feature of brief psychotic disorder is a disturbance that involves at least one of the following positive psychotic symptoms: delusions, hallucinations, disorganized speech (e.g., frequent derailment or incoherence), or grossly abnormal psychomotor behavior, including catatonia (Criterion A). An episode of the disturbance lasts at least 1 day but less than 1 month, and the individual eventually has a full return to the premorbid level of functioning (Criterion B).

Individuals with brief psychotic disorder typically experience emotional turmoil or overwhelming confusion. They may have rapid shifts from one intense affect to another. Although the disturbance is brief, the level of impairment may be severe, and supervision may be required to ensure that nutritional and hygienic needs are met and that the individual is protected from the consequences of poor judgment, cognitive impairment, or acting on the basis of delusions. There appears to be an increased risk of suicidal behavior, particularly during the acute episode.

2.13—Brief Psychotic Disorder; Schizophrenia / Differential Diagnosis; Associated Features; Culture-Related Diagnostic Issues (pp. 109–111)

2.14   A 32-year-old man presents to the emergency department distressed and agitated. He reports that his sister has been killed in a car accident on a trip to South America. When asked how he found out, he says that he and his sister were very close and he "just knows it." After being put on the phone with his sister, who was comfortably staying with friends while on her trip, the man expressed relief that she was alive. Which of the following descriptions best fits this presentation?

   A. He did not have a delusional belief because it changed in light of new evidence.
   B. He had a grandiose delusion because he believed he could know things happening far away.
   C. He had a nihilistic delusion because it involved an untrue, imagined catastrophe.
   D. He did not have a delusion because in some cultures people believe they can know things about family members outside ordinary communications.

Correct Answer: A. He did not have a delusional belief because it changed in light of new evidence.

Explanation: To be a delusion, a belief must be clearly false and must be fixed—that is, not amenable to change in light of additional information. This man's belief was false but held flexibly, and it was conditional on the evidence, such as talking to his living sister. Thus, it is not a delusion. Although cultural factors should be taken into account in determining whether a belief is delusional, that consideration is not relevant here because the belief is not delusional independent of cultural background.

2.14—Key Features That Define the Psychotic Disorders / Delusions (pp. 101–102)

2.15　Which of the following is *not* a commonly recognized type of delusion?

    A. Persecutory.
    B. Alien abduction.
    C. Somatic.
    D. Grandiose.

Correct Answer: B. Alien abduction.

Explanation: Commonly recognized delusion types include persecutory, referential, somatic, nihilistic, grandiose, and erotomanic, as well as combinations of these types. A delusional belief in alien abduction may be grandiose and may involve somatic and/or erotomanic aspects, but it is not itself a major category of delusional thought.

2.15—Key Features That Define the Psychotic Disorders / Delusions (pp. 101–102)

2.16　A 64-year-old man who had been a widower for 3 months presents to the emergency department on the advice of his primary care physician after he reports to the doctor that he hears his deceased wife's voice calling his name when he looks through old photos and sometimes as he is trying to fall asleep. His primary care physician tells him he is having a psychotic episode and needs to get a psychiatric evaluation. Which of the following statements correctly explains why these experiences should not be considered to be psychotic?

    A. The experience occurs as he is falling asleep.
    B. He can invoke her voice with certain activities.
    C. The voice calls his name.
    D. Both A and B.

Correct Answer: D. Both A and B.

Explanation: If an auditory experience occurs only secondary to a controllable action (such as looking through highly affectively charged photos) or in an altered sensorial state, such as just before falling asleep (*hypnagogic*) or just as one is waking up (*hypnopompic*), it is not classified as a hallucination. Frank auditory hallucinations can involve the voice of someone known to the patient and often includes hearing one's name called.

2.16—Key Features That Define the Psychotic Disorders / Hallucinations (p. 102)

2.17　Which of the following does *not* represent a negative symptom of schizophrenia?

A. Affective flattening.
B. Decreased motivation.
C. Impoverished thought processes.
D. Sadness over loss of functionality.

Correct Answer: D. Sadness over loss of functionality.

Explanation: Patients with schizophrenia may be aware of their functional losses and may feel sadness about this. That emotional response would be the opposite of negative symptoms because it would involve an active and expressive-emotional response. The other symptoms mentioned—affective flattening, decreased motivation, and impoverished thought processes—are all part of the negative or deficit symptoms of schizophrenia. It is thus important to distinguish the uses of the word *negative*. In reference to sad emotions, it has one meaning, but the negative symptoms of schizophrenia mean deficits of normal psychological functioning, including absence of sad feelings.

2.17—Key Features That Define the Psychotic Disorders / Negative Symptoms (pp. 102–103)

2.18   Schizophrenia spectrum and other psychotic disorders are defined by abnormalities in one or more of five domains, four of which are also considered psychotic symptoms. Which of the following is *not* considered a psychotic symptom?

A. Delusions.
B. Hallucinations.
C. Disorganized thinking.
D. Avolition.

Correct Answer: D. Avolition.

Explanation: Avolition is a negative symptom of schizophrenia, not a positive (psychotic) symptom. Avolition is an absence of motivation for goal-oriented behaviors. The term *positive* refers not to something of positive valuation but rather to something that is present and existing, as opposed to a deficit symptom such as the negative symptoms of schizophrenia. The other symptom types listed are considered psychotic.

2.18—Key Features That Define the Psychotic Disorders / Negative Symptoms (pp. 102–103)

2.19   What is the most common type of delusion?

A. Somatic delusion of distorted body appearance.
B. Grandiose delusion.
C. Thought insertion.
D. Persecutory delusion.

Correct Answer: D. Persecutory delusion.

Explanation: Persecutory delusions are the most common form. This may be because such delusions are associated with a dysregulation of existing self-protective and/or social-psychological functionalities, but the reason that these are the most commonly encountered delusion is not yet well understood.

2.19—Key Features That Define the Psychotic Disorders / Delusions (pp. 101–102)

2.20   Which of the following presentations would *not* be classified as disorganized behavior for the purpose of diagnosing schizophrenia spectrum and other psychotic disorders?

   A. Masturbating in public.
   B. Wearing slacks on one's head.
   C. Speaking in tongues during a religious retreat.
   D. Turning to face 180 degrees away from the interviewer when answering questions.

Correct Answer: C. Speaking in tongues during a religious retreat.

Explanation: Disorganized thinking (formal thought disorder) is typically inferred from the individual's speech. The individual may switch from one topic to another (derailment or loose associations). Answers to questions may be obliquely related or completely unrelated (tangentiality). Rarely, speech may be so severely disorganized that it is nearly incomprehensible and resembles receptive aphasia in its linguistic disorganization (incoherence or *word salad*). Because mildly disorganized speech is common and nonspecific, the symptom must be severe enough to substantially impair effective communication. The severity of the impairment may be difficult to evaluate if the person making the diagnosis comes from a different linguistic background than that of the person being examined. For example, some religious groups engage in glossolalia (speaking in tongues); others describe experiences of possession trance (trance states in which personal identity is replaced by an external possessing identity). These phenomena are characterized by disorganized speech. These instances do not represent signs of psychosis unless they are accompanied by other clearly psychotic symptoms. Less severely disorganized thinking or speech may occur during the prodromal and residual periods of schizophrenia.

2.20—Key Features That Define the Psychotic Disorders / Grossly Disorganized or Abnormal Motor Behavior (Including Catatonia) (p. 102)

2.21   Which of the following statements about catatonic motor behaviors is *false*?

   A. Catatonic motor behavior is a type of grossly disorganized behavior that has historically been associated with schizophrenia spectrum and other psychotic disorders.

B. Catatonic motor behaviors may occur in many mental disorders (such as mood disorders) and in other medical conditions.

C. A behavior is considered catatonic only if it involves motoric slowing or rigidity, such as mutism, posturing, or waxy flexibility.

D. Catatonia can be diagnosed independently of another psychiatric disorder.

Correct Answer: C. A behavior is considered catatonic only if it involves motoric slowing or rigidity, such as mutism, posturing, or waxy flexibility.

Explanation: *Catatonic behavior* is a marked decrease in reactivity to the environment. This ranges from resistance to instructions (negativism); to maintaining a rigid, inappropriate or bizarre posture; to a complete lack of verbal and motor responses (mutism and stupor). It can also include purposeless and excessive motor activity without obvious cause (catatonic excitement). Other features are repeated stereotyped movements, staring, grimacing, mutism, and the echoing of speech. Although catatonia has historically been associated with schizophrenia, catatonic symptoms are nonspecific and may occur in other mental disorders (e.g., bipolar or depressive disorders with catatonia) and in medical conditions (catatonic disorder due to another medical condition).

2.21—Key Features That Define the Psychotic Disorders / Grossly Disorganized or Abnormal Motor Behavior (Including Catatonia) (p. 102); Catatonia (pp. 134–137)

2.22   Which of the following statements about negative symptoms of schizophrenia is *false*?

A. Negative symptoms are easily distinguished from medication side effects such as sedation.

B. Negative symptoms include diminished emotional expression.

C. Negative symptoms can be difficult to distinguish from medication side effects such as sedation.

D. Negative symptoms include reduced peer or social interaction.

Correct Answer: A. Negative symptoms are easily distinguished from medication side effects such as sedation.

Explanation: Negative symptoms of schizophrenia refer to the deficit aspects of the illness, in contrast to the "positive" symptoms (in the sense of being notable by their presence, not in the sense of being desirable). Positive symptoms include hallucinations, delusions, disorganized behaviors, and disorganized thinking. Side effects of medication such as sedation and bradykinesia may mimic negative symptoms and be wrongly evaluated as primary negative symptomatology. The primary negative symptoms include diminished emotional expression, reduced interaction with others, and decreased motivation for goal-directed activities.

2.22—Key Features That Define the Psychotic Disorders / Negative Symptoms (pp. 102–103)

2.23   Which of the following statements correctly describes a way in which schizoaffective disorder may be differentiated from bipolar disorder?

   A. In bipolar disorder, psychotic symptoms do not last longer than 1 month.
   B. In bipolar disorder, psychotic symptoms always co-occur with mood symptoms.
   C. Schizoaffective disorder never includes full-blown episodes of major depression.
   D. In bipolar disorder, psychotic symptoms are always mood congruent.

Correct Answer: B. In bipolar disorder, psychotic symptoms always co-occur with mood symptoms.

Explanation: Distinguishing schizoaffective disorder from depressive and bipolar disorders with psychotic features is often difficult. Schizoaffective disorder can be distinguished from a depressive or bipolar disorder with psychotic features by the presence of prominent delusions and/or hallucinations for at least 2 weeks in the absence of a major mood episode. In contrast, in depressive or bipolar disorders with psychotic features, the psychotic features occur primarily during the mood episode(s).

2.23—Schizoaffective Disorder / Differential Diagnosis (p. 125)

2.24   Which of the following symptom combinations, if present for 1 month, would meet Criterion A for schizophrenia?

   A. Prominent auditory and visual hallucinations.
   B. Grossly disorganized behavior and avolition.
   C. Disorganized speech and diminished emotional expression.
   D. Paranoid and grandiose delusions.

Correct Answer: C. Disorganized speech and diminished emotional expression.

Explanation: To meet DSM-5-TR Criterion A, two (or more) of the following symptoms must be present for a significant portion of time during a 1-month period (or less if successfully treated): 1) delusions, 2) hallucinations, 3) disorganized speech (e.g., frequent derailment or incoherence), 4) grossly disorganized or catatonic behavior, and 5) negative symptoms (i.e., diminished emotional expression or avolition). At least one of the two symptoms must be the clear presence of delusions (A1), hallucinations (A2), or disorganized speech (A3). Thus, two forms of hallucinations or two types of delusions alone in the absence of other symptoms would be insufficient to meet Criterion A. The combination of grossly disorganized behavior (although considered a psychotic symptom) with negative symptoms is also insufficient to meet Criterion A.

2.24—Schizophrenia / diagnostic criteria (pp. 113–114)

2.25   Which of the following statements about violent or suicidal behavior in schizophrenia is *false*?

A. About 5%–6% of individuals with schizophrenia die by suicide.
B. Persons with schizophrenia frequently assault strangers in a random fashion.
C. Compared with the general population, persons with schizophrenia are more frequently victims of violence.
D. Youth, male sex, and substance abuse are factors that increase the risk for suicide among persons with schizophrenia.

Correct Answer: B. Persons with schizophrenia frequently assault strangers in a random fashion.

Explanation: Hostility and aggression can be associated with schizophrenia, although spontaneous or random assault is uncommon. Aggression is more frequent for younger males and for individuals with a past history of violence, nonadherence to treatment, substance abuse, and impulsivity. It should be noted that the vast majority of persons with schizophrenia are not aggressive and are more frequently victimized than are individuals in the general population.

Approximately 5%–6% of individuals with schizophrenia die by suicide, about 20% attempt suicide on one or more occasions, and many more have significant suicidal ideation. Suicidal behavior is sometimes in response to command hallucinations to harm oneself or others. Suicide risk remains high over the whole life span for males and females, although it may be especially high for younger males with comorbid substance use. Other risk factors include having depressive symptoms or feelings of hopelessness and being unemployed, and the risk is also higher in the period after a psychotic episode or hospital discharge.

2.25—Schizophrenia / Associated Features (p. 116); Association With Suicidal Thoughts or Behavior (p. 119)

2.26   Which of the following statements about childhood-onset schizophrenia is *true*?

A. Childhood-onset schizophrenia tends to resemble poor-outcome adult schizophrenia, with gradual onset and prominent negative symptoms.
B. Disorganized speech patterns in childhood are usually indicative of schizophrenia.
C. Because of the childhood capacity for imagination, delusions and hallucinations in childhood-onset schizophrenia are more elaborate than those in adult-onset schizophrenia.

D. In a child presenting with disorganized behavior, schizophrenia should be ruled out before other childhood diagnoses are considered.

Correct Answer: A. Childhood-onset schizophrenia tends to resemble poor-outcome adult schizophrenia, with gradual onset and prominent negative symptoms.

Explanation: The essential features of schizophrenia are the same in childhood, but it is more difficult to make the diagnosis. Delusions and hallucinations may be less elaborate in children than in adults; visual hallucinations are more common and should be distinguished from normal fantasy play. Disorganized speech occurs in many disorders with childhood onset (e.g., autism spectrum disorder), as does disorganized behavior (e.g., attention-deficit/hyperactivity disorder). These symptoms should not be attributed to schizophrenia without due consideration of the more common disorders of childhood. Childhood-onset cases tend to resemble poor-outcome adult cases, with gradual onset and prominent negative symptoms. Children who later receive the diagnosis of schizophrenia are more likely to have experienced nonspecific emotional-behavioral disturbances and psychopathology, intellectual and language alterations, and subtle motor delays.

2.26—Schizophrenia / Development and Course (pp. 117–118)

2.27 Which of the following statements about sex differences in schizophrenia is *true*?

A. Women with schizophrenia tend to have fewer psychotic symptoms than do men over the course of the illness.
B. A first onset of schizophrenia after age 40 is more likely in women than in men.
C. Psychotic symptoms in women tend to burn out with age to a greater extent than they do in men.
D. Negative symptoms and affective flattening are more frequently observed in women with schizophrenia than in men with the disorder.

Correct Answer: B. A first onset of schizophrenia after age 40 is more likely in women than in men.

Explanation: The lifetime prevalence of schizophrenia appears to be approximately 0.3%–0.7%, although there is reported variation by race/ethnicity, across countries, and by geographic origin for immigrants and children of immigrants. The sex ratio differs across samples and populations: for example, an emphasis on negative symptoms and longer duration of disorder (associated with poorer outcome) shows higher incidence rates for males, whereas definitions allowing for the inclusion of more mood symptoms and brief presentations (associated with better outcome) show equivalent risks for both sexes.

A number of features distinguish the clinical expression of schizophrenia in females and males. The general incidence of schizophrenia tends to be slightly lower in females, particularly among treated cases. The age at onset is later in females, with a second midlife peak. Symptoms tend to be more affect-laden among females, and there are more psychotic symptoms, as well as a greater propensity for psychotic symptoms to worsen in later life. Other symptom differences include less frequent negative symptoms and disorganization. Finally, social functioning tends to remain better preserved in females. There are, however, frequent exceptions to these general caveats.

2.27—Schizophrenia / Prevalence (pp. 116–117); Sex and Gender-Related Diagnostic Issues (p. 119)

2.28   A 19-year-old college student is brought to the emergency department by her family over her objection. Three months ago, she suddenly started feeling "odd," and she came home from college because she could not concentrate. Two weeks after she came home, she began hearing voices telling her that she is "a sinner" and must repent. Although never a religious person, she now believes she must repent, but she does not know how, and she feels confused. She is managing her activities of daily living despite the ongoing auditory hallucinations and delusions, and she is affectively reactive on examination. Which diagnosis best fits this presentation?

A. Schizophreniform disorder, with good prognostic features, provisional.
B. Schizophreniform disorder, without good prognostic features, provisional.
C. Schizophreniform disorder, with good prognostic features.
D. Schizophreniform disorder, without good prognostic features.

Correct Answer: A. Schizophreniform disorder, with good prognostic features, provisional.

Explanation: Schizophreniform disorder is diagnosed under two conditions: 1) when an episode of illness lasts between 1 and 6 months and the individual has already recovered, and 2) when an individual is symptomatic for less than the 6 months' duration required for the diagnosis of schizophrenia but has not yet recovered (as in this vignette). One then adds the qualifier *provisional* because it is uncertain whether the individual will recover from the disturbance within the 6-month period. If the disturbance persists beyond 6 months, the diagnosis should be changed to schizophrenia. In either case, schizophreniform disorder takes the specifier *with good prognostic features* if at least two of the following features are present: 1) onset of prominent psychotic symptoms within 4 weeks of the first noticeable change in usual behavior or functioning; 2) confusion or perplexity; 3) good premorbid social and occupational functioning; and 4) absence of blunted or flat affect. This vignette demonstrates all four of these features. Because we have enough information to make the diagnosis of schizophreniform disorder, unspecified schizophrenia spectrum and other psychotic disorder would be incorrectly applied.

2.28—Schizophreniform Disorder / diagnostic criteria (pp. 111–112); Diagnostic Features (p. 112)

2.29 A 24-year-old college student is brought to the emergency department by the college health service team. A few weeks ago, he was involved in a car accident in which one of his friends was critically injured and died in his arms. The man has not come out of his room or showered for the last 2 weeks. He has eaten only minimally, claimed that aliens have targeted him for abduction, and asserted that he could hear their radio transmissions. Nothing seems to convince him that this abduction will not happen or that the transmissions are not real. Which of the following diagnoses (and justifications) is most appropriate?

A. Brief psychotic disorder with a marked stressor because the symptoms began after the tragic car accident.
B. Brief psychotic disorder without a marked stressor because the content of the psychosis is unrelated to the accident.
C. Unspecified schizophrenia spectrum and other psychotic disorder because more information is needed.
D. Schizophreniform disorder because there are psychotic symptoms but not yet a full-blown schizophrenia picture.

Correct Answer: C. Unspecified schizophrenia spectrum and other psychotic disorder because more information is needed.

Explanation: The diagnosis of *brief psychotic disorder* requires that there be psychotic symptoms lasting more than 1 day but less than 1 month and that the patient has shown a full recovery. In this vignette, we do not know how long the symptoms will last or whether the patient will fully recover. If the patient's symptoms remit in less than 1 month and he shows full recovery, one could diagnose *brief psychotic disorder with a marked stressor.* There is no requirement that the content of the psychotic symptoms match the events that constitute the stressor, as long as the temporal sequence holds. The diagnosis of *delusional disorder* requires 1 month of symptoms and does not usually involve bizarre delusions, nor does it involve the functional deficits seen here. *Schizophreniform disorder* requires 1 month of symptoms. If these symptoms continue for a month and functional deficits persist, the diagnosis could be schizophreniform disorder, and the disorder could possibly progress to schizophrenia after 6 months. We do not yet know the future trajectory of these psychotic symptoms and therefore can justify only the diagnosis of unspecified schizophrenia spectrum and other psychotic disorder. The *unspecified schizophrenia spectrum and other psychotic disorder* category is used in situations in which the clinician chooses not to specify the reason that the criteria are not met for a specific schizophrenia spectrum and other psychotic disorder, and it includes presentations in which there is insufficient information to make a more specific diagnosis (e.g., in emergency department settings).

2.29—Unspecified Schizophrenia Spectrum and Other Psychotic Disorder (p. 138)

CHAPTER 3

Bipolar and Related Disorders

3.1 A 32-year-old patient reports 1 week of feeling unusually irritable. During this time, he has increased energy and activity, sleeps less, and finds it difficult to sit still. He also is more talkative than usual and is easily distractible, to the point of finding it difficult to complete his work assignments. A physical examination and laboratory workup are negative for any medical cause of his symptoms, and he takes no medications. What diagnosis best fits this clinical picture?

A. Manic episode.
B. Hypomanic episode.
C. Bipolar I disorder, with mixed features.
D. Cyclothymic disorder.

Correct Answer: A. Manic episode.

Explanation: In DSM-5-TR, the definition of a manic episode requires a distinct, abnormal mood that can be persistently elevated, expansive, or irritable, along with increased activity for at least 1 week. The person must also experience at least three (four if the mood is only irritable) of the following symptoms: 1) inflated self-esteem or grandiosity, 2) decreased need for sleep, 3) more talkative than usual or pressure to keep talking, 4) flight of ideas or subjective experience that thoughts are racing, 5) distractibility, 6) increase in goal-directed activity or psychomotor agitation, and 7) excessive involvement in activities that have a high potential for painful consequences.

3.1—Bipolar I Disorder / diagnostic criteria (pp. 139–140)

3.2 A 28-year-old patient reports 1 week of increased activity associated with an elevated mood, a decreased need for sleep, and inflated self-esteem. She does not object to her current state ("I'm getting more work done than ever before!"). A physical examination and laboratory work are unrevealing for any medical cause of her symptoms. She had taken fluoxetine for a major depressive episode but self-discontinued it 2 months ago because she felt that her mood was stable. Which diagnosis best fits this clinical picture?

A. Bipolar I disorder.
B. Bipolar II disorder.
C. Cyclothymic disorder.
D. Substance/medication-induced bipolar disorder.

Correct Answer: B. Bipolar II disorder.

Explanation: This patient most likely meets criteria for bipolar II disorder, current episode hypomanic, which is defined as a current or past hypomanic episode in an individual with a previous history of at least one major depressive episode. The lack of a current or past manic episode rules out bipolar I disorder, and the time course and absence of numerous episodes of hypomania rule out cyclothymic disorder. Although antidepressants can precipitate manic episodes, the long period since medication discontinuation (more than 5 half-lives) makes this episode unlikely to be medication induced.

3.2—Bipolar II Disorder / Differential Diagnosis (pp. 157–158)

3.3   Approximately what percentage of individuals who experience a single manic episode will go on to have recurrent mood episodes?

A. 90%.
B. 50%.
C. 25%.
D. 10%.

Correct Answer: A. 90%.

Explanation: Bipolar disorders are highly recurrent, and more than 90% of individuals who have a single manic episode go on to have recurrent mood episodes.

3.3—Bipolar I Disorder / Development and Course (p. 146)

3.4   Which of the following factors is most associated with manic relapse in bipolar I disorder?

A. Childhood adversity.
B. Recent life stress.
C. Initial episode of manic polarity.
D. Suicide attempt.

Correct Answer: C. Initial episode of manic polarity.

Explanation: Polarity of the first episode tends to be associated with predominant polarity of future episodes and clinical features (e.g., depressive onset is associated with greater density of depressive episodes and suicidal behavior). Childhood adversity is associated with poorer prognosis and a worse clinical picture that may include medical or psychiatric comorbidities, suicide, and associated psychotic features. More proximally, recent life stress and other negative life events increase depressive relapse risk in individuals diagnosed with bipolar disorder, whereas manic relapse appears to be specifically linked to goal-attainment life events (e.g., getting married, completing a degree).

3.4—Bipolar I Disorder / Development and Course; Risk and Prognostic Factors (pp. 146–147)

3.5   Which of the following is more common in men than women with bipolar I disorder?

   A. Rapid cycling.
   B. Lethal suicide.
   C. Earlier onset.
   D. Mixed symptoms.

Correct Answer: B. Lethal suicide.

Explanation: Whereas suicide attempts are higher in women, lethal suicide is more common in men with bipolar disorder. Although bipolar I disorder affects men and women equally, mixed and rapid-cycling symptoms are more common in women. Women with bipolar I disorder have a younger average age of onset. Compared with men, women with bipolar disorder are more likely to experience comorbid eating disorders. In the United States, mean age at onset of DSM-5-TR bipolar I disorder is 22 years and slightly younger for women (21.5 years) than for men (23.0 years).

3.5—Bipolar I Disorder / Development and Course; Association With Suicidal Thoughts or Behavior; Sex- and Gender-Related Diagnostic Issues (pp. 146–148)

3.6   A patient with a history of bipolar I disorder presents with a new-onset manic episode and is successfully treated with medication adjustment. He notes chronic depressive symptoms that, on reflection, long preceded the manic episodes. He describes these symptoms as "feeling down"; having decreased energy; and, more often than not, having no motivation. He does not endorse other depressive symptoms; however, the current symptoms have been sufficient to negatively affect his marriage. Which diagnosis best fits this presentation?

   A. Other specified bipolar and related disorder.
   B. Bipolar I disorder, current or most recent episode depressed.
   C. Cyclothymic disorder.
   D. Bipolar I disorder and persistent depressive disorder (dysthymia).

Correct Answer: D. Bipolar I disorder and persistent depressive disorder (dysthymia).

Explanation: This patient's presentation does not meet the full criteria for a major depressive episode and thus would not qualify for a diagnosis of bipolar I disorder, current or most recent episode depressed. If the patient meets criteria for persistent depressive disorder (dysthymia) *and* bipolar I disorder, both should be diagnosed. The presence of a manic episode makes bipolar II disorder, cyclothymic disorder, and other specified bipolar and related disorder inappropriate.

3.6—Bipolar I Disorder / Differential Diagnosis (pp. 148–149)

3.7   In which of the following ways do manic episodes differ from attention-deficit/hyperactivity disorder (ADHD)?

A. Manic episodes are more strongly associated with impulsivity.
B. Manic episodes have clearer symptomatic onsets and offsets.
C. Manic episodes are more likely to show a chronic course.
D. Manic episodes first appear at an earlier age.

Correct Answer: B. Manic episodes have clearer symptomatic onsets and offsets.

Explanation: ADHD is characterized by persistent symptoms of inattention, hyperactivity, and impulsivity, which may resemble the symptoms of a manic episode (e.g., distractibility, increased activity, impulsive behavior), and have onset by age 12. In contrast, the symptoms of mania in bipolar I disorder occur in distinct episodes and typically begin in late adolescence or early adulthood.

3.7—Bipolar I Disorder / Differential Diagnosis (p. 149)

3.8   A patient with a history of bipolar disorder reports experiencing 1 week of elevated and expansive mood. Evidence of which of the following would suggest that the patient is experiencing a hypomanic, rather than manic, episode?

A. Prominent irritability.
B. Increased productivity at work.
C. Psychotic symptoms.
D. Good insight into the illness.

Correct Answer: B. Increased productivity at work.

Explanation: The primary factor that differentiates manic and hypomanic episodes is that manic episodes cause marked impairment in social or occupational functioning or necessitate hospitalization to prevent harm to self or others, or there are psychotic features (Criterion C of bipolar I disorder). In hypomania, "The episode is not severe enough to cause marked impairment in social or occupational functioning or to necessitate hospitalization" (Criterion

E of bipolar II disorder). Both types of episodes can cause irritability or decreased need for sleep. A loss of insight may lead to significant consequences during a manic episode, but it is not included in the diagnostic criteria.

3.8—Bipolar I / diagnostic criteria (pp. 139–141)

3.9   A 25-year-old graduate student presents to a psychiatrist complaining of feeling down and "not enjoying anything." Her symptoms began about a month ago, along with insomnia and poor appetite. She has little interest in activities and is having difficulty attending to her schoolwork. She recalls a similar episode 1 year ago that lasted about 2 months before improving without treatment. She also reports several episodes of increased energy over the past 2 years. The episodes usually last 1–2 weeks, during which time she is very productive, feels more social and outgoing, tends to sleep less, and still feels energetic during the day. Friends tell her that she speaks more rapidly during these episodes but that they do not see it as off-putting. They tell her that she seems more outgoing and clever. She has no medical problems, does not take any medications, and denies using drugs or alcohol. What is the most likely diagnosis?

A. Bipolar I disorder, current episode depressed.
B. Cyclothymic disorder.
C. Bipolar II disorder, current episode depressed.
D. Major depressive disorder.

Correct Answer: C. Bipolar II disorder, current episode depressed.

Explanation: With her current major depressive episode combined with a past history of elevated mood and activity, this patient likely has a bipolar disorder. Because her periods of mood elevation do not cause distress or impairment, they are probably hypomanic episodes, hence a diagnosis of bipolar II disorder. The lack of any current hypomanic symptoms rules out a mixed episode of the illness. The presence of major depressive episodes rules out cyclothymic disorder, and her hypomanic episodes rule out major depressive disorder. This vignette is illustrative of the clinical observation that patients with bipolar II disorder generally present for treatment only when they experience depressive symptoms.

3.9—Bipolar II Disorder / Diagnostic Features (pp. 153–155)

3.10   How do the depressive episodes associated with bipolar II disorder differ from those associated with bipolar I disorder?

A. They are lengthier than those associated with bipolar I disorder.
B. They are less disabling than those associated with bipolar I disorder.
C. They are less severe than those associated with bipolar I disorder.
D. They are rarely a reason for the patient to seek treatment.

Correct Answer: A. They are lengthier than those associated with bipolar I disorder.

Explanation: The recurrent major depressive episodes associated with bipolar II disorder are typically more frequent and lengthier than those associated with bipolar I disorder. The depressive episodes can be very severe and disabling; because of this, DSM-5-TR stresses that bipolar II disorder should not be considered a "milder" form of bipolar I disorder. Bipolar II patients are more likely to seek treatment when depressed than during hypomanic episodes.

3.10—Bipolar II Disorder / Diagnostic Features (pp. 153–155)

3.11 How does the course of bipolar II disorder differ from the course of bipolar I disorder?

   A. It is less episodic than the course of bipolar I disorder.
   B. It is more chronic than the course of bipolar I disorder.
   C. It involves longer asymptomatic periods than the course of bipolar I disorder.
   D. It involves a much lower number of lifetime mood episodes than the course of bipolar I disorder.

Correct Answer: B. It is more chronic than the course of bipolar I disorder.

Explanation: Despite the substantial differences in duration and severity between manic and hypomanic episodes, bipolar II disorder is not a "milder form" of bipolar I disorder. Compared with individuals with bipolar I disorder, individuals with bipolar II disorder have greater chronicity of illness and spend, on average, more time in the depressive phase of their illness, which can be severe and/or disabling.

The number of lifetime episodes (both hypomanic and major depressive episodes) tends to be higher for bipolar II disorder than for major depressive disorder or bipolar I disorder. The interval between mood episodes in the course of bipolar II disorder tends to decrease as the individual ages. Although the hypomanic episode is the feature that defines bipolar II disorder, depressive episodes are more enduring and disabling over time.

3.11—Bipolar II Disorder / Diagnostic Features (p. 154); Development and Course (p. 155)

3.12 Which of the following features confers a worse prognosis for a patient with bipolar II disorder?

   A. Younger age.
   B. Higher educational level.
   C. Rapid-cycling pattern.
   D. Married marital status.

Correct Answer: C. Rapid-cycling pattern.

Explanation: A rapid-cycling pattern is associated with a poorer prognosis. Return to previous level of social function for individuals with bipolar II disorder is more likely for individuals of younger age and with less severe depression, suggesting adverse effects of prolonged illness on recovery. More education, fewer years of illness, and being married are independently associated with functional recovery in individuals with bipolar disorder, even after diagnostic type (I vs. II), current depressive symptoms, and presence of psychiatric comorbidity are taken into account.

3.12—Bipolar II Disorder / Risk and Prognostic Factors (p. 156)

3.13   Women with bipolar II disorder are more likely than men to experience which of the following?

   A. More severe illness course.
   B. Hypomania with mixed depressive features.
   C. More manic episodes.
   D. Onset with depressive symptoms.

Correct Answer: B. Hypomania with mixed depressive features.

Explanation: Patterns of illness and comorbidity seem to differ by sex, with females being more likely than males to report hypomania with mixed depressive features and a rapid-cycling course. No major sex differences have been found in several clinical variables, including rates of depressive episodes, age at and polarity of onset, symptoms, and severity of the illness.

3.13—Bipolar II Disorder / Sex- and Gender-Related Diagnostic Issues (pp. 156–157)

3.14   Which of the following is associated with postpartum hypomania?

   A. The late postpartum period.
   B. Preserved sleep.
   C. Postpartum depression.
   D. Infanticide.

Correct Answer: C. Postpartum depression.

Explanation: Childbirth may be a specific trigger for a hypomanic episode, which can occur in 10%–20% of females in nonclinical populations and most typically in the early postpartum period. Distinguishing hypomania from the elated mood and reduced sleep that normally accompany the birth of a child may be challenging. Postpartum hypomania may foreshadow the onset of a depression that occurs in about half of females who experience postpartum "highs."

3.14—Bipolar II Disorder / Sex- and Gender-Related Diagnostic Issues (pp. 156–157)

3.15   A 42-year-old woman with a history of panic disorder presents to the emergency department, brought in by her family after 2 days of abnormal behavior. They report that she has not slept for the past 2 days, is speaking unusually rapidly, and has been irritable. The patient reports feeling "incredible" despite running out of her long-term benzodiazepine prescription 3 days ago. On exam she repeatedly paces back and forth while demanding immediate discharge from the emergency department. What is the most likely diagnosis?

   A. Panic disorder.
   B. Bipolar II disorder.
   C. Benzodiazepine intoxication.
   D. Substance/medication-induced bipolar and related disorder.

Correct Answer: D. Substance/medication-induced bipolar and related disorder.

Explanation: The diagnosis of substance/medication-induced bipolar and related disorder is based on a prominent and persistent mood disturbance that predominates the clinical picture and is characterized by abnormally elevated, expansive, or irritable mood and increased energy (Criterion A). There must be evidence from history, physical examination, or laboratory findings that these symptoms developed after exposure to or withdrawal from a substance or medication capable of producing them (Criterion B). The disturbance should not be better explained by a bipolar or related disorder that is not substance/medication-induced (Criterion C).

3.15—Substance/Medication-Induced Bipolar and Related Disorder / diagnostic criteria (p. 162)

3.16   A 36-year-old man presents to a psychiatry clinic for intake. He describes a history of several months-long periods throughout his lifetime with sustained low mood, increased sleep, decreased appetite, poor energy, and worsening ability to concentrate at work. He also notes that he has had many periods of uncharacteristically happy moods with excellent energy despite sleeping only 2–4 hours. These periods have never lasted longer than 3 days and typically last only 1–2 days before his mood returns to normal. What is the appropriate diagnosis for this patient?

   A. Bipolar I disorder.
   B. Other specified bipolar and related disorder.
   C. Cyclothymia.
   D. Bipolar II disorder.

Correct Answer: B. Other specified bipolar and related disorder.

Explanation: Other specified bipolar and related disorder is diagnosed when a patient experiences symptoms characteristic of a bipolar and related disorder and related distress or impairment but does not meet full criteria for any of the disorders in the bipolar and related disorders diagnostic class. This diagnosis is made when the clinician chooses to communicate the specific reason that the presentation does not meet criteria (e.g., "short-duration hypomanic episodes and major depressive episodes").

3.16—Other Specified Bipolar and Related Disorder (pp. 168–169)

3.17   In which of the following aspects does cyclothymic disorder differ from bipolar I disorder?

    A. Duration.
    B. Severity.
    C. Age at onset.
    D. Pervasiveness.

Correct Answer: B. Severity.

Explanation: The essential feature of cyclothymic disorder is a chronic, fluctuating mood disturbance involving numerous periods of hypomanic symptoms and periods of depressive symptoms that are distinct from each other. The hypomanic symptoms are of insufficient number, severity, pervasiveness, or duration to meet full criteria for a hypomanic episode, and the depressive symptoms are of insufficient number, severity, pervasiveness, or duration to meet full criteria for a major depressive episode (Criterion A). During the initial 2-year period (1 year for children or adolescents), the symptoms must be persistent (present more days than not), and any symptom-free intervals must last no longer than 2 months (Criterion B). The diagnosis of cyclothymic disorder is made only if the criteria for a major depressive, manic, or hypomanic episode have never been met (Criterion C).

3.17—Cyclothymic Disorder / Diagnostic Features (p. 160)

CHAPTER 4

Depressive Disorders

4.1 A 41-year-old patient without any previous mood disorder history reports two recent periods of sustained sadness, lack of interest in her hobbies, worsened concentration, increased fatigue, and decreased productivity at work. She notes that each of these periods began after a cocaine binge. The mood episodes persisted almost 2 weeks after the cocaine use stopped. After each period, the patient returned to her typical euthymic state without treatment. What is the most appropriate diagnosis?

A. Substance/medication-induced depressive disorder.
B. Premenstrual dysphoric disorder.
C. Major depressive disorder.
D. Unspecified bipolar disorder.

Correct Answer: A. Substance/medication-induced depressive disorder.

Explanation: Substance/medication-induced depressive disorder is defined by a prominent and persistent mood disturbance with evidence from history, physical examination, or laboratory findings that the mood symptoms developed soon after substance intoxication or withdrawal, and the involved substance or medication is capable of producing these symptoms. The neurochemical changes associated with intoxication and withdrawal states for some substances can be relatively protracted; thus, intense depressive symptoms can last for a longer period after the cessation of substance use and still be consistent with a diagnosis of a substance/medication-induced depressive disorder.

4.1—Substance/Medication-Induced Depressive Disorder / diagnostic criteria (p. 201); Diagnostic Features (pp. 203–204)

4.2 A 47-year-old woman with diagnosed major depressive disorder (MDD) presents to your office with new psychiatric complaints. Women are more likely to experience which of the following comorbid disorders?

A. Substance/medication-induced depressive disorder.
B. Generalized anxiety disorder.

C. Alcohol use disorder.

D. Cocaine use disorder.

Correct Answer: B. Generalized anxiety disorder.

Explanation: Other disorders with which major depressive disorder frequently co-occurs are substance-related disorders, panic disorder, generalized anxiety disorder, posttraumatic stress disorder, obsessive-compulsive disorder, anorexia nervosa, bulimia nervosa, and borderline personality disorder. Whereas women are more likely than men to report comorbid anxiety disorders, bulimia nervosa, and somatoform disorder (somatic symptom and related disorders), men are more likely to report comorbid alcohol and substance abuse.

4.2—Major Depressive Disorder / Comorbidity (p. 192)

4.3   What diagnostic provision is made for depressive symptoms following the death of a loved one?

A. Depressive symptoms lasting less than 2 months after the loss of a loved one are excluded from receiving a diagnosis of major depressive episode (MDE).

B. To qualify for a diagnosis of MDE, the depression must start no less than 12 weeks following the loss.

C. To qualify for a diagnosis of MDE, the depressive symptoms in such individuals must include suicidal ideation.

D. Depressive symptoms following the loss of a loved one are not excluded from receiving an MDE diagnosis if the symptoms otherwise fulfill the diagnostic criteria.

Correct Answer: D. Depressive symptoms following the loss of a loved one are not excluded from receiving an MDE diagnosis if the symptoms otherwise fulfill the diagnostic criteria.

Explanation: In DSM-5-TR, there is no exclusion criterion for an MDE within the first 2 months after the death of a loved one. Bereavement is the experience of losing a loved one to death. It generally triggers a grief response that may be intense and may involve many features that overlap with symptoms characteristic of an MDE, such as sadness, difficulty sleeping, and poor concentration. Features that help differentiate a bereavement-related grief response from an MDE include the following: the predominant affects in grief are feelings of emptiness and loss, whereas in an MDE they are persistent depressed mood and a diminished ability to experience pleasure. Moreover, the dysphoric mood of grief is likely to decrease in intensity over days to weeks and occurs in waves that tend to be associated with thoughts or reminders of the deceased, whereas the depressed mood in an MDE is more persistent and not tied to specific thoughts or preoccupations. It is important to note that in a vulnerable individual (e.g., someone with a past history of major depressive disorder), bereavement may trigger not only a grief response but also the development of an episode of depression or the worsening of an existing episode.

Bereavement may induce great suffering, but it does not typically induce an episode of major depressive disorder. When bereavement and an MDE do occur together, the depressive symptoms and functional impairment tend to be more severe and the prognosis is worse compared with bereavement that is not accompanied by major depressive disorder.

4.3—Depressive Disorders / chapter introduction (p. 177); Major Depressive Disorder / Differential Diagnosis (p. 192)

4.4   How does grief differ from a major depressive episode (MDE)?

A. Grief is often characterized by an inability to experience happiness or pleasure.
B. In grief, dysphoria is typically constant, whereas in an MDE sadness commonly comes as "pangs" that come in waves over days or weeks.
C. The thought content associated with grief is generally self-critical or pessimistic ruminations.
D. In grief, when the bereaved individual thinks about death and dying, such thoughts are generally focused on the deceased and possibly about "joining" the deceased, whereas in MDE such thoughts are focused on ending one's own life because of feeling worthless, undeserving of life, or unable to cope with the pain of depression.

Correct Answer: D. In grief, when the bereaved individual thinks about death and dying, such thoughts are generally focused on the deceased and possibly about "joining" the deceased, whereas in MDE such thoughts are focused on ending one's own life because of feeling worthless, undeserving of life, or unable to cope with the pain of depression.

Explanation: In distinguishing grief from an MDE, it is useful to consider that in grief the predominant affect is feelings of emptiness and loss, whereas in an MDE it is persistent depressed mood and the inability to anticipate happiness or pleasure. The dysphoria in grief is likely to decrease in intensity over days to weeks and occurs in waves, the so-called pangs of grief. These waves tend to be associated with thoughts or reminders of the deceased. The depressed mood of an MDE is more persistent and not tied to specific thoughts or preoccupations. The pain of grief may be accompanied by positive emotions and humor that are uncharacteristic of the pervasive unhappiness and misery characteristic of an MDE. The thought content associated with grief generally features a preoccupation with thoughts and memories of the deceased rather than the self-critical or pessimistic ruminations seen in an MDE. In grief, self-esteem is generally preserved, whereas in an MDE feelings of worthlessness and self-loathing are common. If self-derogatory ideation is present in grief, it typically involves perceived failings vis-à-vis the deceased (e.g., not visiting frequently enough, not telling the deceased how much he or she was loved). If a bereaved individual thinks about death and dying, such thoughts are generally focused on the deceased and possibly about "joining" the deceased, whereas in an MDE such thoughts are focused on ending one's own life because of feeling worthless, undeserving of life, or unable to cope with the pain of depression.

4.4—Major Depressive Disorder / diagnostic criteria (pp. 183–184)

4.5   Which of the following is a risk factor for developing substance/medication-induced depressive disorder?

A. Female sex.
B. High socioeconomic status.
C. Recent life stressors.
D. Remission from substance abuse.

Correct Answer: C. Recent life stressors.

Explanation: Risk factors for substance-induced depressive disorder include a history of antisocial personality disorder, schizophrenia, and bipolar disorder; a history of stressful life events in the past 12 months; a history of prior drug-induced depressions; and a family history of substance use disorders. In addition, neurochemical changes associated with alcohol and other drugs of abuse often contribute to depressive and anxiety symptoms during withdrawal that subsequently influence ongoing substance use and reduce the likelihood of remission of substance use disorders. The course of substance-induced depressive disorder may be worsened by social-structural adversity associated with poverty, racism, and marginalization. Among individuals with a substance use disorder, the risk for developing a substance-induced depressive disorder appears to be similar in men and women.

4.5—Substance/Medication-Induced Depressive Disorder / Risk and Prognostic Factors (p. 204) / Sex- and Gender-Related Diagnostic Issues (p. 205)

4.6   A 50-year-old man presents with persistently depressed mood lasting for several weeks that interferes with his ability to work. He has insomnia and fatigue, feels guilty, has thoughts he would be better off dead, and has begun researching ways to die without anyone knowing it was a suicide. His wife informs you that on most days during this period he has also displayed odd behaviors, including speaking rapidly, requesting sex several times a day, and writing extensively about ideas for a "better internet." These behaviors are marked changes from his typical behavior. Which diagnosis best fits this patient?

A. Manic episode, with mixed features.
B. Major depressive episode.

C. Major depressive episode, with mixed features.
D. Major depressive episode, with atypical features.

Correct Answer: C. Major depressive episode, with mixed features.

Explanation: The specifier *with mixed features* is defined by the presence of at least three manic/hypomanic symptoms during the majority of days of the current or most recent major depressive episode (MDE). These symptoms must be observable by others and represent a change from the person's usual behavior. By definition, these symptoms must be insufficient to satisfy criteria for a manic episode, otherwise the diagnosis should be bipolar I or bipolar II disorder. The symptoms should be present during the majority of days during the MDE. Mixed features associated with an MDE have been found to be a significant risk factor for the development of bipolar I or bipolar II disorder. As a result, it is clinically useful to note the presence of this specifier for treatment planning and monitoring of response to treatment.

4.6—Specifiers for Depressive Disorders / With mixed features (p. 211)

4.7   A 45-year-old woman with classic features of schizophrenia has experienced chronic, co-occurring symptoms of feeling "down in the dumps," having a poor appetite, and hopelessness during her episodes of active psychosis. These depressive symptoms occurred only during her psychotic episodes and only during the 4-year period when she was experiencing active symptoms of schizophrenia. After her psychotic episodes were successfully controlled by medication, no further symptoms of depression were present. At no time has the patient met full criteria for major depressive episode. What is the appropriate DSM-5-TR diagnosis?

A. Schizophrenia.
B. Schizoaffective disorder.
C. Persistent depressive disorder (dysthymia).
D. Schizophrenia and persistent depressive disorder (dysthymia).

Correct Answer: A. Schizophrenia.

Explanation: Depressive symptoms are a common associated feature of chronic psychotic disorders (e.g., schizoaffective disorder, schizophrenia, delusional disorder). A separate diagnosis of persistent depressive disorder is not made if the symptoms occur only during the course of the psychotic disorder (including residual phases).

4.7—Persistent Depressive Disorder / Differential Diagnosis (p. 196)

4.8   Which depressive disorder diagnoses were new to DSM-5 and continued in DSM-5-TR?

A. Subsyndromal depressive disorder, premenstrual dysphoric disorder, and mixed anxiety and depressive disorder.

B. Disruptive mood dysregulation disorder, premenstrual dysphoric disorder, and persistent depressive disorder.

C. Disruptive mood dysregulation disorder, premenstrual dysphoric disorder, and subsyndromal depressive disorder.

D. Disruptive mood dysregulation disorder, postmenopausal dysphoric disorder, and persistent depressive disorder.

Correct Answer: B. Disruptive mood dysregulation disorder, premenstrual dysphoric disorder, and persistent depressive disorder.

Explanation: Several new diagnoses first appeared in the DSM-5 "Depressive Disorders" chapter. After careful scientific review of the evidence, premenstrual dysphoric disorder (PMDD) was moved from Appendix B ("Criteria Sets and Axes Provided for Further Study") of DSM-IV to Section II of DSM-5. Almost 20 years of additional research on this condition have confirmed a specific and treatment-responsive form of depressive disorder that begins some time following ovulation and remits within a few days of menses and has a marked impact on functioning.

In order to address concerns about the potential for the overdiagnosis of and treatment for bipolar disorder in children, a new diagnosis, disruptive mood dysregulation disorder (DMDD), referring to the presentation of children with persistent irritability and frequent episodes of extreme behavioral dyscontrol, was added to the depressive disorders for children up to age 12 years. Its placement in this chapter reflects the finding that children with this symptom pattern typically develop unipolar depressive disorders or anxiety disorders, rather than bipolar disorders, as they mature into adolescence and adulthood.

A more chronic form of depression, persistent depressive disorder, can be diagnosed when the mood disturbance continues for at least 2 years in adults or 1 year in children. This diagnosis, which was new in DSM-5, includes the DSM-IV diagnostic categories of chronic major depression and dysthymia.

4.8—Depressive Disorders / chapter introduction (p. 177)

4.9   A patient in a current major depressive episode reports experiencing no pleasure from positive everyday experiences that would usually be enjoyable. He also notes waking up early in the morning with terminal insomnia, feeling worse in the morning than at other times of the day, and having excessive guilt over minor mistakes. Which of the following is the appropriate diagnosis and specifier for this patient?

A. Major depressive disorder, with anxious distress.

B. Major depressive disorder, with atypical features.

C. Major depressive disorder, with melancholic features.

D. Major depressive disorder, with mixed features.

Correct Answer: C. Major depressive disorder, with melancholic features.

Explanation: The specifier *with melancholic features* is applied if, during the current or most recent major depressive episode, a patient meets the following criteria: Criterion A specifies that one of the following must be present during the most severe period of the current episode: 1) loss of pleasure in all, or almost all, activities or 2) lack of reactivity to usually pleasurable stimuli (does not feel much better, even temporarily, when something good happens). Criterion B specifies that three (or more) of the following must be present: 1) a distinct quality of depressed mood characterized by profound despondency, despair, and/or moroseness or by so-called empty mood; 2) depression that is regularly worse in the morning; 3) early morning awakening (i.e., at least 2 hours before usual awakening); 4) marked psychomotor agitation or retardation; 5) significant anorexia or weight loss; 6) excessive or inappropriate guilt.

4.9—Depressive Disorders / Specifiers for Depressive Disorders (pp. 211–212)

4.10   A 39-year-old woman describes becoming quite depressed in the winter last year when her company closed for the season and then experiencing spontaneous remission without treatment in the following spring. She recalls experiencing multiple other major depressive episodes (MDEs) over the past decade during spring and summer months, although none were related to her occupation. Would this patient be eligible for a diagnosis of major depressive disorder, *with seasonal pattern*?

   A. The patient *does not* qualify for this diagnosis because this specifier requires that depressive episode with seasonal features must start in the fall.
   B. The patient *does not* qualify for this diagnosis because this specifier requires onset and remission over at least a 2-year period without any nonseasonal episodes during this period.
   C. The patient *does* qualify for this diagnosis because she experienced a spontaneous remission of a depressive episode with a seasonal relationship.
   D. The patient *does* qualify for this diagnosis because her symptoms are related to a specific psychosocial stressor.

Correct Answer: B. The patient does not qualify for this diagnosis because this specifier requires onset and remission over at least a 2-year period without any nonseasonal episodes during this period.

Explanation: The *with seasonal pattern* specifier requires A) a regular temporal relationship between the onset of MDEs and a particular time of the year (e.g., in the fall or winter). The diagnosis excludes cases in which there is an obvious effect of seasonally related psychosocial stressors (e.g., regularly being unemployed every winter). B) Full remissions also occur at a characteristic time of the year (e.g., depression disappears in the spring). C) In the past 2 years, two MDEs must have occurred that demonstrate the temporal seasonal relationships, and no nonseasonal MDEs occurred during that same period. D) Seasonal MDEs must substantially outnumber the nonseasonal MDEs that may have occurred over the individual's lifetime. The specifier *with seasonal pattern* can be applied to the pattern of MDEs in bipolar I disorder, bipolar II disorder, or major depressive disorder, recurrent.

4.10—Depressive Disorders / Specifiers for Depressive Disorders (p. 214)

4.11   Which of the following demographic groups has the highest depression prevalence?

   A. Reproductive age females.
   B. Reproductive age males.
   C. Elderly males.
   D. Female children.

Correct Answer: A. Reproductive age females.

Explanation: The 12-month prevalence of major depressive disorder in the United States is approximately 7%, with marked differences by age group such that the prevalence in 18- to 29-year-old individuals is threefold higher than the prevalence in individuals age 60 years or older. The most reproducible finding in the epidemiology of major depressive disorder has been a higher prevalence in females, an effect that peaks in adolescence and then stabilizes. Women experience approximately twofold higher rates than do men, especially between menarche and menopause. Women report more atypical symptoms of depression characterized by hypersomnia, increased appetite, and leaden paralysis compared with men.

4.11—Major Depressive Disorder / Prevalence (pp. 187–188)

4.12   Which of the following statements is associated with an increased risk of recurrence in major depressive disorder?

   A. Older age.
   B. Severe symptoms.
   C. Recent first episode.
   D. Longer duration of remission.

Correct Answer: B. Severe symptoms.

Explanation: Recovery from a major depressive episode begins within 3 months of onset for 40% of individuals with major depression and within 1 year for 80% of individuals. Recency of onset is a strong determinant of the likelihood of near-term recovery, and many individuals who have been depressed for only several months can be expected to recover spontaneously. Features associated with lower recovery rates, other than current episode duration, include psychotic features, prominent anxiety, personality disorders, and symptom severity.

The risk of recurrence becomes progressively lower over time as the duration of remission increases. The risk is higher in individuals whose preceding episode was severe, in younger individuals, and in individuals who have already experienced multiple episodes. The persistence of even mild depressive symptoms during remission is a powerful predictor of recurrence.

4.12—Major Depressive Disorder / Development and Course (p. 188)

4.13 Which of the following is an accurate diagnostic marker for major depressive disorder (MDD)?

A. Pro-inflammatory cytokine levels.
B. Neurotrophic factor genetic variants.
C. Hypothalamic-pituitary-gonadal hyperactivity.
D. None of the above.

Correct Answer: D. None of the above.

Explanation: Although an extensive literature exists describing neuroanatomical, neuroendocrinological, and neurophysiological correlates of MDD, no laboratory test has yielded results of sufficient sensitivity and specificity to be used as a diagnostic tool for this disorder. Until recently, hypothalamic-pituitary-adrenal axis hyperactivity had been the most extensively investigated abnormality associated with major depressive episodes, and it appears to be associated with melancholia, psychotic features, and risks for eventual suicide. Molecular studies have also implicated peripheral factors, including genetic variants in neurotrophic factors and pro-inflammatory cytokines. Additionally, functional MRI studies provide evidence for functional abnormalities in specific neural systems supporting emotion processing, reward seeking, and emotion regulation in adults with major depression.

4.13—Major Depressive Disorder / Associated Features (p. 187)

4.14 In major depressive disorder, which of the following is more common in men than women?

A. Suicide completion.
B. Associated gastrointestinal symptoms.
C. Hypersomnia.
D. Treatment responsiveness.

Correct Answer: A. Suicide completion.

Explanation: There are no clear differences between men and women in treatment response or functional consequences. There is some evidence for sex and gender differences in phenomenology and course of illness. Women tend to experience more disturbances in appetite and sleep, including atypical features such as hyperphagia and hypersomnia, and are more likely to experience interpersonal sensitivity and gastrointestinal symptoms. Men with depression, however, may be more likely than depressed women to report greater frequencies and intensities of maladaptive self-coping and problem-solving strategies, including alcohol or other drug misuse, risk-taking, and poor impulse control. Women attempt suicide at a higher rate than men do, whereas men are more likely to complete suicide. The difference in suicide rate between men and women with depressive disorders is smaller than in the population as a whole, however.

4.14—Major Depressive Disorder / Sex- and Gender-Related Diagnostic Issues; Association With Suicidal Thoughts or Behavior (p. 190)

4.15   A 12-year-old youth has been experiencing episodes of temper outbursts that are out of proportion to the situation several times per week over the past year. She frequently screams at anyone in her vicinity and occasionally breaks nearby objects during these episodes. Which of the following aspects of this patient's presentation precludes a diagnosis of disruptive mood dysregulation disorder (DMDD)?

A. Outburst frequency.
B. Aggression toward others.
C. Age at symptom onset.
D. Age at diagnosis.

Correct Answer: C. Age at symptom onset.

Explanation: Criterion A for DMDD specifies severe recurrent temper outbursts manifested verbally (e.g., verbal rages) and/or behaviorally (e.g., physical aggression toward people or property) that are grossly out of proportion in intensity or duration to the situation or provocation. Criterion B specifies that temper outbursts must be inconsistent with developmental level, and Criterion C states that temper outbursts occur, on average, three or more times per week. Per Criterion G the diagnosis can be made between ages 6 and 18, and per Criterion H the symptoms should begin before the patient is 10 years old.

4.15—Disruptive Mood Dysregulation Disorder / diagnostic criteria (p. 178)

4.16   Which of the following features distinguishes disruptive mood dysregulation disorder (DMDD) from bipolar disorder in children?

A. Age at onset.
B. Chronicity.
C. Irritability.
D. Severity.

Correct Answer: B. Chronicity.

Explanation: The core feature of DMDD is chronic, severe, persistent irritability. This severe irritability has two prominent clinical manifestations, the first of which is frequent temper outbursts. These outbursts typically occur in response to frustration and can be verbal or behavioral (the latter in the form of aggression against property, self, or others).

The clinical presentation of DMDD must be carefully distinguished from presentations of other, related conditions, particularly pediatric bipolar disorder. DMDD was added to DSM-5 to address the considerable concern about the appropriate classification and treatment of children who present with chronic, persistent irritability relative to children who present with classic (i.e., episodic) bipolar disorder.

In DSM-5-TR, the term *bipolar disorder* is explicitly reserved for episodic presentations of bipolar symptoms. DSM-IV did not include a diagnosis designed to capture youth whose hallmark symptoms consist of very severe, nonepisodic irritability, whereas DSM-5-TR, with the inclusion of DMDD, provides a distinct category for such presentations.

4.16—Disruptive Mood Dysregulation Disorder / Diagnostic Features (pp. 178–179)

4.17 Children with disruptive mood dysregulation disorder are most likely to develop which of the following disorders in adulthood?

A. Bipolar I disorder.
B. Unipolar depressive disorders.
C. Antisocial personality disorder.
D. Borderline personality disorder.

Correct Answer: B. Unipolar depressive disorders.

Explanation: Approximately half of children with severe, chronic irritability will have a presentation that continues to meet criteria for the condition 1 year later, although those children whose symptoms no longer meet the threshold for the diagnosis often have persistent, clinically impairing irritability. Rates of conversion from severe, nonepisodic irritability to bipolar disorder are very low. Instead, children with chronic irritability are at risk of developing unipolar depressive and/or anxiety disorders in adulthood.

4.17—Disruptive Mood Dysregulation Disorder / Development and Course (p. 179)

4.18 An irritable 8-year-old child has a history of nearly daily temper outbursts both at home and at school over the past 2 years. These outbursts are age-inappropriate and severe. Between outbursts, what characteristic mood is required to qualify this child for a diagnosis of disruptive mood dysregulation disorder?

A. Irritability.
B. Depression.
C. Euthymia.
D. Lability.

Correct Answer: A. Irritability.

Explanation: Criterion D of disruptive mood dysregulation disorder requires that the mood between temper outbursts is persistently irritable or angry most of the day, nearly every day, and observable by others (e.g., parents, teachers, peers).

4.18—Disruptive Mood Dysregulation Disorder / diagnostic criteria (p. 178)

4.19   According to DSM-5-TR diagnostic criteria, disruptive mood dysregulation disorder (DMDD) can be assigned in combination with which of the following diagnoses?

A. Oppositional defiant disorder (ODD).
B. Bipolar II disorder.
C. Intermittent explosive disorder (IED).
D. Attention-deficit/hyperactivity disorder (ADHD).

Correct Answer: D. Attention-deficit/hyperactivity disorder (ADHD).

Explanation: By rule, the diagnosis of DMDD cannot coexist with ODD, IED, or bipolar disorder, though it can coexist with others, including major depressive disorder, ADHD, conduct disorder, and substance use disorders. Individuals whose symptoms meet criteria for both DMDD and ODD should be given the diagnosis of DMDD only. If an individual has ever experienced a manic or hypomanic episode, the diagnosis of DMDD should not be assigned. Because chronically irritable children and adolescents typically present with complex histories, the diagnosis of DMDD must be made while considering the presence or absence of multiple other conditions. The differential diagnosis of DMDD from both bipolar disorder and ODD requires careful consideration. DMDD differs from bipolar disorder in that the former is chronic, whereas the latter is episodic. DMDD differs from ODD in that very severe irritability is required in the former but not the latter. DMDD is characterized by the presence of chronic irritability between outbursts, whereas IED is characterized by the relative absence of mood disturbance between outbursts.

4.19—Disruptive Mood Dysregulation Disorder / diagnostic criteria (p. 178); Differential Diagnosis (pp. 181–182)

4.20 Which of the following factors is associated with a decreased risk of death by suicide?

A. Marriage.
B. Firearm ownership.
C. Impaired cognition.
D. Anhedonia.

Correct Answer: A. Marriage.

Explanation: The possibility of suicidal behavior exists at all times during major depressive episodes. The most consistently described risk factor is a past history of suicide attempts or threats, but it should be remembered that most deaths by suicide are not preceded by nonfatal attempts. Anhedonia has a particularly strong association with suicidal ideation. Other features associated with an increased risk for death by suicide include being single, living alone, social disconnectedness, early life adversity, availability of lethal methods such as a firearm, sleep disturbance, cognitive and decision-making deficits, and having prominent feelings of hopelessness. Women attempt suicide at a higher rate than men, but men are more likely to complete suicide.

4.20—Major Depressive Disorder / Association With Suicidal Thoughts or Behavior (p. 190)

4.21 A 9-year-old boy is brought in for evaluation because of explosive outbursts when he is frustrated with schoolwork. The parents report that their son is well behaved and pleasant at other times. Which diagnosis best fits this clinical picture?

A. Disruptive mood dysregulation disorder (DMDD).
B. Bipolar disorder.
C. Intermittent explosive disorder (IED).
D. Major depressive disorder.

Correct Answer: C. Intermittent explosive disorder (IED).

Explanation: Children with IED present with instances of severe temper outbursts much like those in children with DMDD. However, unlike children with DMDD, children with IED do not exhibit persistent disruption in mood between outbursts. Thus, the two diagnoses are mutually exclusive and cannot be made in the same child. For children with outbursts and intercurrent, persistent irritability, the diagnosis of DMDD should be made. For children with outbursts but no such irritability, the diagnosis of IED should be made.

4.21—Disruptive Mood Dysregulation Disorder / Differential Diagnosis (p. 182)

4.22   A 14-year-old boy describes himself as feeling irritable the vast majority of the time for the past year. He remembers feeling better while he was at camp for 4 weeks during the summer; however, his mood complaints returned when he came home and have continued since. He reports poor concentration and feelings of hopelessness but denies suicidal ideation or changes in his appetite or sleep. What is the most appropriate diagnosis?

A. Major depressive disorder.
B. Disruptive mood dysregulation disorder.
C. Depressive episodes with short-duration hypomania.
D. Persistent depressive disorder, with early onset.

Correct Answer: D. Persistent depressive disorder (dysthymia), with early onset.

Explanation: The essential feature of persistent depressive disorder is a depressed mood that occurs for most of the day, for more days than not, for at least 2 years, or at least 1 year for children and adolescents (Criterion A). This disorder represents a consolidation of DSM-IV-defined chronic major depressive disorder and dysthymic disorder. In children and adolescents, mood can be irritable rather than depressed. In addition to Criterion A, at least two of the six symptoms from Criterion B (appetite changes, sleep changes, low energy, low self-esteem, poor concentration, hopelessness) must be present. Because these symptoms have become a part of the individual's day-to-day experience, particularly in the case of early onset (e.g., "I've always been this way"), they may not be reported unless the individual is directly prompted. During the 2-year period (1 year for children or adolescents), any symptom-free intervals last no longer than 2 months (Criterion C).

4.22—Persistent Depressive Disorder / Diagnostic Features (p. 194)

4.23   A 30-year-old woman reports 3 years of ongoing depressed mood, accompanied by loss of pleasure in all activities, ruminations that she would be better off dead, feelings of guilt about "bad things" she has done, and thoughts about quitting work because of her inability to focus. Although she has never been treated for depression, she feels so distressed at times that she wonders if she should be hospitalized. She denies drug or alcohol use, and her medical workup is completely normal, including laboratory tests for vitamins. The consultation was prompted by further worsening of her mood over the past several weeks. What is the most appropriate diagnosis?

A. Major depressive disorder (MDD).
B. Persistent depressive disorder, with persistent major depressive episode.
C. Cyclothymia.
D. MDD, with melancholic features.

Correct Answer: B. Persistent depressive disorder, with persistent major depressive episode.

Explanation: The essential feature of persistent depressive disorder is a depressed mood that occurs for most of the day, for more days than not, for at least 2 years (Criterion A). This disorder represents a consolidation of DSM-IV-defined chronic major depressive disorder and dysthymic disorder. Major depression may precede persistent depressive disorder, and major depressive episodes may occur during persistent depressive disorder. Individuals whose symptoms meet MDD criteria for 2 years should be given a diagnosis of persistent depressive disorder as well as MDD.

If there is a depressed mood plus two or more symptoms meeting criteria for a persistent depressive episode for 2 years or more, then the diagnosis of persistent depressive disorder is made. The diagnosis depends on the 2-year duration, which distinguishes the disorder from episodes of depression that do not last 2 years. If the symptom criteria are sufficient for a diagnosis of a major depressive episode at any time during this period, then the diagnosis of major depression should be noted, but it is coded not as a separate diagnosis but rather as a specifier with the diagnosis of persistent depressive disorder. If the individual's symptoms currently meet full criteria for a major depressive episode, then the specifier *with intermittent major depressive episodes, with current episode* would be applied. If—as in the patient described in the vignette—the major depressive episode has persisted for at least a 2-year duration and remains present, then the specifier *with persistent major depressive episode* is used. When full major depressive episode criteria are not currently met but there has been at least one previous episode of major depression in the context of at least 2 years of persistent depressive symptoms, then the specifier *with intermittent major depressive episodes, without current episode* is used. If the individual has not experienced an episode of major depression in the past 2 years, then the specifier *with pure dysthymic syndrome* is used.

4.23—Persistent Depressive Disorder / Diagnostic Features (p. 194); Differential Diagnosis (pp. 195–196)

4.24   A 67-year-old woman presents with new depressive symptoms that began approximately 3 weeks after she experienced a cerebrovascular accident (CVA). The symptoms have continued for 2 months. Along with daily depressed mood, she reports middle insomnia, poor appetite, trouble concentrating, and lack of interest in sex. Per her neurologist, she has very limited residual symptoms from her CVA. Despite the lack of residual deficits, she describes frequent absence from and poor performance at work. She denies any active plans to attempt suicide but admits that she "wishes for death" as her mood has worsened. The patient and her husband both deny that she had any previous history of even a mild depressive episode. What is the most likely diagnosis?

   A. Major depressive disorder.
   B. Persistent depressive disorder.
   C. Depressive disorder due to another medical condition.
   D. Substance/medication-induced depressive disorder.

Correct Answer: C. Depressive disorder due to another medical condition.

Explanation: The essential feature of depressive disorder due to another medical condition is a prominent and persistent period of depressed mood or markedly diminished interest or pleasure in all, or almost all, activities that predominates in the clinical picture (Criterion A) and that is thought to be related to the direct physiological effects of another medical condition (Criterion B). In determining whether the mood disturbance is due to another medical condition, the clinician must first establish the presence of such a condition. Furthermore, the clinician must establish that the mood disturbance is etiologically related to the other medical condition through a physiological mechanism. A careful and comprehensive assessment of multiple factors is necessary to make this judgment. Although there are no infallible guidelines for determining whether the relationship between the mood disturbance and another medical condition is etiological, several considerations provide some guidance in this area. One consideration is the presence of a temporal association between the onset, exacerbation, or remission of another medical condition and that of the mood disturbance. A second consideration is the presence of features that are atypical of independent depressive disorders (e.g., atypical age at onset or course or absence of family history).

4.24—Depressive Disorder Due to Another Medical Condition / Diagnostic Features (pp. 206–207)

4.25 A 17-year-old high school senior complains to her gynecologist about periods of pronounced irritability, sadness, conflicts with her classmates, increased appetite, decreased energy, feeling bloated, and decreased concentration. She feels that these symptoms generally start about 3–4 days prior to the onset of menses and disappear within a week. She cannot recall many menstrual cycles without these symptoms since menarche at age 12, but she has never kept any notes or records about them. Her gynecologist asks you to consult on the case. On the basis of her symptoms, which is the most appropriate diagnosis for this patient?

A. Premenstrual syndrome.
B. Major depressive disorder.
C. Premenstrual dysphoric disorder, provisional.
D. The patient has no DSM-5 diagnosis.

Correct Answer: C. Premenstrual dysphoric disorder, provisional.

Explanation: The essential features of premenstrual dysphoric disorder are the expression of mood lability, irritability, dysphoria, and anxiety symptoms that occur repeatedly during the premenstrual phase of the cycle and remit around the onset of menses or shortly thereafter. These symptoms may be accompanied by behavioral and physical symptoms. Premenstrual syndrome differs from premenstrual dysphoric disorder in that premenstrual syndrome requires neither a minimum of five symptoms nor mood-related symptomatology, and it is generally considered to be less severe than premenstrual dysphoric disorder.

If the symptoms of premenstrual dysphoric disorder have not been confirmed by prospective daily ratings of at least two symptomatic cycles, *provisional* should be noted after the name of the diagnosis (i.e., premenstrual dysphoric disorder, provisional).

4.25—Premenstrual Dysphoric Disorder / Recording Procedures; Diagnostic Features (p. 198)

4.26   The presence of which of the following excludes a diagnosis of premenstrual dysphoric disorder?

   A. Labile affect.
   B. Continuous symptoms.
   C. Physical pain.
   D. Delusions.

Correct Answer: B. Continuous symptoms.

Explanation: The essential features of premenstrual dysphoric disorder are the expression of mood lability, irritability, dysphoria, and anxiety symptoms that occur repeatedly during the premenstrual phase of the cycle and remit around the onset of menses or shortly thereafter. These symptoms may be accompanied by behavioral and physical symptoms. Typically, symptoms peak around the time of the onset of menses. Although it is not uncommon for symptoms to linger into the first few days of menses, the individual must have a symptom-free period in the follicular phase after the menstrual period begins. Delusions and hallucinations have been described in the late luteal phase of the menstrual cycle but are rare.

4.26—Premenstrual Dysphoric Disorder / Associated Features (p. 198); Diagnostic Markers (p. 199).

4.27   A 29-year-old woman complains of sad mood every month in anticipation of her very painful menses. The pain begins with the start of her flow and continues for several days. She does not experience pain during other times of the month. She has tried a variety of treatments, none of which have given her relief. What is the appropriate diagnosis?

   A. Premenstrual dysphoric disorder.
   B. Premenstrual syndrome.
   C. Dysmenorrhea.
   D. Persistent depressive disorder.

Correct Answer: C. Dysmenorrhea.

Explanation: Dysmenorrhea is a syndrome of painful menses, but this is distinct from a syndrome characterized by affective changes. Symptoms of dysmenorrhea begin with the onset of menses, whereas symptoms of premenstrual dysphoric disorder, by definition, begin before the onset of menses, even if they linger into the first few days of menses.

4.27—Premenstrual Dysphoric Disorder / Differential Diagnosis (pp. 199–200)

4.28 A 23-year-old woman reports that during every menstrual cycle she experiences breast swelling, bloating, hypersomnia, an increased craving for sweets, poor concentration, and a feeling that she cannot handle her normal responsibilities. She notes that she also feels somewhat more sensitive emotionally and may become tearful when hearing a sad story. She takes no oral medication but does use a drospirenone/ethinyl estradiol patch. What diagnosis best fits this clinical picture?

    A. Premenstrual dysphoric disorder (PMDD).
    B. Dysthymia.
    C. Premenstrual syndrome.
    D. Substance/medication-induced depressive disorder.

Correct Answer: C. Premenstrual syndrome.

Explanation: Premenstrual syndrome differs from PMDD in that a minimum of five symptoms is not required and there is no stipulation of affective symptoms for individuals with premenstrual syndrome. This condition may be more common than PMDD, although the estimated prevalence of premenstrual syndrome varies. Premenstrual syndrome shares with PMDD the feature of symptom expression during the premenstrual phase of the menstrual cycle, but it is generally considered to be less severe than PMDD. Individuals who experience physical or behavioral symptoms in the premenstruum, without the required affective symptoms, likely meet criteria for premenstrual syndrome and not for PMDD.

4.28—Premenstrual Dysphoric Disorder / Differential Diagnosis (pp. 199–200)

4.29 Which of the following is an established risk factor for the development of persistent depressive disorder?

    A. Older age.
    B. Borderline personality disorder.
    C. Schizophrenia.
    D. College degree.

Correct Answer: B. Borderline personality disorder.

Explanation: Persistent depressive disorder often has an early and insidious onset (i.e., in childhood, adolescence, or early adult life) and, by definition, a chronic course. Borderline personality disorder is a particularly robust risk factor for persistent depressive disorder. When persistent depressive disorder and borderline personality disorder coexist, the covariance of the corresponding features over time suggests the operation of a common mechanism. Early onset (i.e., before age 21 years) is associated with a higher likelihood of comorbid personality disorders and substance use disorders.

4.29—Persistent Depressive Disorder / Development and Course (p. 194)

4.30   A 31-year-old woman with no history of mood symptoms reports that she experiences distressing mood lability and irritability starting about 4 days before the onset of menses. She feels "on edge," cannot concentrate, has little enjoyment from any of her activities, experiences bloating, and notes swelling of her breasts. The patient reports that these symptoms started 6 months ago when she began taking oral contraceptives for the first time. If she stops the oral contraceptives and her symptoms remit, what would the diagnosis be?

   A. Premenstrual dysphoric disorder.
   B. Premenstrual syndrome.
   C. Major depressive episode.
   D. Substance/medication-induced depressive disorder.

Correct Answer: D. Substance/medication-induced depressive disorder.

Explanation: Some women who present with moderate to severe premenstrual symptoms may be using hormonal treatments, including hormonal contraceptives. If such symptoms occur after initiation of exogenous hormone use, the symptoms may be attributable to the use of hormones rather than to the underlying condition of premenstrual dysphoric disorder. If the woman stops hormones and the symptoms disappear, then this is consistent with substance/medication-induced depressive disorder.

4.30—Premenstrual Dysphoric Disorder / Differential Diagnosis (pp. 199–200)

4.31   A 37-year-old woman describes a several year history of episodic sadness. Each individual period lasts no longer than 10 days and is accompanied by pronounced anhedonia, insomnia, a loss of appetite, and profound hopelessness. She denies any other psychiatric symptoms. She cannot identify any related life events or stressors. A comprehensive laboratory evaluation is normal. Which of the following would be the most appropriate diagnosis?

   A. Cyclothymia.
   B. Major depressive disorder.

C. Other specified depressive disorder, recurrent brief depression.

D. Premenstrual dysphoric disorder.

Correct Answer: C. Other specified depressive disorder, recurrent brief depression.

Explanation: Other specified depressive disorder applies to presentations in which symptoms characteristic of a depressive disorder that cause clinically significant distress or impairment in social, occupational, or other important areas of functioning predominate but do not meet the full criteria for any of the disorders in the depressive disorders diagnostic class and do not meet criteria for adjustment disorder with depressed mood or adjustment disorder with mixed anxiety and depressed mood. The *other specified depressive disorder* category is used in situations in which the clinician chooses to communicate the specific reason that the presentation does not meet the criteria for any specific depressive disorder. Examples of this disorder include recurrent brief depression: concurrent presence of depressed mood and at least four other symptoms of depression for 2–13 days at least once per month (not associated with the menstrual cycle) for at least 12 consecutive months in an individual whose presentation has never met criteria for any other depressive or bipolar disorder and does not currently meet active or residual criteria for any psychotic disorder.

4.31—Other Specified Depressive Disorder (pp. 209–210)

CHAPTER 5

Anxiety Disorders

5.1   Which of the following disorders is included in the "Anxiety Disorders" chapter of DSM-5-TR?

A. Obsessive-compulsive disorder.
B. Posttraumatic stress disorder.
C. Acute stress disorder.
D. Separation anxiety disorder.

Correct Answer: D. Separation anxiety disorder.

Explanation: The DSM-5-TR "Anxiety Disorders" chapter contains a number of additions and deletions that first appeared in the changes from DSM-IV to DSM-5. A number of anxiety disorders classified in DSM-IV as disorders usually first diagnosed in infancy, childhood, or adolescence, including separation anxiety disorder and selective mutism, were included among the DSM-5 anxiety disorders. Several DSM-IV disorders from the "Anxiety Disorders" chapter, including obsessive-compulsive disorder, posttraumatic stress disorder, and acute stress disorder, were removed from that section in DSM-5 and remain so in DSM-5-TR. This reorganization was the result of a scientific review that concluded that these were distinct disorders that were not sufficiently described by the presence of anxiety symptoms.

5.1—chapter introduction (pp. 215–216)

5.2   A 9-year-old boy cannot go to sleep without having a parent in his room. While falling asleep, he frequently awakens to check that a parent is still there. One parent usually stays until the boy falls asleep. If he wakes up alone during the night, he starts to panic and gets up to find his parents. He also reports frequent nightmares in which he or his parents are harmed. He occasionally calls out that he saw a strange figure peering into his dark room. The parents usually wake in the morning to find the boy asleep on the floor of their room. They once tried to leave him with a relative so they could go on a vacation; however, he became so distressed in anticipation of this that they canceled their plans. What is the most likely diagnosis?

A. Specific phobia.
B. Nightmare disorder.

C. Delusional disorder.
D. Separation anxiety disorder.

Correct Answer: D. Separation anxiety disorder.

Explanation: The essential feature of separation anxiety disorder is excessive fear or anxiety concerning separation from home or attachment figures. The anxiety exceeds what may be expected given the individual's developmental level (Criterion A). Individuals with separation anxiety disorder have symptoms that meet at least three of the following criteria: They experience recurrent excessive distress when separation from home or major attachment figures is anticipated or occurs (Criterion A1). They worry about the well-being or death of attachment figures (Criterion A2), particularly when separated from them, and they need to know the whereabouts of their attachment figures and want to stay in touch with them. They also worry about untoward events to themselves, such as getting lost, being kidnapped, or having an accident, that would keep them from ever being reunited with their major attachment figure (Criterion A3). Individuals with separation anxiety disorder are reluctant or refuse to go out by themselves because of separation fears (Criterion A4). They have persistent and excessive fear or reluctance about being alone or without major attachment figures at home or in other settings. Children with separation anxiety disorder may be unable to stay in or go into a room by themselves and may display "clinging" behavior, staying close to or "shadowing" the parent around the house or requiring someone to be with them when going to another room in the house (Criterion A5). They have persistent reluctance or refusal to go to sleep without being near a major attachment figure or to sleep away from home (Criterion A6). Children with this disorder often have difficulty at bedtime and may insist that someone stay with them until they fall asleep. During the night, they may make their way to their parents' bed (or that of a significant other, such as a sibling). Children may be reluctant or refuse to attend camp, to sleep at friends' homes, or to go on errands.

5.2—Separation Anxiety Disorder / Diagnostic Features (pp. 217–218)

5.3   Which of the following is considered a culture-specific symptom of panic attacks?

A. Derealization.
B. Headaches.
C. Fear of going crazy.
D. Shortness of breath.

Correct Answer: B. Headaches.

Explanation: All of the symptoms listed may occur as part of a panic attack. Cultural interpretations may influence the determination of panic attacks as expected or unexpected. Culture-specific symptoms (e.g., tinnitus, neck soreness, headache, uncontrollable screaming or crying) may be seen; however, such symptoms should not count as one of the four required symptoms.

The rate of fears about mental and somatic symptoms of anxiety appears to vary across cultural contexts and may influence the rate of panic attacks and panic disorder. Also, cultural expectations may influence the classification of panic attacks as expected or unexpected. For example, a Vietnamese individual who has a panic attack after walking out into a windy environment (*trúng gió*; "hit by the wind") may attribute the panic attack to exposure to wind as a result of the cultural syndrome that links these two experiences, resulting in classification of the panic attack as expected. Various other cultural concepts of distress are associated with panic disorder, including *ataque de nervios* ("attack of nerves") among Latin Americans and *khyâl* (wind) attacks and "soul loss" among Cambodians. *Ataque de nervios* may involve trembling, uncontrollable screaming or crying, aggressive or suicidal behavior, and depersonalization or derealization, which may be experienced longer than the few minutes typical of panic attacks.

Some clinical presentations of *ataque de nervios* fulfill criteria for conditions other than panic attack (e.g., functional neurological symptom disorder). These concepts of distress have an impact on the symptoms and frequency of panic disorder, including the individual's attribution of unexpectedness because cultural concepts of distress may create fear of certain situations, ranging from interpersonal arguments (associated with *ataque de nervios*) to types of exertion (associated with *khyâl* attacks) to atmospheric wind (associated with *trúng gió* attacks). Clarification of the details of cultural attributions may aid in distinguishing expected and unexpected panic attacks.

5.3—Panic disorder / diagnostic criteria (pp. 235–236) and Culture-Related Diagnostic Issues (p. 239)

5.4   Which of the following statements best describes how panic attacks differ from panic disorder?

A. Panic attacks require fewer symptoms for a definitive diagnosis.
B. Panic attacks are discrete, occur suddenly, and are usually less severe.
C. Panic attacks are invariably unexpected.
D. Panic attacks represent symptoms that can occur with a variety of other disorders.

Correct Answer: D. Panic attacks represent symptoms that can occur with a variety of other disorders.

Explanation: *Panic attacks* feature prominently within the anxiety disorders as a particular type of fear response. Panic attacks are not limited to anxiety disorders but rather can be seen in other mental disorders as well. In panic disorder, the individual experiences recurrent unexpected panic attacks and is persistently concerned or worried about having more panic attacks or changes their behavior in maladaptive ways because of the panic attacks (e.g., avoidance of exercise or of unfamiliar locations). Panic attacks are abrupt surges of intense fear or intense discomfort that reach a peak within minutes, accompanied by physical and/or cognitive symptoms. Limited-symptom panic attacks include fewer than four symptoms. Panic attacks may be expected, such as in response to a typically feared object or situation, or unexpected, meaning that the panic attack occurs for no apparent reason. Panic attacks function as a marker and prognostic factor for severity of diagnosis, course, and comorbidity across an array of disorders, including, but not limited to, anxiety, substance use, depressive, and psychotic disorders. The specifier *with panic attacks* may therefore be used for panic attacks that occur in the context of any anxiety disorder, as well as other mental disorders (e.g., depressive disorders, posttraumatic stress disorder).

5.4—chapter introduction (pp. 215–216)

5.5   The determination of whether a panic attack is expected or unexpected is ultimately best made by which of the following?

   A. Careful clinical judgment.
   B. Whether the patient associates it with external stress.
   C. The presence or absence of nocturnal panic attacks.
   D. Ruling out possible culture-specific syndromes.

Correct Answer: A. Careful clinical judgment.

Explanation: The term *unexpected* refers to a panic attack for which there is no obvious cue or trigger at the time of occurrence—that is, the attack appears to occur from out of the blue, such as when the individual is relaxing or emerging from sleep (nocturnal panic attack). In contrast, *expected* panic attacks are those for which there is an obvious cue or trigger, such as a situation in which panic attacks have typically occurred. The determination of whether panic attacks are expected or unexpected is made by the clinician, who makes this judgment on the basis of a combination of careful questioning as to the sequence of events preceding or leading up to the attack and the individual's own judgment of whether the attack seemed to occur for no apparent reason. Cultural interpretations may influence the assignment of panic attacks as expected or unexpected (see section "Culture-Related Diagnostic Issues" for this disorder). In the United States and Europe, approximately half of individuals with panic disorder have expected panic attacks as well as unexpected panic attacks.

5.5—Panic Disorder / Diagnostic Features (p. 236)

5.6   Which of the following forms of panic disorder can be triggered by interpersonal arguments?

   A. *Khyâl* attacks.
   B. *Trúng gió* attacks.

C. *Ataque de nervios.*

D. Soul loss.

Correct Answer: C. *Ataque de nervios.*

Explanation: The rate of fears about mental and somatic symptoms of anxiety appears to vary across cultural contexts and may influence the rate of panic attacks and panic disorder. Also, cultural expectations may influence the classification of panic attacks as expected or unexpected. For example, a Vietnamese individual who has a panic attack after walking out into a windy environment (*trúng gió;* "hit by the wind") may attribute the panic attack to exposure to wind as a result of the cultural syndrome that links these two experiences, resulting in classification of the panic attack as expected. Various other cultural concepts of distress are associated with panic disorder, including *ataque de nervios* ("attack of nerves") among Latin Americans and *khyâl* attacks and "soul loss" among Cambodians. *Ataque de nervios* may involve trembling, uncontrollable screaming or crying, aggressive or suicidal behavior, and depersonalization or derealization, which may be experienced longer than the few minutes typical of panic attacks. Some clinical presentations of *ataque de nervios* fulfill criteria for conditions other than panic attack (e.g., functional neurological symptom disorder). These concepts of distress have an impact on the symptoms and frequency of panic disorder, including the individual's attribution of unexpectedness, because cultural concepts of distress may create fear of certain situations, ranging from interpersonal arguments (associated with *ataque de nervios*) to types of exertion (associated with *khyâl* attacks) to atmospheric wind (associated with *trúng gió* attacks). Clarification of the details of cultural attributions may aid in distinguishing expected and unexpected panic attacks.

Panic disorder is not diagnosed if the panic attacks are judged to be a direct physiological consequence of a substance. Intoxication with central nervous system stimulants (e.g., cocaine, amphetamine-type substances, caffeine) or cannabis and withdrawal from central nervous system depressants (e.g., alcohol, barbiturates) can precipitate a panic attack.

5.6—Panic Disorder / Cultural-Related Diagnostic Issues (p. 239)

5.7   A 50-year-old man reports occasional episodes in which he suddenly and unexpectedly awakens from sleep feeling a surge of intense fear that peaks within minutes. He feels short of breath and experiences heart palpitations and sweating. His medical history is significant only for hypertension, which is well controlled with hydrochlorothiazide. As a result of these symptoms, he has begun to have anticipatory anxiety associated with going to sleep. What is the most likely explanation for his symptoms?

A. Anxiety disorder due to another medical condition (hypertension).

B. Substance/medication-induced anxiety disorder.

C. Nocturnal panic attacks.

D. Sleep terrors.

Correct Answer: C. Nocturnal panic attacks.

Explanation: Panic disorder is characterized by recurrent unexpected panic attacks (Criterion A). A *panic attack* is an abrupt surge of intense fear or intense discomfort that reaches a peak within minutes and during which time 4 or more of a list of 13 physical and cognitive symptoms occur. The term *recurrent* means more than one unexpected panic attack. A *nocturnal* panic attack (i.e., waking from sleep in a state of panic) differs from panicking after fully waking from sleep. In the United States, nocturnal panic attack has been estimated to occur at least one time in roughly one-quarter to one-third of individuals with panic disorder, of whom the majority also have daytime panic attacks. Individuals with both daytime and nocturnal panic attacks tend to have more severe panic disorder overall.

5.7—Panic Disorder / diagnostic criteria; Diagnostic Features (pp. 236–237)

5.8   Which of the following is predictive of suicidal behavior in patients with panic disorder?

A. Derealization.
B. Nausea.
C. Anxiety due to another medical condition.
D. Illness anxiety disorder.

Correct Answer: B. Nausea.

Explanation: Panic attacks and a diagnosis of panic disorder in the past 12 months are related to a higher rate of suicidal behavior and suicidal thoughts in the past 12 months even when comorbidity and a history of childhood abuse and other suicide risk factors are taken into account. Approximately 25% of primary care patients with panic disorder report suicidal thoughts. Panic disorder may increase risk for future suicidal behaviors but not deaths.

Epidemiological survey data of panic attack symptoms show that the cognitive symptoms of panic (e.g., derealization) may be associated with suicidal thoughts, whereas physical symptoms (e.g., dizziness, nausea) may be associated with suicidal behaviors.

5.8—Panic Disorder / Association With Suicidal Thoughts or Behavior (p. 240)

5.9   A 65-year-old woman reports being housebound despite being in good physical health. She fell several years ago while shopping but was not injured. Physical examination reveals no problems with mobility or balance. She experiences panic every time she leaves her house unaccompanied. Her distress is absent when she is home; however, she avoids taking the bus to shop for groceries without a companion. What is the most likely diagnosis?

A. Specific phobia, situational type.

B. Social anxiety disorder (social phobia).

C. Posttraumatic stress disorder.

D. Agoraphobia.

Correct Answer: D. Agoraphobia.

Explanation: The essential feature of agoraphobia is marked fear or anxiety triggered by the real or anticipated exposure to a wide range of situations (Criterion A). The diagnosis requires endorsement of symptoms occurring in at least two of the following five situations: 1) using public transportation, such as automobiles, buses, trains, ships, or planes; 2) being in open spaces, such as parking lots, marketplaces, or bridges; 3) being in enclosed spaces, such as shops, theaters, or cinemas; 4) standing in line or being in a crowd; or 5) being outside the home alone.

5.9—Agoraphobia / diagnostic criteria; Diagnostic Features (pp. 246–247)

5.10   A 32-year-old man has regularly experienced panic attacks with palpitations, nausea, headaches, shortness of breath, dizziness, derealization, and fear of dying when out of his home alone. These episodes occur when he stands in line to take the bus and while he is on the bus. He now works only from home for fear of experiencing these attacks, despite loss of income due to remote work. What is the most appropriate diagnosis?

A. Panic disorder with agoraphobia.

B. Agoraphobia with panic attacks.

C. Specific phobia, situational type.

D. Two separate disorders: panic disorder and agoraphobia.

Correct Answer: D. Two separate disorders: panic disorder and agoraphobia.

Explanation: This man has panic disorder and agoraphobia. Agoraphobia is diagnosed irrespective of the presence of panic disorder. If an individual's presentation meets criteria for panic disorder and agoraphobia, both diagnoses should be assigned.

5.10—Agoraphobia / diagnostic criteria / Diagnostic Features (pp. 241–247)

5.11   A 35-year-old man lost a high-paying job because it required frequent long-range traveling. Two years earlier he had been on a particularly turbulent flight. He was convinced that the pilot minimized the risk and that the plane almost crashed. His coworker repeatedly told him that her experience of the flight was that it was only mildly uncomfortable. He flew again 1 month later, and despite having a smooth flight, the anticipation of turbulence was so distressing that he experienced overwhelming anxiety during the flight. He has not flown since and becomes extremely anxious when the possibility of flying is raised. What is the most appropriate diagnosis?

A. Agoraphobia.
B. Posttraumatic stress disorder (PTSD).
C. Specific phobia, situational type.
D. Social anxiety disorder (social phobia).

Correct Answer: C. Specific phobia, situational type.

Explanation: A key feature of specific phobia is that the fear or anxiety is circumscribed to the presence of a particular situation or object (Criterion A), which may be termed the *phobic stimulus.* The categories of feared situations or objects are provided as specifiers. Many individuals fear objects or situations from more than one category or phobic stimulus. For the diagnosis of specific phobia, the response must differ from normal, transient fears that commonly occur in the population. To meet the criteria for a diagnosis, the fear or anxiety must be intense or severe (i.e., "marked") (Criterion A). The amount of fear experienced may vary with proximity to the feared object or situation and may occur in anticipation of or in the actual presence of the object or situation. Also, the fear or anxiety may take the form of a full or limited symptom panic attack (i.e., expected panic attack). Another characteristic of specific phobias is that fear or anxiety is evoked nearly every time the individual comes into contact with the phobic stimulus (Criterion B). Thus, an individual who becomes anxious only occasionally when confronted with the situation or object (e.g., becomes anxious when flying only on one out of every five airplane flights) would not be diagnosed with specific phobia. However, the degree of fear or anxiety expressed may vary (from anticipatory anxiety to a full panic attack) across different occasions of encountering the phobic object or situation because of various contextual factors, such as the presence of others, duration of exposure, and other threatening elements (e.g., turbulence on a flight).

Situational specific phobia may resemble agoraphobia in its clinical presentation, given the overlap in feared situations (e.g., flying, enclosed places, elevators). If an individual fears only one of the agoraphobic situations, then specific phobia, situational, may be diagnosed.

If the situations are feared because of negative evaluation, social anxiety disorder should be diagnosed instead of specific phobia. Individuals with specific phobia may experience panic attacks when confronted with their feared situation or object. A diagnosis of specific phobia would be given if the panic attacks occur only in response to the specific object or situation, whereas a diagnosis of panic disorder would be given if the individual also experiences panic attacks that are unexpected (i.e., not in response to the specific phobia object or situation). If the phobia develops following a traumatic event, PTSD should be considered as a diagnosis. However, traumatic events can precede the onset of PTSD and specific phobia. In this case, a diagnosis of specific phobia would be assigned only if all of the criteria for PTSD are not met.

5.11—Specific Phobia / diagnostic criteria; Diagnostic Features (pp. 224–226) and Differential Diagnosis (pp. 228–229)

5.12 Which of the following types of specific phobia is most likely to be associated with vasovagal fainting?

A. Animal type.
B. Natural environment type.
C. Blood-injection-injury type.
D. Situational type.

Correct Answer: C. Blood-injection-injury type.

Explanation: Individuals with specific phobia typically experience an increase in physiological arousal in anticipation of or during exposure to a phobic object or situation. However, the physiological response to the feared situation or object varies. Whereas individuals with situational, natural environment, and animal specific phobias are likely to show sympathetic nervous system arousal, individuals with blood-injection-injury specific phobia often demonstrate a vasovagal fainting or near-fainting response that is marked by initial brief acceleration of heart rate and elevation of blood pressure followed by a deceleration of heart rate and a drop in blood pressure.

5.12—Specific Phobia / Associated Features (p. 226)

5.13 Although onset of a specific phobia can occur at any age, specific phobias most typically develop during which age period?

A. Childhood.
B. Late adolescence to early adulthood.
C. Middle age.
D. Old age.

Correct Answer: A. Childhood.

Explanation: Specific phobia usually develops in early childhood, with the majority of cases developing prior to age 10 years. Median age at onset is between 7 and 11 years, with the mean at about 10 years. Situational specific phobias tend to have a later age at onset than natural environment, animal, or blood-injection-injury specific phobias. Specific phobias that develop in childhood and adolescence are likely to wax and wane during that period. However, phobias that do persist into adulthood are unlikely to remit for the majority of individuals.

5.13—Specific Phobia / Development and Course (pp. 226–227)

5.14   In social anxiety disorder, the object of an individual's fear is the potential for which of the following?

    A. Social or occupational impairment.
    B. Harm to self or others.
    C. Scrutiny by others.
    D. Separation from objects of attachment.

Correct Answer: C. Scrutiny by others.

Explanation: The essential feature of social anxiety disorder is a marked, or intense, fear or anxiety of social situations in which the individual may be scrutinized by others. In children the fear or anxiety must occur in peer settings and not just during interactions with adults (Criterion A). When exposed to such social situations, the individual fears that they will be negatively evaluated. The individual is concerned that they will be judged as anxious, weak, crazy, stupid, boring, intimidating, dirty, or unlikable. The individual fears that they will act or appear in a certain way or show anxiety symptoms, such as blushing, trembling, sweating, stumbling over one's words, or staring, that will be negatively evaluated by others.

5.14—Social Anxiety Disorder / Diagnostic Features (pp. 230–231)

5.15   When called on at school, a 7-year-old boy will only nod or write in response. The family of the child is surprised to hear this from the teacher because the boy speaks normally when at home with his parents. The child has achieved appropriate developmental milestones, and a medical evaluation indicates that he is healthy. The boy is unable to give any explanation for his behavior, but the parents are concerned that it will affect his school performance. What diagnosis best fits this child's symptoms?

    A. Separation anxiety disorder.
    B. Autism spectrum disorder.
    C. Agoraphobia.
    D. Selective mutism.

Correct Answer: D. Selective mutism.

Explanation: When encountering other individuals in social interactions, children with selective mutism do not initiate speech or reciprocally respond when spoken to by others. Lack of speech occurs in social interactions with children or adults. Children with selective mutism will speak in their home in the presence of immediate family members but often not even in front of close friends or second-degree relatives, such as grandparents or cousins. The disturbance is most often marked by high social anxiety. Children with selective mutism often refuse to speak at school, leading to academic or educational impairment because teachers often find it difficult to assess skills such as reading. The lack of speech may interfere with social communication, although children with this disorder sometimes use nonspoken or nonverbal means (e.g., grunting, pointing, writing) to communicate and may be willing or eager to perform or engage in social encounters when speech is not required (e.g., nonverbal parts in school plays).

5.15—Selective Mutism / Diagnostic Features (p. 222)

5.16 Social anxiety disorder differs from normative shyness in that the disorder leads to which of the following?

A. Social or occupational dysfunction.
B. Higher probability of long-term relationships.
C. Higher probability of being associated with immigrant status.
D. Anxiety at home but not in school for children.

Correct Answer: A. Social or occupational dysfunction.

Explanation: Shyness (i.e., social reticence) is a common personality trait and is not by itself pathological. In some societies, shyness is even evaluated positively. However, when there is a significant adverse impact on social, occupational, and other important areas of functioning, a diagnosis of social anxiety disorder should be considered, and when full diagnostic criteria for social anxiety disorder are met, the disorder should be diagnosed. Only a minority (12%) of self-identified shy individuals in the United States have symptoms that meet diagnostic criteria for social anxiety disorder. Immigrant status is associated with lower rates of social anxiety disorder in both Latinx and non-Latinx white groups. Age at onset of social anxiety disorder does not differ by gender. Women with social anxiety disorder report a greater number of social fears and comorbid major depressive disorder and other anxiety disorders, whereas men are more likely to fear dating; have oppositional defiant disorder, conduct disorder, or antisocial personality disorder; and use alcohol and illicit drugs to relieve symptoms of the disorder.

5.16—Social Anxiety Disorder / diagnostic criteria / Differential Diagnosis / Culture-Related Diagnostic Issues / Sex- and Gender-Related Issues (pp. 229–233)

5.17 In addition to anxiety and worry, individuals with generalized anxiety disorder are most likely to experience which of the following symptoms?

A. Dizziness.
B. Tachycardia.

C. Muscle tension.
D. Shortness of breath.

Correct Answer: C. Muscle tension.

Explanation: The anxiety and worry of generalized anxiety disorder are accompanied by at least three of the following additional symptoms: restlessness or feeling keyed up or on edge, being easily fatigued, difficulty concentrating or mind going blank, irritability, muscle tension, and disturbed sleep, although only one additional symptom is required in children. Trembling, twitching, feeling shaky, and muscle aches or soreness may be associated with muscle tension. Many individuals with generalized anxiety disorder also experience somatic symptoms (e.g., sweating, nausea, diarrhea) and an exaggerated startle response. Symptoms of autonomic hyperarousal (e.g., accelerated heart rate, shortness of breath, dizziness) are less prominent in generalized anxiety disorder than in other anxiety disorders, such as panic disorder. Other conditions that may be associated with stress (e.g., irritable bowel syndrome, headaches) frequently accompany generalized anxiety disorder.

5.17—Generalized Anxiety Disorder / Diagnostic Features / Associated Features (p. 251)

5.18   Which of the following characteristics is suggestive of generalized anxiety disorder in children who have the disorder?

A. Complaining of feeling restless.
B. Being lax with schoolwork.
C. Often being late for appointments.
D. Seeking frequent reassurance from others.

Correct Answer: D. Seeking frequent reassurance from others.

Explanation: In children and adolescents with generalized anxiety disorder, the anxieties and worries often concern the quality of their performance or competence at school or in sporting events, even when their performance is not being evaluated by others. They may have excessive concerns about punctuality. They may also worry about catastrophic events, such as earthquakes or nuclear war. Children with the disorder may be overly conforming, perfectionistic, and unsure of themselves and may tend to redo tasks because of excessive dissatisfaction with less-than-perfect performance. They may be overzealous in seeking reassurance and approval and require excessive reassurance about their performance and other things they are worried about.

Everyday worries are much less likely to be accompanied by physical symptoms (e.g., restlessness, feeling keyed up or on edge). Individuals with generalized anxiety disorder report subjective distress as a result of constant worry and related impairment in social, occupational, or other important areas of functioning.

5.18—Generalized Anxiety Disorder / Diagnostic Features / Development and Course (pp. 251–252)

5.19   What is the primary difference in the clinical expression of generalized anxiety disorder across age groups?

A. Content of worry.
B. Degree of worry.
C. Patterns of comorbidity.
D. Predominance of cognitive versus somatic symptoms.

Correct Answer: A. Content of worry.

Explanation: The clinical expression of generalized anxiety disorder is relatively consistent across the life span. The primary difference across age groups is in the content of the individual's worry. The content of an individual's worry tends to be age appropriate.

5.19—Generalized Anxiety Disorder / Development and Course (p. 252)

5.20   In what aspect of generalized anxiety disorder do men and women most commonly differ?

A. Course.
B. Symptom profile.
C. Degree of impairment.
D. Patterns of comorbidity.

Correct Answer: D. Patterns of comorbidity.

Explanation: In clinical settings, generalized anxiety disorder is diagnosed somewhat more frequently in women than in men (about 55%–60% of those presenting with the disorder are women). In epidemiological studies, approximately two-thirds are women. Women and men who experience generalized anxiety disorder appear to have similar symptoms but demonstrate different patterns of comorbidity consistent with gender differences in the prevalence of disorders. In women, comorbidity is confined largely to the anxiety disorders and unipolar depression, whereas in men, comorbidity is more likely to extend to the substance use disorders as well.

5.20—Generalized Anxiety Disorder / Sex- and Gender-Related Diagnostic Issues (p. 253)

5.21 Which of the following is more suggestive of nonpathological anxiety as opposed to anxiety that qualifies for a diagnosis of generalized anxiety disorder?

A. Anxiety and worry that interfere significantly with functioning.
B. Anxiety and worry that last for months to years.
C. Anxiety and worry in response to a clear precipitant.
D. Anxiety and worry focused on a wide range of life circumstances.

Correct Answer: C. Anxiety and worry in response to a clear precipitant.

Explanation: Several features distinguish generalized anxiety disorder from nonpathological anxiety. First, the worries associated with generalized anxiety disorder are excessive and typically interfere significantly with psychosocial functioning, whereas the worries of everyday life are not excessive and are perceived as more manageable and may be put off when more pressing matters arise. Second, the worries associated with generalized anxiety disorder are more pervasive, pronounced, and distressing; have longer duration; and frequently occur without precipitants. The greater the range of life circumstances about which a person worries (e.g., finances, children's safety, job performance), the more likely their symptoms are to meet criteria for generalized anxiety disorder. Third, everyday worries are much less likely to be accompanied by physical symptoms (e.g., restlessness, feeling keyed up or on edge). Individuals with generalized anxiety disorder report subjective distress as a result of constant worry and related impairment in social, occupational, or other important areas of functioning.

5.21—Generalized Anxiety Disorder / Diagnostic Features (p. 251)

5.22 A 26-year-old man is brought to the emergency department suffering from a sudden, severe surge of panic. He has no history of panic disorder, but he reports taking several doses of an over-the-counter cold medication earlier that day. Which of the following clinical features, if present in this case, would help to confirm a diagnosis of substance/medication-induced anxiety disorder?

A. Symptoms that are mild and do not impair functioning.
B. Symptoms that do not develop for a long time after the substance or medication use.
C. Symptoms that are in excess of what would be expected for the substance or medication.
D. Lack of any prior history of anxiety disorder or panic symptoms.

Correct Answer: D. Lack of any prior history of anxiety disorder or panic symptoms.

Explanation: The essential features of substance/medication-induced anxiety disorder are prominent symptoms of panic or anxiety (Criterion A) that are judged to be due to the effects of a substance (e.g., a drug of abuse, a medication, a toxin exposure). The panic or anxiety symptoms must have developed during or soon after substance intoxication or withdrawal or after exposure to or withdrawal from a medication, and the substances or medications must be capable of producing the symptoms (Criterion B2). Substance/medication-induced anxiety disorder due to a prescribed treatment for a mental disorder or another medical condition must have its onset while the individual is receiving the medication (or during withdrawal, if withdrawal is associated with the medication). Once the treatment is discontinued, the panic or anxiety symptoms will usually improve or remit within days to several weeks to a month (depending on the half-life of the substance or medication and the presence of withdrawal). The diagnosis of substance/medication-induced anxiety disorder should not be given if the onset of the panic or anxiety symptoms precedes the substance/medication intoxication or withdrawal or if the symptoms persist for a substantial period of time (i.e., usually longer than 1 month) from the time of severe intoxication or withdrawal. If the panic or anxiety symptoms persist for substantial periods of time, other causes for the symptoms should be considered.

Diagnosis of substance/medication-induced anxiety disorder should be made instead of a diagnosis of substance intoxication or substance withdrawal only when the symptoms in Criterion A are predominant in the clinical picture and are sufficiently severe to warrant independent clinical attention.

5.22—Substance / Medication-Induced Anxiety Disorder / diagnostic criteria, Diagnostic Features, and Differential Diagnosis (pp. 255–258)

5.23   In which of the following circumstances would a diagnosis of substance/medication-induced anxiety disorder be appropriate rather than a diagnosis of substance withdrawal?

A. Significant anxiety symptoms are present.
B. Anxiety was not present prior to stopping the medication.
C. Anxiety is present that is sufficiently severe to warrant independent clinical attention.
D. Anxiety is present only during bouts of delirium.

Correct Answer: C. Anxiety is present that is sufficiently severe to warrant independent clinical attention.

Explanation: Anxiety symptoms commonly occur in substance intoxication and substance withdrawal. The diagnosis of substance-specific intoxication or substance-specific withdrawal will usually suffice to categorize the symptom presentation. Panic or anxiety symptoms are characteristic of alcohol withdrawal, but a diagnosis of substance/medication-induced anxiety disorder either with onset during intoxication or with onset during withdrawal should be made instead of a diagnosis of substance intoxication or substance withdrawal when the panic or anxiety symptoms are predominant in the clinical picture and are sufficiently severe to warrant clinical attention.

The diagnosis of substance/medication-induced anxiety disorder should be made instead of a diagnosis of substance intoxication or substance withdrawal only when the symptoms in Criterion A are predominant in the clinical picture and are sufficiently severe to warrant independent clinical attention.

5.23—Substance/Medication-Induced Anxiety Disorder/Differential Diagnosis (p. 258)

5.24   A 60-year-old man has just been diagnosed with congestive heart failure and pulmonary edema. He describes himself as intensely anxious and reports feeling as if he cannot breathe, which he describes as "a panic attack." Which of the following features would support a diagnosis of anxiety disorder due to another medical condition rather than adjustment disorder with anxiety?

A. The patient says he does not know why he is anxious because knowing his diagnosis does not worry him.
B. The patient has no anxiety-associated physical symptoms.
C. The patient is focused on what it means that he has a cardiac disorder.
D. The patient is delirious.

Correct Answer: A. The patient says he does not know why he is anxious because knowing his diagnosis does not worry him.

Explanation: The essential feature of anxiety disorder due to another medical condition is clinically significant anxiety that is judged to be best explained as a physiological effect of another medical condition. Symptoms can include prominent anxiety symptoms or panic attacks (Criterion A). The judgment that the symptoms are best explained by the associated physical condition must be based on evidence from the history, physical examination, or laboratory findings (Criterion B). Additionally, it must be judged that the symptoms are not better accounted for by another mental disorder (Criterion C)—in particular, adjustment disorder with anxiety, in which the stressor is the medical condition. In this case, an individual with adjustment disorder is especially distressed about the meaning or the consequences of the associated medical condition. By contrast, there is often a prominent physical component to the anxiety (e.g., shortness of breath) when the anxiety is due to another medical condition. The diagnosis is not made if the anxiety symptoms occur only during the course of a delirium (Criterion D). The anxiety symptoms must cause clinically significant distress or impairment in social, occupational, or other important areas of functioning (Criterion E).

In determining whether the anxiety symptoms are attributable to another medical condition, the clinician must first establish the presence of the medical condition. Furthermore, it must be established that anxiety symptoms can be etiologically related to the medical condition through a physiological mechanism before making a judgment that this is the best explanation for the symptoms in a specific individual. A careful and comprehensive assessment of multiple factors is necessary to make this judgment. Several aspects of the clinical presentation should be considered: 1) the presence of a clear temporal association between the onset, exacerbation, or remission of the medical condition and the anxiety symptoms; 2) the presence of features that are atypical of an independent anxiety disorder (e.g., atypical age at onset or course); and 3) evidence in the literature that a known physiological mechanism (e.g., hyperthyroidism) causes anxiety. In addition, the disturbance must not be better explained by an independent anxiety disorder, a substance/medication-induced anxiety disorder, or another mental disorder (e.g., adjustment disorder).

A number of medical conditions are known to include anxiety as a symptomatic manifestation. Examples include endocrine disease (e.g., hyperthyroidism, pheochromocytoma, hypoglycemia, hyperadrenocortisolism), cardiovascular disorders (e.g., congestive heart failure, pulmonary embolism, arrhythmia such as atrial fibrillation), respiratory illness (e.g., chronic obstructive pulmonary disease, asthma, pneumonia), metabolic disturbances (e.g., vitamin B_{12} deficiency, porphyria), and neurological illness (e.g., neoplasms, vestibular dysfunction, encephalitis, seizure disorders).

5.24—Anxiety Disorder Due to Another Medical Condition / Diagnostic Features (p. 259); Differential Diagnosis (pp. 260–261)

5.25 Which of the following anxiety disorders is most associated with a transition from suicidal thoughts to suicide attempts?

A. Separation anxiety disorder.
B. Agoraphobia.
C. Selective mutism.
D. Generalized anxiety disorder.

Correct answer: D. Generalized anxiety disorder.

Explanation: Individuals with anxiety may be more likely to have suicidal thoughts, attempt suicide, and die from suicide than are those without anxiety. Panic disorder, generalized anxiety disorder, and specific phobia have been identified as the anxiety disorders most strongly associated with a transition from suicidal thoughts to suicide attempt.

5.25—Anxiety Disorders / chapter introduction (pp. 215–216)

CHAPTER 6

Obsessive-Compulsive and Related Disorders

6.1   How are compulsions defined in obsessive-compulsive disorder (OCD)?

   A. Compulsions in OCD are typically goal-directed, fulfilling a realistic purpose.
   B. Compulsions include paraphilias (sexual compulsions) and addictive behaviors such as gambling or substance use.
   C. Compulsions involve repetitive and persistent thoughts, images, or urges.
   D. Compulsions in OCD are aimed at reducing the distress triggered by obsessions.

Correct Answer: D. Compulsions in OCD are aimed at reducing the distress triggered by obsessions.

Explanation: *Obsessions* are repetitive and persistent thoughts (e.g., of contamination), images (e.g., of violent or horrific scenes), or urges (e.g., to stab someone). *Compulsions* (or rituals) are repetitive behaviors (e.g., washing, checking) or mental acts (e.g., counting, repeating words silently) that the individual feels driven to perform in response to an obsession or according to rules that must be applied rigidly. Most individuals with OCD have both obsessions and compulsions. Compulsions are typically performed in response to an obsession (e.g., thoughts of contamination leading to washing rituals or that something is incorrect leading to repeating rituals until it feels "just right"). The aim is to reduce the distress triggered by obsessions or to prevent a feared event (e.g., becoming ill). However, these compulsions either are not connected in a realistic way to the feared event (e.g., arranging items symmetrically to prevent harm to a loved one) or are clearly excessive (e.g., showering for hours each day). Compulsions are not done for pleasure, although some individuals experience relief from anxiety or distress.

   Certain behaviors are sometimes described as "compulsive," including sexual behavior (in the case of paraphilias), gambling (i.e., gambling disorder), and substance use (e.g., alcohol use disorder). However, these behaviors differ from the compulsions of OCD in that the person usually derives pleasure from the activity and may wish to resist it only because of its deleterious consequences.

6.1—Obsessive-Compulsive Disorder / diagnostic criteria (p. 265); Diagnostic Features (pp. 266–267); Differential Diagnosis (pp. 270–271)

6.2   A 52-year-old man with raw, chapped hands is referred to a psychiatrist by his primary care doctor. The man reports that he washes his hands repeatedly, spending up to 4 hours a day, using abrasive cleansers and scalding hot water. Although he admits that his hands are uncomfortable, he is entirely convinced that unless he washes in this manner he will become gravely ill. A medical workup is unrevealing, and the man takes no medications. What is the most appropriate diagnosis?

A. Delusional disorder, somatic type.
B. Illness anxiety disorder.
C. Obsessive-compulsive disorder (OCD), with absent insight.
D. Factitious disorder.

Correct Answer: C. Obsessive-compulsive disorder (OCD), with absent insight.

Explanation: Obsessive-compulsive and related disorders that have a cognitive component (i.e., OCD, body dysmorphic disorder, and hoarding disorder) include a specifier for indicating the individual's degree of insight with respect to disorder-related beliefs. Individuals with OCD vary in the degree of insight they have about the accuracy of the beliefs that underlie their obsessive-compulsive symptoms. Many individuals have good or fair insight (e.g., the individual believes that the house definitely will not, probably will not, or might or might not burn down if the stove is not checked 30 times). Some have poor insight (e.g., the individual believes that the house will probably burn down if the stove is not checked 30 times), and a few (4% or less) have absent insight or delusional beliefs (e.g., the individual is convinced that the house will burn down if the stove is not checked 30 times).

Some individuals with OCD have poor insight or even delusional OCD beliefs. However, they have obsessions and compulsions (distinguishing their condition from delusional disorder) and do not have other features of schizophrenia or schizoaffective disorder (e.g., hallucinations or disorganized speech). For individuals whose OCD symptoms warrant the *with absent insight/delusional beliefs* specifier, these symptoms should not be diagnosed as a psychotic disorder.

In DSM-5-TR, if the delusional belief is limited to the obsessions and compulsions, a separate psychotic disorder diagnosis is not required. Individuals with illness anxiety disorder worry about having an illness; however, they do not have the classic obsessions and compulsions found in OCD.

Dermatitis artefacta (also referred to as factitious dermatitis) is a term used in dermatology to refer to medically unexplained, presumably self-induced skin lesions that the individual denies any role in creating. Cases in which there is evidence of deception on the individual's part concerning the skin lesions can be diagnosed as either malingering (if the skin picking is motivated by external incentives) or factitious disorder (if the skin picking occurs in the absence of obvious external rewards). In the absence of deception, excoriation disorder can be diagnosed if there are repeated attempts to decrease or stop skin picking.

6.2—Obsessive-Compulsive Disorder / Specifiers (p. 266) and Differential Diagnosis (pp. 270–271); Excoriation (Skin-Picking) Disorder / Differential Diagnosis (p. 287)

6.3   In obsessive-compulsive disorder (OCD), which of the following is more likely to be seen in men than women?

A. Comorbid tics.
B. Later age of onset.
C. Obsession with cleaning.
D. Hormonal symptom associations.

Correct Answer: A. Comorbid tics.

Explanation: Men have an earlier age at onset of OCD than women, often in childhood, and are more likely to have comorbid tic disorders. Onset in girls is more typically in adolescence; among adults, OCD is slightly more common in women than in men. Gender differences in the pattern of symptom dimensions have been reported, with, for example, women more likely to have symptoms in the cleaning dimension and men more likely to have symptoms in the forbidden thoughts and symmetry dimensions. Onset or exacerbation of OCD, as well as symptoms that can interfere with the mother-infant relationship (e.g., aggressive obsessions such as intrusive violent thoughts of harming the infant, leading to avoidance of the infant), has been reported in the peripartum period. Some women also report exacerbation of OCD symptoms premenstrually.

6.3—Obsessive-Compulsive Disorder / Sex- and Gender-Related Diagnostic Issues (pp. 268–269)

6.4   A 63-year-old woman has been saving financial documents and records for decades, placing papers in piles throughout her apartment to the point where it has become unsafe. She acknowledges that the piles are a concern; however, she says that the papers include important documents and she is afraid to throw them away. She recalls a previous instance when her taxes were audited and she needed certain documents to avoid a penalty. She describes repetitive worries about a new audit with an inability to ignore these worries. She feels somewhat reassured by her growing pile of legal paperwork but notes concern because her landlord is threatening to evict her unless she removes the piles of papers. What is the most likely diagnosis?

A. Nonpathological collecting behavior.
B. Hoarding disorder.

C. Obsessive-compulsive disorder (OCD).
D. Dementia (major neurocognitive disorder).

Correct Answer: C. Obsessive-compulsive disorder (OCD).

Explanation: Hoarding disorder symptoms focus exclusively on the persistent difficulty discarding or parting with possessions, marked distress associated with discarding items, and excessive accumulation of objects. However, if an individual has obsessions that are typical of OCD (e.g., concerns about incompleteness or harm) and these obsessions lead to compulsive accumulation (e.g., acquiring all objects in a set to attain a sense of completeness or not discarding old newspapers because they may contain information that could prevent harm), a diagnosis of OCD should be given instead.

Hoarding disorder is not diagnosed if the symptoms are judged to be a direct consequence of typical obsessions or compulsions, such as fears of contamination or harm or feelings of incompleteness in OCD. Feelings of incompleteness (e.g., losing one's identity; having to document and preserve all life experiences) are the most frequent OCD symptoms associated with this form of hoarding.

6.4—Obsessive-Compulsive Disorder / Differential Diagnosis (pp. 270–271); Hoarding Disorder / Differential Diagnosis (pp. 280–281)

6.5   Which of the following is a protective factor for suicide risk associated with obsessive-compulsive disorder (OCD)?

A. Male gender.
B. Religious obsessions.
C. Substance abuse.
D. Comorbid anxiety disorder.

Correct Answer: D. Comorbid anxiety disorder.

Explanation: A systematic literature review of suicidal ideation and suicide attempts in clinical samples of individuals with OCD from multiple countries found a mean rate of lifetime suicide attempts of 14.2%, a mean rate of lifetime suicidal ideation of 44.1%, and a mean rate of current suicidal ideation of 25.9%. Predictors of greater suicide risk were severity of OCD, the symptom dimension of unacceptable thoughts, severity of comorbid depressive and anxiety symptoms, and past history of suicidality. Another international systematic review of 48 studies found a moderate to high significant association between suicidal ideation or suicide attempts and OCD.

A cross-sectional study of 582 outpatients with OCD from Brazil found that 36% reported lifetime suicidal thoughts, 20% had made suicide plans, 11% had already attempted suicide, and 10% presented with current suicidal thoughts.

The sexual/religious dimension of OCD and comorbid substance use disorders were associated with suicidal thoughts and suicide plans, impulse-control disorders were associated with current suicidal thoughts and with suicide plans and attempts, and lifetime comorbid major depressive disorder and posttraumatic stress disorder were associated with all aspects of suicidal behaviors.

In a study using Swedish national registry data involving 36,788 individuals with OCD and matched general population control subjects, individuals with OCD had a higher risk of suicide death (OR=9.8) and suicide attempt (OR=5.5), and the increased risk for both outcomes remained substantial even after adjusting for psychiatric comorbidities. Comorbid personality or substance use disorder increased suicide risk, whereas female gender, higher parental education, and a comorbid anxiety disorder were protective factors.

6.5—Obsessive-Compulsive Disorder / Association With Suicidal Thoughts or Behavior (p. 269)

6.6   Which of the following is required for a diagnosis of body dysmorphic disorder (BDD)?

A. An apparent physical defect noticeable by a physician.
B. Repetitive behaviors or thoughts related to concerns about one's appearance.
C. Unhealthy weight loss with the goal of improving one's appearance.
D. Preservation of baseline social, occupational, and general function.

Correct Answer: B. Repetitive behaviors or thoughts related to concerns about one's appearance.

Explanation: Individuals with BDD (formerly known as dysmorphophobia) are preoccupied with one or more perceived defects or flaws in their physical appearance (Criterion A), which they believe is ugly, unattractive, abnormal, or deformed. The perceived flaws are not observable or appear only slight to other individuals. The preoccupations are intrusive, unwanted, time-consuming (occurring, on average, 3–8 hours per day), and usually difficult to resist or control. Excessive repetitive behaviors or mental acts (e.g., comparing) are performed in response to the preoccupation (Criterion B). The individual feels driven to perform these behaviors, which are not pleasurable and may increase anxiety and dysphoria. The preoccupation must cause clinically significant distress or impairment in social, occupational, or other important areas of functioning (Criterion C); usually both distress and impairment are present. BDD must be differentiated from an eating disorder. In BDD, insight may range from good to poor to absent/delusional.

6.6—Body Dysmorphic Disorder / diagnostic criteria (pp. 271–272); Diagnostic Features (pp. 272–273)

6.7   A 25-year-old man is concerned that he looks "weak" and "puny" despite the fact that to neutral observers he appears very muscular. When confronted about his belief, he thinks he is being humored and that people are in fact making fun of his small size behind his back. He has tried a number of strategies to increase muscle mass, including exercising excessively and using anabolic steroids; however, he remains dissatisfied with his appearance. What is the most likely diagnosis?

A. Delusional disorder, somatic type.
B. Body dysmorphic disorder (BDD), with muscle dysmorphia.
C. Body identity integrity disorder.
D. *Koro*.

Correct Answer: B. Body dysmorphic disorder (BDD), with muscle dysmorphia.

Explanation: Muscle dysmorphia, a form of BDD occurring almost exclusively in men and adolescent boys, consists of preoccupation with the idea that one's body is too small or insufficiently lean or muscular. Individuals with this form of the disorder actually have a normal-looking body or are even very muscular. They may also be preoccupied with other body areas, such as skin or hair. A majority (but not all) of these individuals diet, exercise, and/or lift weights excessively, sometimes causing bodily damage. Some use potentially dangerous anabolic-androgenic steroids and other substances to try to make their body bigger and more muscular.

Appearance-related ideas or delusions of reference (i.e., thinking that other people take special notice in a negative way because of one's appearance) are common in BDD. However, unlike schizophrenia or schizoaffective disorder, BDD involves prominent appearance preoccupations and related repetitive behaviors; disorganized behavior and other psychotic symptoms are absent (except for appearance beliefs, which may be delusional).

Body integrity dysphoria (which is included in ICD-11 but not DSM-5) involves a persistent desire to become an amputee in order to correct a mismatch between the individual's sense of how their body should be configured and their actual anatomical configuration. In contrast to BDD, the individual does not feel that the limb to be amputated is ugly or defective in any way, just that it should not be there. *Koro*, a culturally related disorder that usually occurs in epidemics in Southeast Asia, consists of a fear that the penis (labia, nipples, or breasts in females) is shrinking or retracting and will disappear into the abdomen, often accompanied by a belief that death will result. *Koro* differs from body dysmorphic disorder in several ways, including a focus on death rather than preoccupation with perceived ugliness.

6.7—Body Dysmorphic Disorder / Specifiers (p. 272); Differential Diagnosis (pp. 275–277)

6.8   A 19-year-old woman is referred to a psychiatrist by her internist after she admits to him that she recurrently pulls hair from her eyebrows to the point that she has scarring and there is little or no eyebrow hair left. She states that her natural eyebrows are "bushy" and "repulsive" and that she "looks like a caveman." A photograph of the woman before she began pulling her eyebrow hair shows a normal-looking teenager. What is the most appropriate diagnosis?

A. Trichotillomania (hair-pulling disorder).
B. Delusional disorder, somatic type.
C. Body dysmorphic disorder (BDD).
D. Obsessive-compulsive disorder (OCD).

Correct Answer: C. Body dysmorphic disorder (BDD).

Explanation: The preoccupations and repetitive behaviors of BDD differ from obsessions and compulsions in OCD in that the former focus only on physical appearance. These disorders have other differences, such as poorer insight, more frequent depression, and higher rates of suicidal ideation in BDD. When hair removal (plucking, pulling, or other types of removal) is intended to improve perceived defects in the appearance of facial, head, or body hair, BDD is diagnosed rather than trichotillomania (hair-pulling disorder). Appearance-related ideas or delusions of reference (i.e., thinking that other people take special notice in a negative way because of the individual's appearance) are common in BDD. However, unlike schizophrenia or schizoaffective disorder, BDD involves prominent appearance preoccupations and related repetitive behaviors; disorganized behavior and other psychotic symptoms are absent (except for appearance beliefs, which may be delusional). BDD differs from normal appearance concerns in being characterized by excessive appearance-related preoccupations and repetitive behaviors that are time-consuming, are usually difficult to resist or control, and cause clinically significant distress or impairment in functioning

6.8—Body Dysmorphic Disorder / Differential Diagnosis (pp. 275–277)

6.9   A 48-year-old man presents to a psychiatrist along with his husband, stating that he pressured him to seek help. He explains that he likes to collect wine, and he does not see a problem with this; he claims that many of the wines are quite valuable and a potential investment. On further questioning, he admits that he rarely drinks the wines because it "never seems the right time." He has never sold or given away any wine because he finds it hard to part with the bottles. He has filled multiple rooms of his house for storage of the wine, which, along with the financial hardship, is his husband's primary concern. The husband notes that when the patient attempts to discard or sell any of the wine, he bursts into tears. The patient admits that many of the wine bottles have probably spoiled because he cannot afford to properly store the wine and the bottles have sat for years on shelves. What is the most appropriate diagnosis?

A. Narcissistic personality disorder .
B. Obsessive-compulsive disorder (OCD).

C. Delusional disorder.
D. Hoarding disorder, excessive acquisition type.

Correct Answer: D. Hoarding disorder, excessive acquisition type.

Explanation: The essential feature of hoarding disorder is persistent difficulty discarding or parting with possessions, regardless of their actual value (Criterion A). The term *persistent* indicates a long-standing difficulty rather than more transient life circumstances that may lead to excessive clutter, such as inheriting property. The difficulty in discarding possessions noted in Criterion A refers to any form of discarding, including throwing away, selling, giving away, or recycling. Individuals with hoarding disorder purposefully save possessions and experience distress (e.g., anxiety, frustration, regret, sadness, guilt) when facing the prospect of discarding them. Individuals accumulate large numbers of items that fill up and clutter active living areas to the extent that their intended use is no longer possible (Criterion C). Criterion C emphasizes the "active" living areas of the home rather than more peripheral areas, such as garages, attics, or basements, that are sometimes cluttered in homes of individuals without hoarding disorder. Symptoms (i.e., difficulty discarding and/or clutter) must cause clinically significant distress or impairment in social, occupational, or other important areas of functioning, including maintaining a safe environment for self and others (Criterion D).

Approximately 80%–90% of individuals with hoarding disorder also display excessive acquisition in which they collect, buy, or steal objects that are not needed and for which there is no space. In such cases, this is indicated with a specifier. Although persons with OCD may hoard items, they usually experience distress at their inability to throw the objects away, or their storage of the possessions serves some other purpose related to their obsessions (e.g., worrying that they will throw out something important).

6.9—Hoarding Disorder / Specifiers; Diagnostic Features (p. 278)

6.10 A diagnosis of hoarding disorder can still be given even if which of the following is suspected to contribute to the presentation?

A. Prader-Willi syndrome.
B. Focal brain damage.
C. Neurocognitive dysfunction.
D. Family history.

Correct Answer: D. Family history.

Explanation: Hoarding behavior is familial, with about 50% of individuals who hoard reporting having a relative who also hoards. Twin studies indicate that approximately 50% of the variability in hoarding behavior is attributable to additive genetic factors.

Hoarding disorder is not diagnosed if the symptoms are judged to be a direct consequence of another medical condition (Criterion E), such as traumatic brain injury, surgical resection for treatment of a tumor or seizure control, cerebrovascular disease, infections of the CNS (e.g., herpes simplex encephalitis), or neurogenetic conditions such as Prader-Willi syndrome. Damage to the anterior ventromedial prefrontal and cingulate cortices has been particularly associated with the excessive accumulation of objects. Hoarding disorder is not diagnosed if the accumulation of objects is judged to be a direct consequence of a degenerative disorder, such as neurocognitive disorder associated with frontotemporal degeneration or Alzheimer's disease. In such cases, onset of the accumulating behavior is typically gradual and follows onset of the neurocognitive disorder. The accumulating behavior may be accompanied by self-neglect and severe domestic squalor, alongside other neuropsychiatric symptoms.

6.10—Hoarding Disorder / Risk and Prognostic Factors (p. 279); Differential Diagnosis (pp. 280–281)

6.11   Hoarding disorder has the highest prevalence in which population?

A. Men.
B. Adolescents.
C. Elderly adults.
D. Reproductive age women.

Correct Answer: C. Elderly adults.

Explanation: Nationally representative prevalence studies of hoarding disorder are not available. Community surveys estimate the point prevalence of clinically significant hoarding in the United States and Europe to range between 1.5% and 6%. In a meta-analysis of 12 studies across high-income countries, a prevalence of 2.5% was found, with no gender difference identified. This contrasts with clinical samples, which consist predominantly of women. In one population-based study in the Netherlands, hoarding symptoms appeared to be almost three times more prevalent in older adults (older than 65 years) compared with younger adults (ages 30–40 years).

6.11—Hoarding Disorder / Prevalence (p. 279)

6.12   Which of the following would be inconsistent with a diagnosis of trichotillomania (hair-pulling disorder)?

A. Acceptance of hair-pulling behavior as normative.
B. Episodic hair pulling.
C. Failed attempts to reduce hair pulling.
D. Hair pulling in areas covered by clothing.

Correct Answer: A. Acceptance of hair-pulling behavior as normative.

Explanation: The essential feature of trichotillomania (hair-pulling disorder) is the recurrent pulling out of one's own hair (Criterion A). Hair pulling may occur from any region of the body in which hair grows; the most common sites are the scalp, eyebrows, and eyelids, and less common sites are axillary, facial, pubic, and perirectal regions. Hair-pulling sites may vary over time. Hair pulling may occur in brief episodes scattered throughout the day or during less frequent but more sustained periods that can continue for hours, and such hair pulling may endure for months or years. Criterion A requires that hair pulling lead to hair loss, although individuals with this disorder may pull hair in a widely distributed pattern (i.e., pulling single hairs from all over a site) such that hair loss may not be clearly visible. In addition, individuals may attempt to conceal or camouflage hair loss (e.g., by using makeup, scarves, or wigs). Individuals with trichotillomania have made repeated attempts to decrease or stop hair pulling (Criterion B). Criterion C indicates that hair pulling causes clinically significant distress or impairment in social, occupational, or other important areas of functioning. The term *distress* includes negative affects that may be experienced by individuals with hair pulling, such as feeling a loss of control, embarrassment, and shame. Significant impairment may occur in several different areas of functioning (e.g., social, occupational, academic, and leisure), in part because of avoidance of work, school, or other public situations.

6.12—Trichotillomania (Hair-Pulling Disorder) / Diagnostic Features (pp. 281–282)

6.13   Which of the following is *not* associated with trichotillomania (hair-pulling disorder)?

A. Broken hair follicles.
B. Alopecia.
C. Dental damage.
D. Bezoar.

Correct Answer: B. Alopecia.

Explanation: Most individuals with trichotillomania admit to hair pulling; thus, dermatopathological diagnosis is rarely required. Skin biopsy and dermoscopy (or trichoscopy) of trichotillomania are able to differentiate the disorder from other causes of alopecia. In trichotillomania, dermoscopy shows a range of characteristic features, including decreased hair density, short vellus hair, and broken hairs with different shaft lengths.

Trichotillomania is associated with distress as well as with social and occupational impairment. There may be irreversible damage to hair growth and hair quality. Infrequent medical consequences of trichotillomania include digit purpura, musculoskeletal injury (e.g., carpal tunnel syndrome; back, shoulder and neck pain), blepharitis, and dental damage (e.g., worn or broken teeth resulting from hair biting). Swallowing of hair (trichophagia) may lead to trichobezoars, with subsequent anemia, abdominal pain, hematemesis, nausea and vomiting, bowel obstruction, and even bowel perforation.

6.13—Trichotillomania (Hair-Pulling Disorder) / Diagnostic Markers; Functional Consequences of Trichotillomania (Hair-Pulling Disorder) (p. 283)

6.14   A 25-year-old man is referred to a psychiatrist by his primary care doctor after mentioning to the doctor that he routinely spends a lot of time pulling out facial hair with tweezers, even after carefully shaving. On evaluation, he admits to frequent pulling of his facial hair, consuming a significant amount of time; he explains that he becomes anxious when looking at himself because his mustache, hairline, and sideburns are asymmetrical. He pulls out hairs in an effort to make his facial hair more symmetrical but is rarely satisfied with the results. He finds this very upsetting but cannot resist the urge to try to "fix" his facial hair. What is the most appropriate diagnosis?

A. Trichotillomania (hair-pulling disorder).
B. Body dysmorphic disorder (BDD).
C. Delusional disorder, somatic type.
D. Obsessive-compulsive disorder (OCD).

Correct Answer: D. Obsessive-compulsive disorder (OCD).

Explanation: Individuals with OCD and symmetry concerns may pull out hairs as part of their symmetry rituals, and individuals with BDD may remove body hair that they perceive as ugly, asymmetrical, or abnormal; in such cases a diagnosis of trichotillomania is not given. Trichotillomania should not be diagnosed when hair removal is performed solely for cosmetic reasons (i.e., to improve physical appearance). Many individuals twist and play with their hair, but this behavior does not usually qualify for a diagnosis of trichotillomania. Some individuals may bite rather than pull hair; again, this does not qualify for a diagnosis of trichotillomania. Individuals with a psychotic disorder may remove hair in response to a delusion or hallucination.

6.14—Trichotillomania (Hair-Pulling Disorder) / Differential Diagnosis (pp. 283–284)

6.15   A 17-year-old girl is brought to a child and adolescent psychiatry clinic for evaluation. Her parents report that over the past 3 years she has developed a worsening habit of digging into her forearms and shins with her fingernails. The patient describes a bothersome feeling, almost like an itch, that is relieved on scratching. She finds it deeply relieving in the moment but is embarrassed about the residual scars, wearing long sleeves in the summer and staying home more often to avoid others seeing her resulting lesions. Despite support from parents, a school counselor, and friends, the habit has only gotten worse in the past year. Laboratory testing is all within normal limits. What is the appropriate diagnosis for this patient?

A. Delusional parasitosis.
B. Dermatitis artefacta.
C. Obsessive-compulsive disorder (OCD).
D. Excoriation (skin-picking) disorder.

Correct Answer: D. Excoriation (skin-picking) disorder

Explanation: The essential feature of excoriation (skin-picking) disorder is recurrent picking at one's own skin (Criterion A). Individuals with excoriation disorder have made repeated attempts to decrease or stop skin picking (Criterion B). Criterion C indicates that skin picking causes clinically significant distress or impairment in social, occupational, or other important areas of functioning. The term *distress* includes negative affects that may be experienced by individuals with skin picking, such as feeling a loss of control, embarrassment, and shame. Significant impairment may occur in several different areas of functioning (e.g., social, occupational, academic, and leisure), in part because of avoidance of social situations.

Skin picking may occur in response to a delusion (i.e., parasitosis) or tactile hallucination (i.e., formication) in a psychotic disorder. Excessive washing compulsions in response to contamination obsessions in individuals with OCD may lead to skin lesions, and skin picking may occur in individuals with body dysmorphic disorder who pick their skin because of appearance concerns; in such cases, excoriation disorder should not be diagnosed. Dermatitis artefacta (also referred to as factitious dermatitis) is a term used in dermatology to refer to medically unexplained, presumably self-induced skin lesions that the individual denies any role in creating. Cases in which there is evidence of deception on the individual's part concerning the skin lesions can be diagnosed as either malingering (if the skin picking is motivated by external incentives) or factitious disorder (if the skin picking occurs in the absence of obvious external rewards). In the absence of deception, excoriation disorder can be diagnosed if there are repeated attempts to decrease or stop skin picking.

6.15—Excoriation (Skin-Picking) Disorder / Diagnostic Features (p. 285); Differential Diagnosis (pp. 286–287)

6.16   Which of the following is a common comorbid condition with trichotillomania (hair-pulling) disorder?

A. Borderline personality disorder.
B. Bipolar disorder.
C. Excoriation (skin-picking) disorder.
D. Generalized anxiety disorder.

Correct Answer: C. Excoriation (skin-picking) disorder.

Explanation: Trichotillomania is often accompanied by other mental disorders, most commonly major depressive disorder and excoriation (skin-picking) disorder. Repetitive body-focused symptoms other than hair pulling or skin picking (e.g., nail biting) occur in the majority of individuals with trichotillomania and may deserve an additional diagnosis of other specified obsessive-compulsive and related disorder (i.e., other body-focused repetitive behavior disorder).

6.16—Trichotillomania (Hair-Pulling) Disorder / Comorbidity (p. 284)

6.17 In excoriation (skin-picking) disorder, which of the following is the most typical motivation for the skin-picking behavior?

A. Inducing pain.
B. Symmetry concerns.
C. Boredom.
D. Fear of infection.

Correct Answer: C. Boredom.

Explanation: Skin picking may be triggered by feelings of anxiety or boredom; may be preceded by an increasing sense of tension (either immediately before picking the skin or when attempting to resist the urge to pick); and may lead to gratification, pleasure, or a sense of relief when the skin or scab has been picked. Some individuals report picking in response to a minor skin irregularity or to relieve an uncomfortable bodily sensation. Pain is not routinely reported to accompany skin picking. Some individuals engage in skin picking that is more focused (i.e., with preceding tension and subsequent relief), whereas others engage in more automatic picking (i.e., without preceding tension and without full awareness), and many have a mix of both behavioral styles. Skin picking does not usually occur in the presence of other individuals, except immediate family members.

6.17—Excoriation (Skin-Picking) Disorder / Associated Features (p. 285)

6.18 A 55-year-old retail worker believes that he has "chronic halitosis" and fears that his bad breath is "scaring away shoppers." He is in danger of losing his job because he so frequently absents himself from the sales floor to brush his teeth and use mouthwash. He constantly chews mint gum, even though his employer has asked him not to. His coworkers regularly reassure him that his breath is fine, but he is convinced that they are just being polite. Although the possibility of losing his job causes him concern, he finds his worries about his breath to be intolerable. He has seen his doctor and dentist, both of whom tell him that he is healthy and does not have malodorous breath. What is the most appropriate diagnosis?

A. Social anxiety disorder (social phobia).
B. Other specified obsessive-compulsive and related disorder
C. Body dysmorphic disorder.
D. Illness anxiety disorder.

Correct Answer: B. Other specified obsessive-compulsive and related disorder.

Explanation: Olfactory reference syndrome is characterized by the individual's persistent preoccupation with the belief that they emit a foul or offensive body odor that is unnoticeable or only slightly noticeable to others; in response to this preoccupation, these individuals often engage in repetitive and excessive behaviors such as repeatedly checking for body odor, showering excessively, or seeking reassurance, as well as excessive attempts to camouflage the perceived odor. These symptoms cause clinically significant distress or impairment in social, occupational, or other important areas of functioning. In traditional Japanese psychiatry this disorder is known as *jikoshu-kyofu*, a variant of *taijin kyofusho.*

6.18—Other Specified Obsessive-Compulsive and Related Disorder (pp. 293–294)

6.19 A 44-year-old woman goes to the emergency department with excoriations down her forearms bilaterally. She describes an overwhelming concern that she has a skin infection based on "itchy" feelings in her arms and states that she finds some relief in repetitive scratching. She is convinced that the scratching and resulting excoriations are helping prevent spread of infection throughout her body. She does not want medical care, but a companion brought her into the emergency department, concerned that her thinking was out of character and concerning. Laboratory testing is positive for amphetamines, and the patient reports last use approximately 4 hours ago. What is the most appropriate diagnosis for this patient?

A. Substance/medication-induced obsessive compulsive and related disorder.
B. Amphetamine withdrawal.
C. Obsessive-compulsive disorder.
D. Delusional disorder.

Correct Answer: A. Substance/medication-induced obsessive compulsive and related disorder.

Explanation: The essential features of substance/medication-induced obsessive-compulsive and related disorder are prominent symptoms of an obsessive-compulsive and related disorder (Criterion A) that are judged to be attributable to the effects of a substance (e.g., drug of abuse, medication). The obsessive-compulsive and related disorder symptoms must have developed during or soon after substance intoxication or withdrawal or after exposure to or withdrawal from a medication or toxin, and the substance or medication must be capable of producing the symptoms (Criterion B). Diagnosis of substance/medication-induced obsessive-compulsive and related disorder should be made instead of a diagnosis of substance intoxication or substance withdrawal only when the symptoms in Criterion A predominate in the clinical picture and are sufficiently severe to warrant independent clinical attention.

6.19—Substance/Medication-Induced Obsessive-Compulsive and Related Disorder / Diagnostic Features (p. 289)

C H A P T E R 7

Trauma- and Stressor-Related Disorders

7.1   How does DSM-5-TR differ from DSM-5 in the diagnoses included in the trauma- and stressor-related disorders category?

    A. In DSM-5-TR, prolonged grief disorder is included as a trauma- and stressor-related disorder diagnosis.
    B. In DSM-5-TR, posttraumatic stress disorder (PTSD) has been placed with the depressive disorders.
    C. In DSM-5-TR, PTSD has been placed in a newly created chapter.
    D. In DSM-5-TR, prolonged grief disorder has been placed with "Other Conditions That May Be a Focus of Clinical Attention."

Correct Answer: C. In DSM-5-TR, PTSD has been placed in a newly created chapter.

Explanation: Trauma- and stressor-related disorders include disorders in which exposure to a traumatic or stressful event is listed explicitly as a diagnostic criterion. These include reactive attachment disorder, disinhibited social engagement disorder, PTSD, acute stress disorder, adjustment disorders, and prolonged grief disorder. Placement of this chapter reflects the close relationship between these diagnoses and disorders in the surrounding chapters on anxiety disorders, obsessive-compulsive and related disorders, and dissociative disorders. Psychological distress following exposure to a traumatic or stressful event is quite variable. In some cases, symptoms can be well understood within an anxiety- or fear-based context. It is clear, however, that many individuals who have been exposed to a traumatic or stressful event exhibit a phenotype in which, rather than anxiety- or fear-based symptoms, the most prominent clinical characteristics are anhedonic and dysphoric symptoms, externalizing angry and aggressive symptoms, or dissociative symptoms. Because of these variable expressions of clinical distress following exposure to catastrophic or aversive events, the aforementioned disorders are grouped under a separate category: trauma- and stressor-related disorders.

7.1—chapter introduction (p. 295); Prolonged Grief Disorder (pp. 322–327)

7.2   Which two trauma- and stressor-related disorders require social neglect as a criterion?

A. Posttraumatic stress disorder and panic disorder.
B. Acute stress disorder and posttraumatic stress disorder.
C. Reactive attachment disorder and disinhibited social engagement disorder.
D. Prolonged grief disorder and reactive attachment disorder.

Correct Answer: C. Reactive attachment disorder and disinhibited social engagement disorder.

Explanation: Social neglect—that is, the absence of adequate caregiving during childhood—is a diagnostic requirement of both reactive attachment disorder and disinhibited social engagement disorder. Although the two disorders share a common etiology, the former is expressed as an internalizing disorder with depressive symptoms and withdrawn behavior, whereas the latter is marked by disinhibition and externalizing behavior.

7.2—chapter introduction (p. 295)

7.3   Which of the following statements about reactive attachment disorder is *true?*

A. It occurs only in children who lack healthy attachments.
B. It occurs only in children who have secure attachments.
C. It occurs only in children who have impaired communication.
D. It occurs in children without a history of severe social neglect.

Correct Answer: A. It occurs only in children who lack attachments.

Explanation: Reactive attachment disorder is characterized by a pattern of markedly disturbed and developmentally inappropriate attachment behaviors, in which a child rarely or minimally turns preferentially to an attachment figure for comfort, support, protection, and nurturance. The essential feature is absent or grossly underdeveloped attachment between the child and putative caregiving adults. Children with reactive attachment disorder are believed to have the capacity to form selective attachments. However, because of limited opportunities during early development, they fail to show the behavioral manifestations of selective attachments.

7.3—Reactive Attachment Disorder / Diagnostic Features (p. 296)

7.4   A 4-year-old boy in day care often displays fear that does not seem to be related to any of his activities. Although frequently distressed, he does not seek contact with any of the staff and does not respond when a staff member tries to comfort him. What additional caregiver-obtained information about this child would be important in deciding whether his symptoms represent reactive attachment disorder or autism spectrum disorder?

A. Age at first appearance of the behavior.
B. Family history about his siblings.
C. History of language delay.
D. Indications that he has experienced severe social neglect.

Correct Answer: D. Indications that he has experienced severe social neglect.

Explanation: Aberrant social behaviors manifest in young children with reactive attachment disorder, but they also are key features of autism spectrum disorder. Specifically, young children with either condition can manifest dampened expression of positive emotions, cognitive and language delays, and impairments in social reciprocity. As a result, reactive attachment disorder must be differentiated from autism spectrum disorder. These two disorders can be distinguished on the basis of differential histories of neglect and the presence of restricted interests or ritualized behaviors, specific deficit in social communication, and selective attachment behaviors. Children with reactive attachment disorder have experienced a history of severe social neglect, although it is not always possible to obtain detailed histories about the precise nature of their experiences, especially in initial evaluations. Children with autism spectrum disorder will only rarely have a history of social neglect. The restricted interests and repetitive behaviors characteristic of autism spectrum disorder are not a feature of reactive attachment disorder. These clinical features manifest as excessive adherence to rituals and routines; restricted, fixated interests; and unusual sensory reactions.

7.4—Reactive Attachment Disorder / Differential Diagnosis (Autism spectrum disorder) (pp. 297–298)

7.5   Which of the following situations would qualify for a disorder specifier of *severe* in a child diagnosed with reactive attachment disorder?

A. The child has been in five foster homes.
B. The child never expresses positive emotions when interacting with caregivers.
C. The disorder has been present for 18 months.
D. The child meets all symptoms of the disorder, with each symptom manifesting at relatively high levels.

Correct Answer: D. The child meets all symptoms of the disorder, with each symptom manifesting at relatively high levels.

Explanation: Reactive attachment disorder is specified as severe when a child exhibits all symptoms of the disorder, with each symptom manifesting at relatively high levels.

7.5—Reactive Attachment Disorder / diagnostic criteria (p. 296)

7.6   A 6-year-old girl has repeatedly approached strangers while in the park with her class. The teacher requests an evaluation of the behavior. The girl has a history of being placed in several different foster homes over the past 3 years. Which diagnosis is suggested from this history?

A. Attention-deficit/hyperactivity disorder (ADHD).
B. Disinhibited social engagement disorder.
C. Autism spectrum disorder.
D. Bipolar I disorder.

Correct Answer: B. Disinhibited social engagement disorder.

Explanation: The essential feature of disinhibited social engagement disorder is a pattern of behavior that involves culturally inappropriate, overly familiar behavior with relative strangers (Criterion A). This behavior must exhibit at least two of the following: 1) reduced or absent reticence in approaching and interacting with unfamiliar adults; 2) overly familiar verbal or physical behavior (that is not consistent with culturally sanctioned and with age-appropriate social boundaries); 3) diminished or absent checking back with adult caregiver after venturing away, even in unfamiliar settings; or 4) willingness to go off with an unfamiliar adult with minimal or no hesitation. These behaviors are not limited to impulsivity (as in ADHD) but include socially disinhibited behavior (Criterion B).

7.6—Disinhibited Social Engagement Disorder / diagnostic criteria (pp. 298–299)

7.7   A 25-year-old woman presents with a history of being accosted on her way home approximately 2 months ago. The attacker told her he had a gun, was going to rape her, and would shoot her if she resisted. He walked her toward an alley. She was sure he would kill her afterward no matter what she did, and therefore she pushed away from him, aware that she might be shot. She was able to escape unharmed. She describes not being able to fall asleep or walk down that street the day after the incident. Subsequently, she resumed her usual activity, with normalization of her sleep, and was able to walk down that street without anxiety. Now, 4 months after the incident, she says she feels highly anxious all of the time, is often tearful, and feels uncomfortable leaving the house but can walk down that street on her way to work. She denies flashbacks or intrusive thoughts about the incident. What is the most likely diagnosis?

A. Posttraumatic stress disorder (PTSD).
B. Acute stress disorder.
C. Adjustment disorder.
D. Dissociative amnesia.

Correct Answer: C. Adjustment disorder.

Explanation: PTSD can occur at any age beginning after the first year of life. Symptoms usually begin within the first 3 months after the trauma, although there may be a delay of months, or even years, before full criteria for the diagnosis are met.

In adjustment disorders, the stressor can be of any severity or type rather than a stressor involving exposure to actual or threatened death, serious injury, or sexual violence as required by PTSD Criterion A. The diagnosis of an adjustment disorder is used when the response to a stressor that meets PTSD Criterion A does not meet all other PTSD criteria (or criteria for another mental disorder). An adjustment disorder is also diagnosed when the symptom pattern of PTSD occurs in response to a stressor that does not meet PTSD Criterion A (e.g., spouse leaving, being fired).

The essential feature of acute stress disorder is the development of characteristic symptoms lasting from 3 days to 1 month following exposure to one or more traumatic events (Criterion A), which are the same type as described in PTSD Criterion A.

7.7—Posttraumatic Stress Disorder / Diagnostic Features (pp. 305–308); Differential Diagnosis (pp. 312–313), and Development and Course (pp. 308–309; Acute Stress Disorder / Diagnostic Features (pp. 315–316)

7.8   After a routine chest X-ray, a 53-year-old man with a history of heavy cigarette use is told that he has a suspicious lesion on his lung. A bronchoscopy leads to a diagnosis of a benign tumor that needs to be resected. The man delays scheduling a follow-up appointment with the surgeon for more than a month and describes feeling as if "all of this is not real." He is tearful and is afraid he will die. He feels intense guilt that his smoking caused the tumor and expresses the thought that he "deserves" to have cancer. What diagnosis best fits this clinical picture?

A. Acute stress disorder.
B. Posttraumatic stress disorder (PTSD).
C. Adjustment disorder.
D. Major depressive disorder.

Correct Answer: C. Adjustment disorder.

Explanation: The essential feature of acute stress disorder is the development of characteristic symptoms lasting from 3 days to 1 month following exposure to one or more traumatic events (Criterion A), which are the same type as described in PTSD Criterion A. This criterion specifies exposure to actual or threatened death, serious injury, or sexual violence in one (or more) of the following ways: 1) directly experiencing the traumatic event(s); 2) witnessing, in person, the event(s) as it occurred to others; 3) learning that the event(s) occurred to a close family member or close friend (in cases of actual or threatened death of a family member or friend, the event[s] must have been violent or accidental); or 4) experiencing repeated or extreme exposure to aversive details of the traumatic event(s) (e.g., first responders collecting human remains, police officers repeatedly exposed to details of child abuse).

In contrast, for adjustment disorders, the stressor can be of any severity rather than of the severity and type required by Criterion A of acute stress disorder. The diagnosis of an adjustment disorder is used when the response to a Criterion A event does not meet the criteria for acute stress disorder (or another specific mental disorder) and when the symptom pattern of acute stress disorder occurs in response to a stressor that does not meet Criterion A for exposure to actual or threatened death, serious injury, or sexual violence (e.g., spouse leaving, being fired). For example, severe stress reactions to life-threatening illnesses that may include some acute stress disorder symptoms may be more appropriately described as an adjustment disorder. Some forms of acute stress response do not include acute stress disorder symptoms and may be characterized by anger, depression, or guilt. These responses are more appropriately described as primarily an adjustment disorder.

7.8—Acute Stress Disorder / Diagnostic Features (pp. 315–316); Differential Diagnosis (pp. 318–319)

7.9   Criterion B for acute stress disorder requires the presence of 9 (or more) of 12 symptoms from any of five categories of response. Which of the following is *not* one of these five categories?

A. Intrusion.
B. Dissociation.
C. Confusion.
D. Avoidance.

Correct Answer: C. Confusion.

Explanation: Criterion B for acute stress disorder requires the presence of 9 (or more) of a total of 12 symptoms from any of the five categories of intrusion, negative mood, dissociation, avoidance, and arousal, beginning or worsening after the traumatic event(s) occurred.

7.9—Acute Stress Disorder / diagnostic criteria (pp. 313–315)

7.10   Which of the following stressful situations would meet Criterion A for the diagnosis of acute stress disorder?

A. Finding out that one's spouse has been fired.
B. Failing an important final examination.
C. Receiving a serious medical diagnosis.
D. Being in the crossfire of a police shootout but not being harmed.

Correct Answer: D. Being in the crossfire of a police shootout but not being harmed.

Explanation: The essential feature of acute stress disorder is the development of characteristic symptoms lasting from 3 days to 1 month following exposure to one or more traumatic events (Criterion A), which are the same type as described in posttraumatic stress disorder Criterion A.

7.10—Acute Stress Disorder / Diagnostic Features (pp. 315–316)

7.11 Following discharge from the hospital, a 22-year-old man describes vivid and intrusive memories of his stay in the ICU. During the ICU stay, he was extremely agitated, requiring antipsychotic treatment for a few days. Now at home, he states that he has memories of people being tortured in the ICU. He dreams of this every night, waking from sleep in a terror. He talks about not feeling like himself after the experience, finding little pleasure in life after what happened to him, and being easily angered by his family; in addition, he avoids his physician out of fear that he will be told he needs to return to the ICU. What is the most likely explanation for this patient's symptoms?

A. He has acute stress disorder because his life was in danger during the ICU stay.
B. He has posttraumatic stress disorder because his life was in danger during the ICU stay.
C. He has a delirium persisting from the ICU stay.
D. He had a delirium in the ICU and now has an adjustment disorder.

Correct Answer: D. He had a delirium in the ICU and now has an adjustment disorder.

Explanation: Flashbacks in acute stress disorder must be distinguished from illusions, hallucinations, and other perceptual disturbances that may occur in schizophrenia, other psychotic disorders, depressive or bipolar disorder with psychotic features, a delirium, substance/medication-induced disorders, and psychotic disorders due to another medical condition. Acute stress disorder flashbacks are distinguished from these other perceptual disturbances by being directly related to the traumatic experience and by occurring in the absence of other psychotic or substance-induced features.

7.11—Acute Stress Disorder / Differential Diagnosis (Psychotic disorders) (p. 318)

7.12 Which of the following experiences would *not* qualify as exposure to a traumatic event (Criterion A) in the diagnosis of acute stress disorder or posttraumatic stress disorder?

A. Hearing that one's brother was killed in combat.
B. Hearing that one's close childhood friend survived a motor vehicle accident but is paralyzed.

C. Hearing that one's child has been kidnapped.

D. Hearing that one's company has suddenly closed.

Correct Answer: D. Hearing that one's company has suddenly closed.

Explanation: The *directly experienced* traumatic events in Criterion A include, but are not limited to, exposure to war as a combatant or civilian, threatened or actual physical assault (e.g., physical attack, robbery, mugging, childhood physical abuse), threatened or actual sexual violence (e.g., forced sexual penetration, alcohol/drug-facilitated sexual penetration, abusive sexual contact, noncontact sexual abuse, sexual trafficking), being kidnapped, being taken hostage, terrorist attack, torture, incarceration as a prisoner of war, natural or human-made disasters, and severe motor vehicle accidents. A life-threatening illness or debilitating medical condition is not necessarily considered a traumatic event. Medical incidents that qualify as traumatic events involve sudden, catastrophic events (e.g., waking during surgery, anaphylactic shock).

Witnessed events include, but are not limited to, observing threatened or serious injury, unnatural death, physical or sexual abuse of another person due to violent assault, domestic violence, accident, war or disaster, or a medical catastrophe in one's child (e.g., a life-threatening hemorrhage).

Indirect exposure through learning about an event is limited to experiences affecting close relatives or friends and experiences that are violent or accidental (e.g., death due to natural causes does not qualify). Such events include violent personal assault, suicide, serious accident, and serious injury. The disorder may be especially severe or long-lasting when the stressor is interpersonal and intentional (e.g., torture, sexual violence).

7.12—Posttraumatic Stress Disorder / Diagnostic Features (pp. 305–308)

7.13   A 31-year-old man narrowly escapes (without injury) from a house fire caused when he dropped a lighter while trying to light his crack pipe. Six weeks later, while smoking crack, he thinks he smells smoke and runs from the building in a panic, shouting, "It's on fire!" Which of the following symptoms or circumstances would rule out a diagnosis of posttraumatic stress disorder (PTSD) for this patient?

A. Having difficulty falling asleep.

B. Being uninterested in going back to work.

C. Inappropriately getting angry at family members.

D. Experiencing symptoms only when smoking crack cocaine.

Correct Answer: D. Experiencing symptoms only when smoking crack cocaine.

Explanation: Although the stressor and symptoms described would qualify this man for a diagnosis of PTSD, Criterion G states that "The disturbance is not attributable to the physiological effects of a substance (e.g., medication or alcohol) or another medical condition."

7.13—Posttraumatic Stress Disorder / diagnostic criteria (pp. 301–304)

7.14   Criterion A4 of posttraumatic stress disorder (PTSD) requires "Experiencing repeated or extreme exposure to aversive details of the traumatic event." Which of the following would *not* qualify as experiencing trauma under this criterion?

   A. A police officer reviewing surveillance videotapes of homicides to identify perpetrators.
   B. A social worker interviewing children who have been sexually abused and obtaining the details of the abuse.
   C. A soldier sifting through the rubble of a collapsed building to retrieve remains of comrades.
   D. A college student at a film festival watching a series of violent movies that contain scenes of graphic violence.

Correct Answer: D. A college student at a film festival watching a series of violent movies that contain scenes of graphic violence.

Explanation: The indirect exposure of professionals to the grotesque effects of war, rape, genocide, or abusive violence inflicted on others occurring in the context of their work duties can also result in PTSD and thus is considered to be a qualifying trauma (Criterion A4). Examples include first responders exposed to serious injury or death and military personnel collecting human remains. Indirect exposure can also occur through photos, videos, verbal accounts, or written accounts (e.g., police officers reviewing crime reports or conducting interviews with crime victims, drone operators, members of the news media covering traumatic events, psychotherapists exposed to details of their patients' traumatic experiences). Criterion A4 does not apply to exposure through electronic media, television, movies, or pictures, unless this exposure is work related.

7.14—Posttraumatic Stress Disorder / diagnostic criteria (pp. 301–303)

7.15   Which of the following is *true* about the risk of developing posttraumatic stress disorder (PTSD) in women and men?

   A. The risk is lower in females in preschool-age populations.
   B. The risk is higher in females across the life span.
   C. The risk is higher in males in elderly populations.
   D. The risk is lower in middle-age females than in middle-age males.

Correct Answer: B. The risk is higher in females across the life span.

Explanation: PTSD is more prevalent among women than among men across the life span. Lifetime prevalence of PTSD ranges from 8.0% to 11.0% for women and 4.1% to 5.4% for men based on two large U.S. population-based studies using DSM-5 criteria. Some of the increased risk for PTSD in women appears to be attributable to a greater likelihood of exposure to childhood sexual abuse, sexual assault, and other forms of interpersonal violence, which carry the highest risk for development of PTSD. Women in the general population also experience PTSD for a longer duration than do men. However, other factors likely contributing to the higher prevalence in women include gender differences in the emotional and cognitive processing of trauma, as well as effects of reproductive hormones. When responses of men and women to specific stressors are compared, gender differences in risk for PTSD persist. On the other hand, PTSD symptom profiles and factor structures are similar between men and women.

7.15—Posttraumatic Stress Disorder / Sex- and Gender-Related Diagnostic Issues (p. 311)

7.16 A 5-year-old child was present when her babysitter was sexually assaulted. Which of the following symptoms would be most suggestive of posttraumatic stress disorder (PTSD) in this child?

A. Playing normally with toys.
B. Having dreams about princesses and castles.
C. Taking the clothing off her dolls while playing.
D. Expressing no fear when talking about the event.

Correct Answer: C. Taking the clothing off her dolls while playing.

Explanation: The clinical expression of reexperiencing can vary across development. Developmental variations in clinical expression inform the use of different criteria in children 6 years and younger and in individuals who are older. Young children may report new onset of frightening dreams without content specific to the traumatic event. Children ages 6 and younger may develop PTSD as a result of severe emotional abuse (e.g., threat of abandonment), which can be perceived as life-threatening. During treatment for life-threatening illness (e.g., cancer, solid organ transplantation), the experience of young children of the severity and intensity of the treatment may contribute to risk of developing posttraumatic stress symptoms; the self-appraisal of threat may also contribute to the risk of developing posttraumatic stress symptoms in adolescents. Before age 6 years, young children are more likely to express reexperiencing symptoms through play that refers directly or symbolically to the trauma (see PTSD criteria for children 6 years and younger, DSM-5-TR pp. 303–304). They may not manifest fearful reactions at the time of the exposure or during reexperiencing. Parents may report a wide range of emotional or behavioral changes in young children. Children may focus on imagined interventions in their play or storytelling.

7.16—Posttraumatic Stress Disorder / Development and Course (pp. 308–309)

7.17   Which of the following statements about risk factors for developing posttraumatic stress disorder (PTSD) is *true*?

A. Sustaining personal injury does not affect the risk of developing PTSD.
B. Severity of the trauma influences the risk of developing PTSD.
C. Dissociation has no impact on the risk of developing PTSD.
D. Perceived life threat is the only risk factor for developing PTSD.

Correct Answer: B. Severity of the trauma influences the risk of developing PTSD.

Explanation: Risk factors for PTSD can operate in many ways, including predisposing individuals to trauma or to extreme emotional responses when exposed to traumatic events. Risk (and protective) factors are generally divided into pretraumatic, peritraumatic, and posttraumatic factors.

Temperamental factors: High-risk factors include childhood emotional problems (e.g., externalizing or anxiety problems) by age 6 years and prior mental disorders (e.g., panic disorder, depressive disorder, PTSD, obsessive-compulsive disorder). Individual differences in premorbid personality may influence the trajectory of response to trauma and treatment outcomes. Personality traits associated with negative emotional responses such as depressed mood and anxiousness represent risk factors for the development of PTSD. Such traits might be captured in measures of negative affectivity (neuroticism) on standardized personality scales. Premorbid trait impulsivity tends to be associated with externalizing manifestations of PTSD and comorbidities of the externalizing spectrum, including substance use disorder or aggressive behavior.

Environmental factors: Risk factors include severity (dose) of the trauma, perceived life threat, personal injury, interpersonal violence (particularly trauma perpetrated by a caregiver or involving a witnessed threat to a caregiver in children), and, for military personnel, being a perpetrator, witnessing atrocities, or killing the enemy. Other risk factors include dissociation, fear, panic, and other peritraumatic responses that occur during the trauma and persist afterward.

7.17—Posttraumatic Stress Disorder / Risk and Prognostic Factors / Pretraumatic factors / Temperamental; Peritraumatic factors / Environmental (pp. 309–310)

7.18   A woman complains of sad mood and feeling hopeless 3 months after her husband files for divorce. She finds it difficult to take care of her home or make meals for her family but has continued to fulfill her responsibilities. She denies suicidal ideation, feels she was a good wife who has "nothing to feel guilty about," and wishes she could "forget about the whole thing." She cannot stop thinking about her situation. Which diagnosis best fits this symptom picture?

A. Adjustment disorder, with depressed mood.
B. Adjustment disorder, with disturbance of conduct.

C. Adjustment disorder, with anxiety.
D. Adjustment disorder, with mixed disturbance of emotions and conduct.

Correct Answer: A. Adjustment disorder, with depressed mood.

Explanation: The presence of emotional or behavioral symptoms in response to an identifiable stressor is the essential feature of adjustment disorders (Criterion A). The stressor may be a single event (e.g., termination of a romantic relationship), or there may be multiple stressors (e.g., marked business difficulties and marital problems). Stressors may be recurrent (e.g., associated with seasonal business crises or unfulfilling sexual relationships) or continuous (e.g., a persistent painful illness with increasing disability, living in a crime-ridden neighborhood). Stressors (e.g., a natural disaster) may affect a single individual, an entire family, or a larger group or community. Some stressors may accompany specific developmental events (e.g., going to school, leaving a parental home, reentering a parental home, getting married, becoming a parent, failing to attain occupational goals, retirement). When low mood, tearfulness, or feelings of hopelessness are predominant, the specifier *with depressed moo*d should be included.

7.18—Adjustment Disorders / diagnostic criteria / Diagnostic Features (pp. 319–320)

7.19   Twelve months after the death of her husband, a 70-year-old woman is seen for symptoms of overwhelming sadness, anger regarding her husband's unexpected death from a heart attack, intense yearning for him to come back, and repeated unsuccessful attempts to begin moving out of her large home (which she can no longer afford) due to inability to sort through and dispose of her husband's belongings. She cannot believe that he has died and expresses the feeling that "a part of me died that day." What is the most appropriate diagnosis?

A. Major depressive disorder.
B. Posttraumatic stress disorder.
C. Adjustment disorder, with depressed mood.
D. Prolonged grief disorder

Correct Answer: D. Prolonged grief disorder.

Explanation: Prolonged grief disorder represents a maladaptive grief reaction that can be diagnosed only after at least 12 months (6 months in children and adolescents) have elapsed since the death of someone with whom the bereaved had a close relationship (Criterion A). The persistent grief response is characterized by intense yearning or longing for the deceased person (often with intense sorrow and frequent crying) or preoccupation with thoughts or memories of the deceased; in children and adolescents, this preoccupation may focus on the circumstances of the death. The intense yearning/longing or the preoccupation has been present most days to a clinically significant degree and has occurred nearly every day for at least the previous month (Criterion B). In addition, since the death, at least three of the following symptoms have been present most days to a clinically significant degree and have occurred nearly every day for at least the past month (Criterion C): identity disruption (e.g., feeling as though part of oneself has died); a marked sense of disbelief about the death; avoidance of reminders that the person is dead; intense emotional pain; difficulty reintegrating into personal relationships and activities; emotional numbness; feeling that life is meaningless as a result of the death; or intense loneliness as a consequence of the death.

The symptoms of prolonged grief disorder must result in clinically significant distress or impairment in social, occupational, or other important areas of functioning (Criterion D). The nature, duration, and severity of the bereavement reaction must clearly exceed expected social, cultural, or religious norms for the individual's culture and context (Criterion E). Although there are variations in how grief can manifest, the symptoms of prolonged grief disorder occur across genders and in diverse social and cultural groups.

7.19—Prolonged Grief Disorder / diagnostic criteria / Diagnostic Features (pp. 322–324)

7.20   A 25-year-old woman with asthma becomes extremely anxious when she gets an upper respiratory infection. She presents to the emergency department with complaints of being unable to breathe. While there, she begins to hyperventilate and then reports feeling extremely dizzy. Her hyperventilation causes her to become fatigued, and when the medical evaluation indicates that she is retaining carbon dioxide, it becomes necessary to admit her. The woman denies any other symptoms beyond anxiety. What is the most appropriate diagnosis?

A. Acute stress disorder.
B. Generalized anxiety disorder.
C. Adjustment disorder with anxiety.
D. Psychological factors affecting other medical conditions.

Correct Answer: D. Psychological factors affecting other medical conditions.

Explanation: In psychological factors affecting other medical conditions, specific psychological entities (e.g., psychological symptoms, behaviors, other factors) exacerbate a medical condition. These psychological factors can precipitate, exacerbate, or put an individual at risk for medical illness, or they can worsen an existing condition. In contrast, an adjustment disorder is a reaction to the stressor (e.g., having a medical illness).

The essential feature of psychological factors affecting other medical conditions is the presence of one or more clinically significant psychological or behavioral factors that adversely affect a medical condition by increasing the risk for suffering, death, or disability (Criterion B). These factors can adversely affect the medical condition by influencing its course or treatment, by constituting an additional well-established health risk factor, or by influencing the underlying pathophysiology to precipitate or exacerbate symptoms or to necessitate medical attention.

Psychological or behavioral factors include psychological distress, patterns of interpersonal interaction, coping styles, and maladaptive health behaviors such as denial of symptoms or poor adherence to medical recommendations. Common clinical examples are anxiety-exacerbating asthma, denial of need for treatment for acute chest pain, and manipulation of insulin by an individual with diabetes wishing to lose weight.

7.20—Adjustment Disorders / Differential Diagnosis (Psychological factors affecting other medical conditions) (p. 322); Somatic Symptom and Related Disorders / Psychological Factors Affecting Other Medical Conditions / Diagnostic Features (p. 365)

7.21   How many Criterion B symptoms are required to be present for the diagnosis of acute stress disorder?

   A. One.
   B. Three.
   C. Five.
   D. Nine.

Correct Answer: D. Nine.

Explanation: Presence of nine (or more) symptoms from any of the five categories of intrusion, negative mood, dissociation, avoidance, and arousal, beginning or worsening after the traumatic event(s) occurred, is needed for diagnosis.

7.21—Acute Stress Disorder / diagnostic criteria (p. 314)

7.22   Criterion B in the DSM-5-TR diagnostic criteria for acute stress disorder requires the presence of symptoms from five different categories: *intrusion, negative mood, dissociative, avoidance,* and *arousal*. Match each of the following symptoms to the appropriate category (each symptom may be placed into only one category).

   A. Recurrent, involuntary, and intrusive distressing memories of the traumatic event(s).
   B. Problems with concentration.
   C. Persistent inability to experience positive emotions (e.g., inability to experience happiness, satisfaction, or loving feelings).
   D. An altered sense of the reality of one's surroundings or oneself (e.g., seeing oneself from another's perspective, being in a daze, time slowing).

E. Efforts to avoid external reminders (people, places, conversations, activities, objects, situations) that arouse distressing memories, thoughts, or feelings about or closely associated with the traumatic event(s).

F. Irritable behavior and angry outbursts (with little or no provocation), typically expressed as verbal or physical aggression toward people or objects.

G. Inability to remember an important aspect of the traumatic event(s) (typically due to dissociative amnesia and not other factors such as head injury, alcohol, or drugs).

H. Recurrent distressing dreams in which the content and/or affect of the dream is related to the event(s).

I. Hypervigilance.

J. Dissociative reactions (e.g., flashbacks) in which the individual feels or acts as if the traumatic event(s) were recurring.

K. Exaggerated startle response.

L. Efforts to avoid distressing memories, thoughts, or feelings about or closely associated with the traumatic event(s).

M. Sleep disturbance (e.g., difficulty falling or staying asleep, restless sleep).

N. Intense or prolonged psychological distress or marked physiological reactions in response to internal or external cues that symbolize or resemble an aspect of the traumatic event(s).

Correct Matches:
Intrusion: A, H, J, N;
Negative Mood: C;
Dissociative: D, G;
Avoidance: E, L;
Arousal: B, F, I, K, M.

Explanation: The clinical presentation of acute stress disorder may vary by individual but typically involves an anxiety response that includes some form of reexperiencing of or reactivity to the traumatic event. Presentations may include intrusion symptoms, negative mood, dissociative symptoms, avoidance symptoms, and arousal symptoms (Criteria B1–B14). In some individuals, a dissociative or detached presentation can predominate, although these individuals typically will also display strong emotional or physiological reactivity in response to trauma reminders. In other individuals, there can be a strong anger response in which reactivity is characterized by irritable or possibly aggressive responses.

7.22—chapter introduction (p. 295); Acute Stress Disorder / diagnostic criteria (pp. 313–315)

7.23 Two months following the death of her son, a 49-year-old woman consults you for psychotherapy. She reports that her son died following a skiing accident on a trip that she gave him as a gift for his 17th birthday. She is preoccupied with the death and blames herself for providing the gift of the trip, but she does not experience yearning for her son. Although she denies any overt suicidal plans, she describes sadness and anxiety related to his death. She has not entered her son's room since his death and has difficulty relating to her husband, feeling anger toward him for agreeing to allow their son to go on the ski trip. She was treated with a selective serotonin reuptake inhibitor at full dose for 3 months after her son's death but reports that the medication had no impact on her symptoms. What is the most appropriate diagnosis?

A. Major depressive disorder.
B. Normal grief.
C. Prolonged grief disorder.
D. Adjustment disorder.

Correct Answer: D. Adjustment disorder.

Explanation: The presence of emotional or behavioral symptoms in response to an identifiable stressor is the essential feature of adjustment disorders (Criterion A). The stressor may be a single event (e.g., a termination of a romantic relationship), or there may be multiple stressors (e.g., marked business difficulties and marital problems). Stressors may be recurrent (e.g., associated with seasonal business crises or unfulfilling sexual relationships) or continuous (e.g., a persistent painful illness with increasing disability; living in a crime-ridden neighborhood). Stressors (e.g., a natural disaster) may affect a single individual, an entire family, or a larger group or community. Some stressors may accompany specific developmental events (e.g., going to school, leaving a parental home, reentering a parental home, getting married, becoming a parent, failing to attain occupational goals, retirement). Adjustment disorders may be diagnosed following the death of a loved one when the intensity, quality, or persistence of grief reactions exceeds what normally might be expected when cultural, religious, or age-appropriate norms are taken into account and the grief reaction does not meet criteria for prolonged grief disorder.

7.23—Adjustment Disorders / Diagnostic Features (p. 320)

CHAPTER 8

Dissociative Disorders

8.1 Which of the following disorders can be comorbid with dissociative identity disorder?

A. Bipolar disorder.
B. Schizophrenia.
C. Posttraumatic stress disorder (PTSD).
D. Factitious disorder.

Correct Answer: C. Posttraumatic stress disorder (PTSD).

Explanation: Disorders that can be comorbid with dissociative identity disorder include PTSD (option C is correct); depressive disorders; substance-related disorders; feeding and eating disorders; obsessive-compulsive disorder; antisocial personality disorder; and other specified personality disorder with avoidant, obsessive-compulsive, or borderline personality traits. Dissociative identity disorder is commonly misdiagnosed as bipolar disorder (option A is incorrect). Individuals with dissociative identity disorder may experience symptoms that can superficially appear similar to those of schizophrenia and other psychotic disorders (option B is incorrect). In factitious disorder, individuals who feign dissociative identity disorder usually do not report the subtle symptoms of intrusion characteristic of the disorder (option D is incorrect).

8.1—Dissociative Identity Disorder / Differential Diagnosis (pp. 335–337); Comorbidity (p. 337)

8.2 Which of the following is considered a dissociative disorder?

A. Acute stress disorder.
B. Posttraumatic stress disorder (PTSD).
C. Traumatic brain injury.
D. Depersonalization/derealization disorder.

Correct Answer: D. Depersonalization/derealization disorder.

Explanation: The dissociative disorders include dissociative identity disorder, dissociative amnesia, depersonalization/derealization disorder (option D is correct), other specified dissociative disorder, and unspecified dissociative disorder. Dissociative disorders are frequently found in the aftermath of a wide variety of psychologically traumatic experiences that result in psychological sequelae, as opposed to the physical impact that can cause traumatic brain injury (option C is incorrect). Dissociative disorders are placed next to, but are not part of, the trauma- and stressor-related disorders, reflecting the close relationship between these diagnostic classes (options A and B are incorrect). Both acute stress disorder and PTSD include dissociative symptoms.

8.2—chapter introduction (pp. 329–330)

8.3   Which of the following statements correctly describes the adjectives *positive* and *negative* when applied to dissociative symptoms?

  A. Negative dissociative symptoms involve loss of continuity in subjective experience.
  B. Positive dissociative symptoms include amnesia.
  C. Negative dissociative symptoms refer to the inability to access information or to control mental functions in a normal fashion.
  D. Negative dissociative symptoms include division of identity.

Correct Answer: C. Negative dissociative symptoms refer to the inability to access information or to control mental functions in a normal fashion.

Explanation: Dissociative symptoms are experienced as unbidden intrusions into awareness and behavior, with accompanying losses of continuity in subjective experience (i.e., *positive* dissociative symptoms [option A is incorrect] such as division of identity [option D is incorrect], depersonalization, and derealization) and/or inability to access information or to control mental functions that normally are readily amenable to access or control (i.e., *negative* dissociative symptoms [option C is correct] such as amnesia [option B is incorrect]).

8.3—chapter introduction (pp. 329–330)

8.4   Which of the following is a *true* statement about depersonalization/derealization disorder?

  A. The 12-month prevalence of depersonalization/derealization disorder is thought to be markedly less than the prevalence of transient depersonalization/derealization symptoms.
  B. The mean age at onset of depersonalization/derealization disorder is 25 years.
  C. During depersonalization or derealization experiences, individuals typically lose reality testing.

D. Sexual abuse is the most common childhood interpersonal trauma in individuals with depersonalization/derealization disorder.

Correct Answer: A. The 12-month prevalence of depersonalization/derealization disorder is thought to be markedly less than the prevalence of transient depersonalization/derealization symptoms.

Explanation: Transient depersonalization/derealization symptoms lasting hours to days are common in the general population. The 12-month prevalence of depersonalization/derealization disorder is thought to be markedly less than the prevalence of transient symptoms. The mean age at onset of depersonalization/derealization disorder is 16 years. Less than 20% of individuals experience onset after age 20 years and only 5% after age 25 years (option B is incorrect). Per Criterion B, during depersonalization or derealization experiences, reality testing remains intact (option C is incorrect). There is a clear association between depersonalization/derealization disorder and childhood interpersonal traumas in a substantial portion of individuals. In particular, emotional abuse and emotional neglect have been most strongly and consistently associated with the disorder. Sexual abuse is a much less common antecedent but can be encountered (option D is incorrect).

8.4—Depersonalization / Derealization Disorder / diagnostic criteria (p. 343); Prevalence (p. 344); Development and Course (pp. 344–345); Risk and Prognostic Factors (p. 345)

8.5   Which of the following symptom presentations is the most common manifestation of Criterion A for non-possession-form dissociative identity disorder?

A. Elaborate personality states with different names, wardrobes, hairstyles, handwritings, and accents.
B. Ego-syntonic abrupt inhibition of speech and action.
C. Alterations in sense of self and agency that the individual experiences as under their control.
D. Experience of the self as multiple simultaneously overlapping and interfering states.

Correct Answer: D. Experience of the self as multiple simultaneously overlapping and interfering states.

Explanation: The defining feature of dissociative identity disorder is the presence of two or more distinct personality states or an experience of possession (Criterion A). The elaboration of dissociative personality states with different names, wardrobes, hairstyles, handwritings, accents, and so forth occurs in only a *minority* of individuals with the non-possession-form dissociative identity disorder and is *not* essential to diagnosis (option A is incorrect). Thoughts and emotions may unexpectedly vanish, and speech and actions are abruptly inhibited. These experiences are frequently reported as ego-dystonic (option B is incorrect). Alterations in sense of self and agency may be accompanied by a feeling that attitudes, emotions, and behaviors—even the individual's own body—are "not mine" or are "not under my control" (option C is incorrect). In general, the individual with dissociative identity disorder experiences themselves as multiple, simultaneously overlapping and interfering states (option D is correct).

8.5—Dissociative Identity Disorder / diagnostic criteria (p. 330); Diagnostic Features (pp. 331–332)

8.6   Which of the following statements best characterizes Criterion B (dissociative amnesia) in dissociative identity disorder?

A. Dissociative amnesia is not typically apparent to others.
B. Minimization or rationalization of amnesia is common.
C. Amnesia is limited to stressful or traumatic events.
D. Dissociative fugues are uncommon.

Correct Answer: B. Minimization or rationalization of amnesia is common.

Explanation: Dissociative amnesia (Criterion B) manifests in several major domains. Dissociative fugues, with amnesia for travel, are common (option D is incorrect). Amnesia in individuals with dissociative identity disorder is not limited to stressful or traumatic events (option C is incorrect). Dissociative amnesia may be apparent to others (option A is incorrect). Minimization or rationalization of amnesia is common (option B is correct).

8.6—Dissociative Identity Disorder / Diagnostic Features (pp. 331–332)

8.7   Which of the following is the most common type of dissociative amnesia?

A. Continuous amnesia.
B. Irreversible amnesia.
C. Localized or selective amnesia.
D. Generalized amnesia.

Correct Answer: C. Localized or selective amnesia for specific events.

Explanation: Dissociative amnesia is conceptualized as a potentially reversible memory retrieval deficit (option B is incorrect). In this way, among others, it differs from the amnesias attributable to neurobiological damage or toxicity that impairs memory storage or retrieval.

    Criterion A notes that dissociative amnesia most often consists of localized or selective amnesia for a specific event or events or generalized amnesia for identity and life history. Most commonly, individuals with dissociative amnesia report *localized amnesia* (a failure to recall events during a circumscribed period of time) and/or *selective amnesia* (in which the individual can recall some, but not all, of the events during a circumscribed period of time) (option C is correct).

Generalized dissociative amnesia involves a complete loss of memory for most or all of the individual's life history (option D is incorrect).

In continuous amnesia (i.e., anterograde dissociative amnesia), an individual forgets each new event as it occurs. In general, the memory deficit in dissociative amnesia is *retrograde* (option A is incorrect).

8.7—Dissociative Amnesia / diagnostic criteria (p. 337); Diagnostic Features (p. 338)

8.8   Which of the following presentations can be specified using the *other specified dissociative disorder* designation?

A. Symptoms characteristic of a dissociative disorder that do not meet the full criteria for any of the disorders in the dissociative disorders diagnostic class.
B. Chronic and recurrent syndromes of mixed dissociative symptoms.
C. Presentations for which there is insufficient information to make a more specific diagnosis.
D. The clinician chooses *not* to specify the reason that the criteria are not met for a specific dissociative disorder.

Correct Answer: B. Chronic and recurrent syndromes of mixed dissociative symptoms.

Explanation: Examples of presentations that can be specified using the *other specified* designation include 1) chronic and recurrent syndromes of mixed dissociative symptoms (option B is correct), 2) identity disturbance due to prolonged and intense coercive persuasion, 3) acute dissociative reactions to stressful events, and 4) dissociative trance. Unspecified dissociative disorder applies to presentations in which symptoms characteristic of a dissociative disorder predominate but do not meet the full criteria for any of the disorders in the dissociative disorders diagnostic class (option A is incorrect). The unspecified dissociative disorder category is used in situations in which the clinician chooses *not* to specify the reason that the criteria are not met for a specific dissociative disorder (option C is incorrect) and includes presentations for which there is insufficient information to make a more specific diagnosis (option D is incorrect).

8.8—Other Specified Dissociative Disorder (pp. 347–348); Unspecified Dissociative Disorder (p. 348)

CHAPTER 9

Somatic Symptom and Related Disorders

9.1　Somatoform disorders in DSM-IV are referred to as somatic symptom and related disorders in DSM-5-TR. Which of the following features characterizes the major diagnosis in this class, somatic symptom disorder?

A.　Absence of a medical explanation for somatic symptoms.
B.　Initial presentation mainly in mental health care rather than medical settings.
C.　Lack of medical comorbidity.
D.　Distressing somatic symptoms plus abnormal thoughts, feelings, and behaviors in response to these symptoms.

Correct Answer: D. Distressing somatic symptoms plus abnormal thoughts, feelings, and behaviors in response to these symptoms.

Explanation: Somatic symptom disorder emphasizes diagnosis made on the basis of positive symptoms and signs (distressing somatic symptoms plus abnormal thoughts, feelings, and behaviors in response to these symptoms; option D is correct) rather than the absence of a medical explanation for somatic symptoms (option A is incorrect). All of the somatic symptom disorders are characterized by the prominent focus on somatic concerns and their initial presentation mainly in medical rather than mental health care settings (option B is incorrect). There is considerable medical comorbidity among individuals with somatic symptom and related disorders (option C is incorrect).

9.1—chapter introduction (pp. 349–351)

9.2　In DSM-IV, a patient with a high level of anxiety about having a disease and many associated somatic symptoms would have been given the diagnosis of hypochondriasis. What DSM-5-TR diagnosis would apply to this patient?

A.　Psychological factors affecting other medical condition.
B.　Illness anxiety disorder.
C.　Somatic symptom disorder.
D.　Functional neurologic symptom disorder.

Correct Answer: C. Somatic symptom disorder.

Explanation: Somatic symptom disorder and illness anxiety disorder offer more clinically useful methods of characterizing individuals who may have been considered in the past for a diagnosis of somatization disorder and hypochondriasis. Furthermore, approximately two-thirds to three-fourths of individuals previously diagnosed with hypochondriasis are subsumed under the diagnosis of somatic symptom disorder (option C is incorrect). However, the remaining one-quarter to one-third of individuals with previously diagnosed hypochondriasis have high health anxiety in the *absence* of somatic symptoms (option B is incorrect), and many such individuals' symptoms would not qualify for an anxiety disorder diagnosis. The DSM-5 diagnosis of illness anxiety disorder is for this latter group of individuals (option B is incorrect). Psychological factors affecting other medical conditions has as its essential feature the presence of one or more clinically significant psychological or behavioral factors that adversely affect a medical condition by increasing the risk for suffering, death, or disability (option A is incorrect). In functional neurological symptom disorder, the key to diagnosis is neurological symptoms that can be demonstrated, on the basis of positive clinical examination features, to be incompatible with recognized pathophysiology (option D is incorrect).

9.2—chapter introduction (pp. 349–351)

9.3 In DSM-III and DSM-IV, a large number of somatic symptoms were needed to qualify for the diagnosis of somatization disorder. How many somatic symptoms are needed to meet symptom criteria for the DSM-5-TR diagnosis of somatic symptom disorder?

A. None.
B. Two or more.
C. One.
D. Any number of symptoms that are continuously present.

Correct Answer: C. One.

Explanation: The diagnosis of somatic symptom disorder requires one or more somatic symptoms that are distressing or result in disruption of daily life (Criterion A; option C is correct and option A is incorrect). Although one somatic symptom may not be continuously present (option D is incorrect), the state of being symptomatic is persistent (typically for more than 6 months) (Criterion C). Severity of somatic symptom disorder can be specified by the number of fulfilled B criteria; in moderate somatic symptom disorder, two or more B criteria are present (option B is incorrect).

9.3—Somatic Symptom Disorder / diagnostic criteria (p. 351); Diagnostic Features (pp. 351–352)

9.4   After an airplane flight, a 60-year-old woman with a history of chronic anxiety develops deep vein thrombophlebitis and a subsequent pulmonary embolism. Over the next year, she focuses relentlessly on sensations of pleuritic chest pain and repeatedly seeks medical attention for this symptom, with concern that it is due to recurrent pulmonary emboli, despite negative test results. Review of systems reveals the presence of chronic back pain and multiple prior consultations for symptoms of culture-negative cystitis. What diagnosis best fits this clinical picture?

A. Illness anxiety disorder.
B. Panic disorder.
C. Generalized anxiety disorder.
D. Somatic symptom disorder.

Correct Answer: D. Somatic symptom disorder.

Explanation: Individuals with somatic symptom disorder typically have multiple current somatic symptoms that are distressing or result in significant disruption of daily life. The symptoms may or may not be associated with another medical condition. Individuals with somatic symptom disorder tend to have very high levels of worry about illness. They appraise their bodily symptoms as unduly threatening, harmful, or troublesome and often think the worst about their health, even when there is evidence to the contrary. There is often a high level of medical care utilization, which rarely alleviates the individual's concerns. Consequently, the individual may seek care from multiple doctors for the same symptoms. If the individual has extensive worries about health but no or minimal somatic symptoms, it may be more appropriate to consider illness anxiety disorder (option A is incorrect). In panic disorder, somatic symptoms and anxiety about health tend to occur in acute episodes, whereas in somatic symptom disorder, anxiety and somatic symptoms are more persistent (option B is incorrect). Individuals with generalized anxiety disorder worry about multiple events, situations, or activities, only one of which may involve their health. The main focus is not usually somatic symptoms or fear of illness as it is in somatic symptom disorder (option C is incorrect).

9.4—Somatic Symptom Disorder / Diagnostic Features (pp. 351–352); Associated Features (p. 352); Differential Diagnosis (pp. 355–356)

9.5   Illness anxiety disorder involves a preoccupation with having or acquiring a serious illness. How severe are the accompanying somatic symptoms?

A. Moderate.
B. Severe.
C. Somatic symptoms are not present.
D. Mild.

Correct Answer: D. Mild.

Explanation: Illness anxiety disorder entails a preoccupation with having or acquiring a serious, undiagnosed medical illness (Criterion A). Somatic symptoms are not present or, if present, are only mild in intensity (option D is correct; options A, B, and C are incorrect).

9.5—Illness Anxiety Disorder / diagnostic criteria (p. 357)

9.6   Over a period of several years, a 50-year-old woman visits her dermatologist's office every few weeks to be evaluated for skin cancer, showing the dermatologist various freckles, nevi, and patches of dry skin. None of the skin findings have ever been abnormal, and the dermatologist has provided repeated reassurance. The patient has no pain, itching, bleeding, or other somatic symptoms. What is the most likely diagnosis?

A. Adjustment disorder.
B. Illness anxiety disorder.
C. Obsessive-compulsive disorder (OCD).
D. Somatic symptom disorder.

Correct Answer: B. Illness anxiety disorder.

Explanation: Illness anxiety disorder entails a preoccupation with having or acquiring a serious, undiagnosed medical illness. Somatic symptoms are not present or, if present, are only mild in intensity (option B is correct). Health-related anxiety is a normal response to serious illness and is not a mental disorder. Such nonpathological health anxiety is clearly related to the medical condition and is typically time limited. If the health anxiety is severe enough to cause clinically significant distress or impairment in one or more important areas of functioning, an adjustment disorder may be diagnosed (option A is incorrect). Individuals with illness anxiety disorder may have intrusive thoughts about having a disease and also may have associated compulsive behaviors (e.g., seeking reassurance). However, in illness anxiety disorder, the preoccupations are usually focused on having a disease, whereas in OCD, the thoughts are intrusive and are usually focused on fears of getting a disease in the future (option C is incorrect). Both somatic symptom disorder and illness anxiety disorder may be characterized by a high level of anxiety about health and excessive health-related behaviors. They are differentiated by the fact that somatic symptom disorder requires the presence of somatic symptoms that are distressing or result in significant disruption of daily life, whereas in illness anxiety disorder, somatic symptoms either are not present or, if present, are only mild in intensity (option D is incorrect).

9.6—Illness Anxiety Disorder / Diagnostic Features (pp. 357–358); Differential Diagnosis (pp. 359–360)

9.7   A 45-year-old man with a family history of early-onset coronary artery disease avoids climbing stairs, eschews exercise, and abstains from sexual activity for fear of provoking a heart attack. He frequently checks his pulse, reads extensively about preventive cardiology, and tries many health food supplements alleged to be good for the heart. When experiencing an occasional twinge of chest discomfort, he rests in bed for 24 hours; however, he does not go to doctors because of fear about hearing bad news. What diagnosis best fits this clinical picture?

A. Generalized anxiety disorder.
B. Major depressive disorder.
C. Illness anxiety disorder.
D. Other medical condition.

Correct Answer: C. Illness anxiety disorder.

Explanation: In a minority of cases of illness anxiety disorder, individuals are too anxious to seek medical attention and avoid medical health care. The anxiety leads to maladaptive avoidance of situations (e.g., visiting sick family members) or activities (e.g., exercise) that these individuals fear might jeopardize their health (option C is correct). The first differential diagnostic consideration is an underlying medical condition. The presence of a medical condition does not rule out the possibility of coexisting illness anxiety disorder (option D is incorrect). If a medical condition is present, the health-related anxiety and disease concerns are clearly disproportionate to its seriousness. In generalized anxiety disorder, individuals worry about multiple events, situations, or activities, only one of which may involve health (option A is incorrect). In illness anxiety disorder, the health anxiety and fears are more persistent and enduring. Some individuals with a major depressive episode ruminate about their health and worry excessively about illness. A separate diagnosis of illness anxiety disorder is not made if these concerns occur only during major depressive episodes (option B is incorrect). If excessive illness worry persists after remission of an episode of major depressive disorder, the diagnosis of illness anxiety disorder should be considered.

9.7—Illness Anxiety Disorder / Diagnostic Features (pp. 357–358); Associated Features (p. 358); Differential Diagnosis (pp. 359–360)

9.8   A 25-year-old woman is hospitalized for evaluation of witnessed episodes that include loss of consciousness, rocking of the head from side to side, and nonsynchronous, bicycling movements of the arms and legs. Per family report, the episodes occur a few times per day and last for 2–5 minutes. Electroencephalography during the episodes does not reveal any ictal activity. Immediately after a fit, the sensorium appears clear. What is the most likely diagnosis?

A. Factitious disorder.
B. Malingering.
C. Somatic symptom disorder.

D. Conversion disorder (functional neurological symptom disorder), with attacks or seizures.

Correct Answer: D. Conversion disorder (functional neurological symptom disorder), with attacks or seizures.

Explanation: The diagnostic criteria of functional neurological symptom disorder include one or more symptoms of altered voluntary motor or sensory function that cause clinically significant distress or impairment in social, occupational, or other important areas of functioning or warrant medical attention. These symptoms are incompatible with recognized neurological or medical conditions and cannot be better explained by another mental disorder. Episodes of apparent unresponsiveness with or without limb movements may resemble epileptic seizures, syncope, or coma. The diagnosis rests on clinical findings that show clear evidence for incompatibility with recognized neurological disease (option D is correct). Functional neurological symptom disorder describes genuinely experienced symptoms that are not intentionally produced (i.e., not feigned). However, definite evidence of feigning (e.g., marked discrepancy between reported and observed activities of daily living) would suggest malingering if the individual's apparent aim is to obtain an obvious external reward (option B is incorrect) or factitious disorder in the absence of such reward (option A is incorrect). Functional neurological symptom disorder may be diagnosed in addition to somatic symptom disorder. Most of the somatic symptoms encountered in somatic symptom disorder cannot be demonstrated to be clearly incompatible with recognized neurological or medical disease, whereas in functional neurological symptom disorder, such incompatibility is required for the diagnosis.

9.8—Functional Neurological Symptom Disorder (Conversion Disorder) / diagnostic criteria (pp. 360–361); Diagnostic Features (pp. 361–362); Differential Diagnosis (pp. 363–364)

9.9   Which of the following presentations is most suggestive of a diagnosis of conversion disorder (functional neurological symptom disorder)?

A. Absence of Hoover's sign.
B. Chronic dystonic movements.
C. Tunnel vision.
D. Tremor with consistent direction and frequency.

Correct Answer: C. Tunnel vision.

Explanation: A tubular visual field (i.e., tunnel vision) and tests that indicate internal inconsistency in visual acuity suggest functional visual symptoms (option C is correct). Examples of examination findings that indicate incompatibility with recognized neurological disease include Hoover's sign, in which weakness of hip extension returns to normal strength with contralateral hip flexion against resistance (option A is incorrect), or an inability to copy simple rhythmical movements because of functional tremor (option D is incorrect). For functional dystonia, individuals typically present with sudden onset (option B is incorrect).

9.9—Functional Neurological Symptom Disorder (Conversion Disorder) / Diagnostic Features (pp. 361–362)

9.10 Why is *la belle indifférence* (apparent lack of concern about the symptom) not included as a diagnostic criterion for conversion disorder (functional neurological symptom disorder)?

    A. It is often associated with dissociative symptoms.
    B. It has poor specificity.
    C. It may be absent in up to 50% of individuals.
    D. It is present only at symptom onset or during attacks.

Correct Answer: B. It has poor specificity.

Explanation: Several associated features can support the diagnosis of functional neurological symptom disorder, although none are specific. The phenomenon of *la belle indifférence* (i.e., apparent lack of concern about the nature or implications of the symptom) has been associated with functional neurological symptom disorder, but it is not specific and should not be used to make the diagnosis (option B is correct). Although assessment for stress and trauma is important, *la belle indifférence* may be absent in up to 50% of individuals (option C is incorrect). Functional neurological symptom disorder is often associated with dissociative symptoms (option A is incorrect), particularly at symptom onset or during attacks (option D is incorrect).

9.10—Functional Neurological Symptom Disorder (Conversion Disorder) / Associated Features (p. 362)

9.11 A 20-year-old man presents with the complaint of acute onset of decreased visual acuity in the left eye. Physical, neurological, and laboratory examinations are entirely normal, including stereopsis testing, fogging test, and brain magnetic resonance imaging. The remainder of the history is negative except for the patient's perseverative focus on facial asymmetry with plans to have plastic surgery soon. Which of the following diagnoses is suggested?

    A. Somatic symptom disorder and panic disorder.
    B. Factitious disorder and malingering.
    C. Body dysmorphic disorder and conversion disorder (functional neurological symptom disorder).
    D. Depressive disorder.

Correct Answer: C. Body dysmorphic disorder and conversion disorder (functional neurological symptom disorder).

Explanation: Most of the somatic symptoms encountered in somatic symptom disorder cannot be demonstrated to be clearly incompatible with recognized neurological or medical disease, whereas in functional neurological symptom disorder, such incompatibility is required for the diagnosis (option A is incorrect and option C is correct). Individuals with body dysmorphic disorder are excessively concerned about a perceived defect in their physical appearance (option C is correct). Functional neurological symptom disorder describes genuinely experienced symptoms that are not intentionally produced (i.e., not feigned). However, definite evidence of feigning (e.g., marked discrepancy between reported and observed activities of daily living) would suggest malingering if the individual's apparent aim is to obtain an obvious external reward or factitious disorder in the absence of such reward (option B is incorrect). In depressive disorders, individuals may report general heaviness of their limbs, whereas the weakness of functional neurological symptom disorder is more focal and prominent. Depressive disorders are also differentiated by the presence of core depressive symptoms (option D is incorrect).

9.11—Functional Neurological Symptom Disorder (Conversion Disorder) / Differential Diagnosis (pp. 363–364)

9.12 A 50-year-old man with hard-to-control hypertension admits regularly "taking a break" from medications because he was brought up with the belief that pills are bad and natural remedies are better. He is well aware that his blood pressure can become dangerously high when he is not taking his medications. Which diagnosis best fits this case?

A. Somatic symptom disorder.
B. Illness anxiety disorder.
C. Adjustment disorder.
D. Psychological factors affecting other medical conditions.

Correct Answer: D. Psychological factors affecting other medical conditions.

Explanation: The diagnosis of psychological factors affecting another medical condition applies when a medical symptom or condition (other than a mental disorder) is present (Criterion A) *and* psychological or behavioral factors adversely affect the medical condition (Criterion B). The psychological or behavioral factors adversely affect the medical condition in one of the following ways: 1) there is a close temporal association between the psychological factors and the development or exacerbation of, or delayed recovery from, the medical condition; 2) the factors interfere with the treatment of the medical condition (e.g., poor adherence); 3) the factors constitute additional well-established health risks for the individual; or 4) the factors influence the underlying pathophysiology, precipitating or exacerbating symptoms or necessitating medical attention (option D is correct). Somatic symptom disorder is characterized by a combination of distressing somatic symptoms and excessive or maladaptive thoughts, feelings, and behavior in response to these symptoms or associated health concerns. The individual may or may not have a diagnosable medical condition. In contrast, in psychological factors affecting other medical conditions, the psychological factors adversely affect a medical condition; the individual's thoughts, feelings, and behavior are not necessarily excessive (option A is incorrect). Illness anxiety disorder is characterized by high illness anxiety that is distressing and/or disruptive to daily life, with minimal somatic symptoms. In psychological factors affecting other medical conditions, anxiety may be a relevant psychological factor affecting a medical condition, but the clinical concern is the adverse effects on the medical condition (option B is incorrect). Abnormal psychological or behavioral symptoms that develop in response to a medical condition are more properly coded as an adjustment disorder (a clinically significant psychological response to an identifiable stressor); option C is incorrect.

9.12—Psychological Factors Affecting Other Medical Conditions / diagnostic criteria (pp. 364–365); Differential Diagnosis (pp. 366–367)

9.13 A 60-year-old man with prostate cancer has bony metastases that cause persistent pain. He is being treated with antiandrogen medications that result in hot flashes. Although (by his own assessment) his pain is well controlled with analgesics, he states that he is unable to work because of his symptoms. Despite reassurance that his medications are controlling his metastatic disease, every instance of pain leads him to worry that he has new bony lesions and is about to die, and he continually expresses fears about his impending death to his wife and children. Which diagnosis best fits this patient's presentation?

A. Panic disorder.
B. Illness anxiety disorder.
C. Somatic symptom disorder.
D. Psychological factors affecting other medical conditions.

Correct Answer: C. Somatic symptom disorder.

Explanation: The diagnosis of somatic symptom disorder requires distressing or impairing somatic symptoms that may or may not be associated with another medical condition but must be accompanied by excessive or disproportionate thoughts, feelings, or behaviors related to the somatic symptoms or associated health concerns (option C is correct). In contrast, the diagnosis of psychological factors affecting other medical conditions requires the presence of a medical condition, as well as psychological factors that adversely affect its course or interfere with its treatment (option D is incorrect). In panic disorder, somatic symptoms and anxiety about health tend to occur in acute episodes, whereas in somatic symptom disorder, anxiety and somatic symptoms are more persistent (option A is incorrect). If the individual has extensive worries about health but no or minimal somatic symptoms, it may be more appropriate to consider illness anxiety disorder (option B is incorrect).

9.13—Somatic Symptom Disorder / Differential Diagnosis (pp. 355–356)

9.14 What is the essential diagnostic feature of factitious disorder?

A. Motivation to assume the sick role.
B. Falsification of medical or psychological signs and symptoms.
C. Obvious external rewards.
D. Absence of a preexisting medical condition.

Correct Answer: B. Falsification of medical or psychological signs and symptoms.

Explanation: The essential feature of factitious disorder is the falsification of medical or psychological signs and symptoms in the individual or others that are associated with the identified deception (option B is correct). The diagnosis of factitious disorder emphasizes the objective identification of falsification of signs and symptoms of illness and not the individual motivations of the falsifier (option A is incorrect). The diagnosis requires demonstrating that the individual is taking surreptitious actions to misrepresent, simulate, or cause signs or symptoms of illness or injury even in the absence of obvious external rewards (option C is incorrect). Although a preexisting medical condition may be present, the deceptive behavior or induction of injury associated with deception causes others to view such individuals as more ill or impaired, and this can lead to excessive clinical intervention (option D is incorrect).

9.14—Factitious Disorder / Diagnostic Features (p. 368)

9.15 When a parent knowingly and deceptively reports signs and symptoms of illness in her preschool-age child, resulting in the child's hospitalization and subjection to numerous tests and procedures, what diagnosis should be recorded for the child?

A. Deception to avoid legal liability.
B. Educational deficits or disabilities.
C. No diagnosis is made for the child.
D. Factitious disorder imposed on another.

Correct Answer: C. No diagnosis is made for the child.

Explanation: When an individual falsifies illness in another (e.g., children, adults, pets), the diagnosis is factitious disorder imposed on another. The perpetrator, not the victim, is given the diagnosis (option C is correct and option

D is incorrect). Individuals with factitious disorder imposed on another sometimes falsely allege the presence of educational deficits or disabilities in their children for which they demand special attention, often at considerable inconvenience to education professionals (option B is incorrect). Caregivers who lie about abuse injuries in dependents solely to protect themselves from liability are not diagnosed with factitious disorder imposed on another because protection from liability is an external reward (option A is incorrect).

9.15—Factitious Disorder / Recording Procedures (p. 368); Associated Features (p. 368); Differential Diagnosis (pp. 369–370)

9.16 A 25-year-old woman with a history of intravenous heroin abuse is admitted to the hospital with infective endocarditis. Blood cultures are positive for several fungal species. Search of the patient's belongings discloses hidden syringes and needles and a small bag of dirt, which, when cultured, yields the same fungal species. Which of the following diagnoses apply?

A. Opioid use disorder and borderline personality disorder.
B. Opioid use disorder and malingering.
C. Opioid use disorder and factitious disorder.
D. Malingering and borderline personality disorder.

Correct Answer: C. Opioid use disorder and factitious disorder.

Explanation: The essential feature of factitious disorder is the falsification of medical or psychological signs and symptoms in the individual or others who are associated with the identified deception. The diagnosis requires demonstrating that the individual is taking surreptitious actions to misrepresent, simulate, or cause signs or symptoms of illness or injury even in the absence of obvious external rewards. Individuals with factitious disorder might, for example, physically injure themselves or induce illness in themselves or another (e.g., by injecting fecal material to produce an abscess or to induce sepsis; option C is correct). Malingering is differentiated from factitious disorder by the intentional reporting of symptoms for personal gain (e.g., money, time off work). In contrast, the diagnosis of factitious disorder requires that the illness falsification is not fully accounted for by external rewards (options B and D are incorrect). Deliberate physical self-harm in the absence of suicidal intent can also occur in association with other mental disorders, such as borderline personality disorder. Factitious disorder requires that the induction of injury occur in association with deception (options A and D are incorrect).

9.16—Factitious Disorder / Diagnostic Features (p. 368); Differential Diagnosis (pp. 369–370)

9.17 After finding a breast lump, a 50-year-old woman with a family history of breast cancer is overwhelmed by feelings of anxiety. Consultation with a breast surgeon, mammogram, and biopsy show the lump to be benign. The surgeon tells her that she requires no treatment; however, she continues to ruminate about the possibility of cancer and surgery that will result in disfigurement. Her sleep is restless, and she is having trouble concentrating at work. After 6 weeks of these symptoms, her primary physician refers her for psychiatric consultation. Her medical and psychiatric history is otherwise negative. Which diagnosis best fits this presentation?

A. Somatic symptom disorder.
B. Illness anxiety disorder.
C. Unspecified somatic symptom and related disorder.
D. Other specified somatic symptom and related disorder.

Correct Answer: D. Other specified somatic symptom and related disorder.

Explanation: The category of *other specified somatic symptom and related disorder* applies to presentations in which symptoms characteristic of a somatic symptom and related disorder that cause clinically significant distress or impairment in social, occupational, or other important areas of functioning predominate but do not meet the full criteria for any of the disorders in the somatic symptom and related disorders diagnostic class. Examples include a brief somatic symptom disorder or brief illness anxiety disorder with duration of symptoms less than 6 months (option D is correct). Criterion C of somatic symptom disorder specifies that the state of being symptomatic is persistent (typically more than 6 months) (option A is incorrect). Criterion E of illness anxiety disorder specifies that illness preoccupation has been present for at least 6 months (option B is incorrect). The category of *unspecified somatic symptom and related disorder* applies to presentations in which symptoms characteristic of a somatic symptom and related disorder that cause clinically significant distress or impairment in social, occupational, or other important areas of functioning predominate but do not meet the full criteria for any of the disorders in the somatic symptom and related disorders diagnostic class. The unspecified somatic symptom and related disorder category should not be used unless there are decidedly unusual situations where there is insufficient information to make a more specific diagnosis (option C is incorrect).

9.17—Other Specified Somatic Symptom and Related Disorder (p. 370)

9.18   After finding a breast lump, a 53-year-old woman with a family history of breast cancer is overwhelmed by feelings of anxiety. Consultation with a breast surgeon, mammogram, and biopsy show the lump to be benign. The surgeon indicates that she requires no treatment; however, she continues to ruminate about the possibility of cancer and surgery that will result in disfigurement. Her sleep is restless, and she is having trouble concentrating at work. After 6 weeks in this state, her primary physician requests that she consult a psychiatrist. On initial evaluation the patient weeps throughout the interview and is so distraught that the evaluator is unable to elicit details of her medical and psychiatric history beyond reviewing the current "crisis." Which diagnosis best fits this presentation?

A. Somatic symptom disorder.
B. Illness anxiety disorder.
C. Unspecified somatic symptom and related disorder.
D. Other specified somatic symptom and related disorder.

Correct Answer: C. Unspecified somatic symptom and related disorder.

Explanation: The category of *unspecified somatic symptom and related disorder* applies to presentations in which symptoms characteristic of a somatic symptom and related disorder that cause clinically significant distress or impairment in social, occupational, or other important areas of functioning predominate but do not meet the full criteria for any of the disorders in the somatic symptom and related disorders diagnostic class. The unspecified somatic symptom and related disorder category should not be used unless there are decidedly unusual situations where there is insufficient information to make a more specific diagnosis (option C is correct). Criterion C of somatic symptom disorder specifies that the state of being symptomatic is persistent (typically more than 6 months); option A is incorrect. Criterion E of illness anxiety disorder specifies that illness preoccupation has been present for at least 6 months (option B is incorrect). The category *other specified somatic symptom and related disorder* applies to presentations in which symptoms characteristic of a somatic symptom and related disorder that cause clinically significant distress or impairment in social, occupational, or other important areas of functioning predominate but do not meet the full criteria for any of the disorders in the somatic symptom and related disorders diagnostic class (option D is incorrect).

9.18—Unspecified Somatic Symptom and Related Disorder (p. 370)

CHAPTER 10

Feeding and Eating Disorders

10.1 A 27-year-old pregnant woman in her first trimester is joined at her OB-GYN appointment by her partner. The partner informs the physician that the patient has been eating odd items such as pieces of paper and cloth over the past 2 months. The patient admits this behavior, noting that it disturbs her. She is upset at having lost weight and denies any desire to do so. What is the most appropriate diagnosis?

  A. Anorexia nervosa.
  B. Unspecified feeding or eating disorder.
  C. Pica
  D. Factitious disorder.

Correct Answer: C. Pica.

Explanation: The essential feature of pica is the eating of one or more nonnutritive, nonfood substances on a persistent basis over a period of at least 1 month (Criterion A) that is severe enough to warrant clinical attention. The term *nonfood* is included because the diagnosis of pica does not apply to ingestion of diet products that have minimal nutritional content. There is typically no aversion to food in general. The eating of nonnutritive, nonfood substances must be developmentally inappropriate (Criterion B) and not part of a culturally supported or socially normative practice (Criterion C).

   Pica can usually be distinguished from the other feeding and eating disorders by the consumption of nonnutritive, nonfood substances. It is important to note, however, that some presentations of anorexia nervosa include ingestion of nonnutritive, nonfood substances, such as paper tissues, as a means of attempting to control appetite. In such cases, when the eating of nonnutritive, nonfood substances is primarily used as a means of weight control, anorexia nervosa should be the primary diagnosis. Some individuals with factitious disorder may intentionally ingest foreign objects as part of the pattern of falsification of physical symptoms. In such instances, there is an element of deception that is consistent with deliberate induction of injury or disease.

10.1—Pica / Diagnostic Features (p. 372); Differential Diagnosis (p. 373)

10.2   Which of the following is a common comorbid diagnosis with rumination disorder?

   A. Anorexia nervosa.
   B. Intellectual disability.
   C. Bulimia nervosa.
   D. Avoidant/restrictive food intake disorder.

Correct Answer: B. Intellectual disability.

Explanation: The essential feature of rumination disorder is the repeated regurgitation of food occurring after feeding or eating over a period of at least 1 month (Criterion A). Previously swallowed food that may be partially digested is brought up into the mouth without apparent nausea, involuntary retching, or disgust. The food may be re-chewed and then ejected from the mouth or re-swallowed. Regurgitation in rumination disorder should be frequent, occurring at least several times per week, typically daily. The behavior is not better explained by an associated gastrointestinal or other medical condition (e.g., gastroesophageal reflux, pyloric stenosis) (Criterion B) and does not occur exclusively during the course of anorexia nervosa, bulimia nervosa, binge-eating disorder, or avoidant/restrictive food intake disorder (Criterion C). If the symptoms occur in the context of another mental disorder (e.g., intellectual developmental disorder [intellectual disability]), they must be sufficiently severe to warrant additional clinical attention (Criterion D) and should represent a primary aspect of the individual's presentation requiring intervention. The disorder may be diagnosed across the life span, particularly in individuals who also have intellectual developmental disorder.

10.2—Rumination Disorder / Diagnostic Features (p. 374)

10.3   Which of the following distinguishes anorexia nervosa from bulimia nervosa?

   A. Binge eating.
   B. Intense fear of gaining weight.
   C. Abnormally low body weight.
   D. Compensatory behaviors.

Correct Answer: C. Abnormally low body weight.

Explanation: Individuals with bulimia nervosa exhibit recurrent episodes of binge eating, engage in inappropriate behavior to avoid weight gain (e.g., self-induced vomiting), and are overly concerned with body shape and weight. However, unlike individuals with anorexia nervosa, binge-eating/purging type, individuals with bulimia nervosa maintain body weight at or above a minimally normal level.

10.4 Which of the following distinguishes binge-eating disorder from bulimia nervosa?

A. Compensatory behaviors.
B. Binge-eating frequency.
C. Binge-eating quantity.
D. Frequent dieting.

Correct Answer: A. Compensatory behaviors.

Explanation: Binge-eating disorder has recurrent binge eating in common with bulimia nervosa but differs from the latter disorder in some fundamental respects. In terms of clinical presentation, the recurrent inappropriate compensatory behavior (e.g., purging, driven exercise) seen in bulimia nervosa is absent in binge-eating disorder. Unlike individuals with bulimia nervosa, individuals with binge-eating disorder typically do not show marked or sustained dietary restriction designed to influence body weight and shape between binge-eating episodes. They may, however, report frequent attempts at dieting.

10.4—Binge-Eating Disorder / Differential Diagnosis (p. 395)

10.5 According to DSM-5-TR criteria, which of the following precludes a diagnosis of avoidant/restrictive food intake disorder (ARFID)?

A. A lifetime anorexia nervosa diagnosis.
B. Significant weight loss.
C. Dependence on enteral feeding.
D. Distorted body image.

Correct Answer: D. Distorted body image.

Explanation: ARFID replaces and extends the DSM-IV diagnosis of feeding disorder of infancy or early childhood to include older children, adolescents, and adults. The main diagnostic feature of avoidant/restrictive food intake disorder is avoidance or restriction of food intake that is associated with one or more of the following consequences: significant weight loss, significant nutritional deficiency (or related health impact), dependence on enteral feeding or oral nutritional supplements, or marked interference with psychosocial functioning (Criterion A).

ARFID does not include avoidance or restriction of food intake related to lack of availability of food (e.g., food insecurity) or to cultural practices (e.g., religious fasting, normal dieting) (Criterion B). The disturbance is not better explained by excessive concern about body weight or shape (Criterion C) or by concurrent medical factors or mental disorders (Criterion D). Although ARFID should not occur exclusively during the course of bulimia or anorexia nervosa (Criterion C), those diagnoses do not preclude a diagnosis of ARFID if appropriate.

10.5—Avoidant/Restrictive Food Intake Disorder / Diagnostic Features (pp. 376–377)

10.6   Which specific pattern of avoidant/restrictive food intake disorder (ARFID) is most likely to appear during infancy?

    A. ARFID based on food characteristics.
    B. ARFID related to aversive experiences.
    C. ARFID with lack of interest in food.
    D. ARFID affecting social functioning.

Correct Answer: C. ARFID with lack of interest in food.

Explanation: Food avoidance or restriction associated with insufficient intake or lack of interest in eating most commonly develops in infancy or early childhood and may persist in adulthood. Likewise, avoidance based on sensory characteristics of food tends to arise in the first decade of life but may persist into adulthood. Avoidance related to aversive consequences can arise at any age. The scant literature regarding long-term outcomes suggests that food avoidance or restriction based on sensory aspects is relatively stable and longstanding, but when persisting into adulthood, such avoidance/restriction can be associated with relatively normal functioning.

10.6—Avoidant/Restrictive Food Intake Disorder / Development and Course (pp. 377–378)

10.7   A 45-year-old woman had a choking episode 3 years ago after eating salad. Since that time she has been afraid to eat a wide range of foods, fearing that she will choke. This fear has affected her functionality and her ability to go to restaurants with friends and has contributed to weight loss. Which diagnosis best fits this clinical picture?

    A. Anorexia nervosa.
    B. Avoidant/restrictive food intake disorder.
    C. Specific phobia.
    D. Adjustment disorder.

Correct Answer: B. Avoidant/restrictive food intake disorder.

Explanation: Food avoidance or restriction may also represent a conditioned negative response associated with food intake following, or in anticipation of, an aversive experience, such as choking; a traumatic investigation, usually involving the gastrointestinal tract (e.g., esophagoscopy); or repeated vomiting. The terms *functional dysphagia* and *globus hystericus* have also been used for such conditions.

Restriction of energy intake relative to requirements that leads to significantly low body weight is a core feature of anorexia nervosa. However, individuals with anorexia nervosa also display a fear of gaining weight or of becoming fat or persistent behavior that interferes with weight gain, as well as specific disturbances in relation to perception and experience of their own body weight and shape. These features are not present in avoidant/restrictive food intake disorder.

Specific phobia, other type, includes as an example "situations that may lead to choking or vomiting," which can represent the primary trigger for the fear, anxiety, or avoidance required for diagnosis. Distinguishing specific phobia from avoidant/restrictive food intake disorder can be difficult when a fear of choking or vomiting has resulted in food avoidance. Although avoidance or restriction of food intake secondary to a pronounced fear of choking or vomiting can be conceptualized as specific phobia, in situations in which the eating problem becomes the primary focus of clinical attention, avoidant/restrictive food intake disorder is the appropriate diagnosis.

10.7—Avoidant/Restrictive Food Intake Disorder / Diagnostic Features (pp. 376–377); Differential Diagnosis (pp. 379–380)

10.8   What are the two subtypes of anorexia nervosa?

A. Restricting type and binge-eating/purging type.
B. Energy-sparing type and binge-eating/purging type.
C. Low-calorie/low-carbohydrate type and restricting type.
D. Restricting type and low-weight type.

Correct Answer: A. Restricting type and binge-eating/purging type.

Explanation: The subtype specifiers describe the primary mode of weight loss used for the past 3 months. In the restricting subtype of anorexia nervosa, weight loss is accomplished primarily through dieting, fasting, and/or excessive exercise; in the binge-eating/purging subtype, it is accomplished through recurrent episodes of binge eating or purging behavior (i.e., self-induced vomiting or the misuse of laxatives, diuretics, or enemas).

Most individuals with the binge-eating/purging type of anorexia nervosa who binge eat also purge through self-induced vomiting or the misuse of laxatives, diuretics, or enemas. Some individuals with this subtype of anorexia nervosa do not binge eat but do regularly purge after the consumption of small amounts of food. Crossover between the subtypes over the course of the disorder is not uncommon; therefore, subtype description should be used to describe current symptoms rather than longitudinal course.

10.8—Anorexia Nervosa / diagnostic criteria (p. 381); Subtypes (p. 382)

10.9   Which of the following is required for the diagnosis of anorexia nervosa?

A. Inability to gain weight despite normal intake.
B. Social, occupational, or functional disturbance.

C. Compensatory purging behaviors.

D. Disturbed body image.

Correct Answer: D. Disturbed body image.

Explanation: There are three essential features of anorexia nervosa: persistent energy intake restriction, intense fear of gaining weight or of becoming fat or persistent behavior that interferes with weight gain, and a disturbance in self-perceived weight or shape. The individual maintains a body weight that is below a minimally normal level for age, sex, developmental trajectory, and physical health (Criterion A). Individuals' body weights frequently meet this criterion following a significant weight loss, but among children and adolescents, there may alternatively be failure to make expected weight gain or to maintain a normal developmental trajectory (i.e., while growing in height) instead of weight loss.

The experience and significance of body weight and shape are distorted in these individuals (Criterion C). Some individuals feel globally overweight. Others realize that they are thin but are still concerned that certain body parts, particularly the abdomen, buttocks, and thighs, are "too fat." They may employ a variety of techniques to evaluate their body size or weight, including frequent weighing, obsessive measuring of body parts, and persistent use of a mirror to check for perceived areas of fat.

10.9—Anorexia Nervosa / Diagnostic Features (pp. 382–383)

10.10 Which of the following laboratory abnormalities is commonly found in individuals with anorexia nervosa?

A. Elevated thyroxine (T_4).

B. Elevated blood urea nitrogen (BUN).

C. Elevated bone density.

D. Elevated phosphate.

Correct Answer: B. Elevated blood urea nitrogen (BUN).

Explanation: Presence of certain laboratory abnormalities may serve to increase diagnostic confidence. The following abnormalities may be observed in anorexia nervosa: Leukopenia is common, with the loss of all cell types but usually with apparent lymphocytosis. Mild anemia can occur, as well as thrombocytopenia and, rarely, bleeding problems. Dehydration may be reflected by an elevated BUN level. Hypercholesterolemia is common. Hepatic enzyme levels may be elevated. Hypomagnesemia, hypozincemia, hypophosphatemia, and hyperamylasemia are occasionally observed. Self-induced vomiting may lead to metabolic alkalosis (elevated serum bicarbonate), hypochloremia, and hypokalemia; laxative abuse may cause a mild metabolic acidosis. Serum T_4 levels are usually in the low-normal range; triiodothyronine (T_3) levels are decreased, whereas reverse T_3 levels are elevated. Females have low serum estrogen levels, whereas males have low levels of serum testosterone. Sinus bradycardia is common, and, rarely, arrhythmias are noted. Significant prolongation of the QTc interval is observed in some individuals. Low bone mineral density, with specific areas of osteopenia or osteoporosis, is often seen. The risk of fracture is significantly elevated.

Electroencephalography: Diffuse abnormalities, reflecting a metabolic encephalopathy, may result from significant fluid and electrolyte disturbances. There is often a significant reduction in resting energy expenditure.

10.10—Anorexia Nervosa / Diagnostic Markers (p. 385)

10.11 Which of the following is commonly comorbid with anorexia nervosa?

A. Major depressive disorder.
B. Narcissistic personality disorder.
C. Schizophrenia.
D. Intellectual disability.

Correct Answer: A. Major depressive disorder.

Explanation: Bipolar, depressive, and anxiety disorders commonly co-occur with anorexia nervosa. Many individuals with anorexia nervosa report the presence of either an anxiety disorder or symptoms of anxiety prior to onset of their eating disorder. Obsessive-compulsive disorder is described in some individuals with anorexia nervosa, especially those with the restricting type. Alcohol use disorder and other substance use disorders may also be comorbid with anorexia nervosa, especially among individuals with the binge-eating/purging type.

10.11—Anorexia Nervosa / Comorbidity (p. 387)

10.12 In which developmental period does bulimia nervosa most commonly begin?

A. Middle adulthood.
B. Early childhood.
C. Adolescence.
D. It is equally distributed across the life cycle.

Correct Answer: C. Adolescence.

Explanation: Bulimia nervosa commonly begins in adolescence or young adulthood. Onset before puberty or after age 40 is uncommon. The binge eating frequently begins during or after an episode of dieting to lose weight. Experiencing multiple stressful life events also can precipitate onset of bulimia nervosa. Disturbed eating behavior persists for at least several years in a high percentage of clinical samples. The course may be chronic or intermittent, with periods of remission alternating with recurrences of binge eating. However, over longer-term follow-up, the symptoms of many individuals appear to diminish with or without treatment, although treatment clearly has impacts on outcome. Periods of remission longer than 1 year are associated with better long-term outcome.

10.12—Bulimia Nervosa / Development and Course (p. 390)

10.13 Which of the following is a common comorbid diagnosis in patients with bulimia nervosa?

A. Stimulant use disorder.
B. Antisocial personality disorder.
C. Avoidant personality disorder.
D. Binge-eating disorder.

Correct Answer: A. Stimulant use disorder.

Explanation: Comorbidity with mental disorders is common in individuals with bulimia nervosa, with most experiencing at least one other mental disorder and many experiencing multiple comorbidities. Comorbidity is not limited to any particular subset but rather occurs across a wide range of mental disorders. There is an increased frequency of depressive symptoms (e.g., low self-esteem) and bipolar and depressive disorders (particularly depressive disorders) in individuals with bulimia nervosa. In many individuals, the mood disturbance begins at the same time as or following the development of bulimia nervosa, and individuals often ascribe their mood disturbances to the bulimia nervosa. However, in some individuals, the mood disturbance clearly precedes the development of bulimia nervosa. There may also be an increased frequency of anxiety symptoms (e.g., fear of social situations) or anxiety disorders. These mood and anxiety disturbances frequently remit following effective treatment of the bulimia nervosa. The lifetime prevalence of substance use disorder, particularly alcohol use disorder or stimulant use disorder, is at least 30% among individuals with bulimia nervosa. Stimulant use often begins in an attempt to control appetite and weight. A substantial percentage of individuals with bulimia nervosa also have personality features that meet criteria for one or more personality disorders, most frequently borderline personality disorder.

10.13—Bulimia Nervosa / Comorbidity (p. 392)

10.14 To meet criteria for a diagnosis of binge-eating disorder, which of the following accurately characterizes an episode of binge eating?

A. It is independent of cultural context.
B. It can go on for up to 6 hours.

C. It occurs at least once a week for 3 months.

D. It may consist of continual snacking.

Correct Answer: C. It occurs at least once a week for 3 months.

Explanation: The essential feature of binge-eating disorder is recurrent episodes of binge eating that must occur, on average, at least once per week for 3 months (Criterion D). An episode of binge eating is defined as eating, in a discrete period of time, an amount of food that is definitely larger than most people would eat in a similar period of time under similar circumstances (Criterion A1). The context in which the eating occurs may affect the clinician's estimation of whether the intake is excessive. For example, a quantity of food that might be regarded as excessive for a typical meal might be considered normal during a celebration or holiday meal. A *discrete period of time* refers to a limited period, usually less than 2 hours. A single episode of binge eating need not be restricted to one setting. For example, an individual may begin a binge in a restaurant and then continue to eat on returning home. Continual snacking on small amounts of food throughout the day would not be considered an eating binge.

10.14—Binge-Eating Disorder / Diagnostic Features (pp. 393–394)

CHAPTER 11

Elimination Disorders

11.1   A 7-year-old boy with moderate developmental delay presents with a chronic history of wetting his clothes during the day about once weekly, even during school. He is now refusing to go to school for fear of wetting his pants and being ridiculed by his classmates. Which of the following statements accurately describes the diagnostic options regarding enuresis in this case?

    A. He should not be diagnosed with enuresis because the frequency is less than twice per week.

    B. He should be diagnosed with enuresis because the incontinence is resulting in impairment of age-appropriate role functioning.

    C. He should not be diagnosed with enuresis because his mental age is likely less than 5 years.

    D. He should be diagnosed with enuresis, diurnal-only subtype.

Correct Answer: C. He should not be diagnosed with enuresis because his mental age is likely less than 5 years.

Explanation: Criterion C requires that an individual be of an age at which consistent continence can be reasonably expected. Although this ordinarily occurs at age 5, in the case of developmental delay, one goes by the child's mental age. In this vignette it is likely that the child has not yet attained a mental age of 5 and is ineligible for the diagnosis even though he has clinically significant distress. Criterion B requires that the incontinence be clinically significant, and this condition can be met by the frequency/duration requirement of twice weekly for 3 months or by the fact that it causes clinically significant distress. In this vignette the latter condition is fulfilled (because the child has clinically significant distress), so Criterion B is met and would not be a reason to withhold the diagnosis. Although the general public may think of nighttime incontinence as a central aspect, enuresis can present as, and can be specified as, nocturnal only, diurnal only, or nocturnal and diurnal (i.e., combined presentation).

11.1—Enuresis / diagnostic criteria (p. 399)

11.2   What is more common in children with enuresis?

A. High self-esteem.
B. Being socially oppressed.
C. Persistence of urinary incontinence into adulthood.
D. Older age.

Correct Answer: B. Being socially oppressed.

Explanation: Boys and members of socially oppressed groups may have a higher prevalence of enuresis, as found in African American children in the United States and Turkish or Moroccan children in the Netherlands. The prevalence of nocturnal enuresis in the community decreases with age; in several geographic settings, including the United States, the Netherlands, and Hong Kong, the range is around 5%–10% among 5-year-olds, 3%–5% among 10-year-olds, and around 1% among individuals 15 years or older. The amount of impairment associated with enuresis is a function of the limitation on the child's social activities (e.g., ineligibility for sleepaway camp) or its effect on the child's self-esteem; the degree of social ostracism by peers; and the anger, punishment, and rejection on the part of caregivers. Diurnal enuresis is uncommon after age 9 years. When enuresis persists into late childhood or adolescence, the incontinence may resolve, but urinary frequency generally persists, and incontinence can recur later in adulthood in women.

11.2—Enuresis / Prevalence; Development and Course (pp. 400–401)

11.3   What is associated with the diurnal-only subtype of enuresis?

A. Male sex.
B. Age >9 years old.
C. Monosymptomatic enuresis.
D. *Voiding postponement*, in which micturition is consciously deferred because of a social reluctance to use the bathroom or to interrupt a play activity.

Correct Answer: D. *Voiding postponement*, in which micturition is consciously deferred because of a social reluctance to use the bathroom or to interrupt a play activity.

Explanation: The nocturnal-only subtype of enuresis is sometimes referred to as *monosymptomatic enuresis*. The diurnal-only subtype of enuresis involves incontinence only during the day and is also referred to as *urinary incontinence*. It is more common in females and is uncommon after age 9. In daytime (diurnal) enuresis, the child defers voiding until incontinence occurs, sometimes because of a reluctance to use the toilet as a result of social anxiety or a preoccupation with school or play activity. The enuretic event most commonly occurs in the early afternoon on school days and may be associated with symptoms of disruptive behavior.

11.3—Enuresis / Associated Features; Development and Course; Sex- and Gender-Related Diagnostic Issues (pp. 400–401)

11.4 Which of the following statements correctly identifies a distinction between primary enuresis and secondary enuresis?

A. Children with secondary enuresis have higher rates of psychiatric comorbidity than do children with primary enuresis.
B. Primary enuresis has a typical onset at age 10, much later than the onset of secondary enuresis.
C. Primary enuresis is never preceded by a period of continence, whereas secondary enuresis is always preceded by a period of continence.
D. Unlike primary enuresis, secondary enuresis tends to persist into late adolescence.

Correct Answer: C. Primary enuresis is never preceded by a period of continence, whereas secondary enuresis is always preceded by a period of continence.

Explanation: In primary enuresis, the individual has never established urinary continence; in secondary enuresis, incontinence develops after a period of established continence. By definition, primary incontinence begins when a child reaches the mental age of 5. Prior to this, there is no expectation of consistent continence, and incontinence of urine is not considered pathological. After age 5, a child has either established continence and lost it or never developed continence, in which case the onset should be considered to be at age 5, regardless of age at presentation. Urinary incontinence secondary to another medical condition is not diagnosed as enuresis because Criterion D rules this out. Secondary enuresis is not associated with higher rates of psychiatric comorbidity, and both forms tend to disappear by late adolescence (when prevalence rates approach 1%).

11.4—Enuresis / Development and Course (p. 400)

11.5 Which of the following statements correctly describes factors related to the etiology and/or onset of enuresis?

A. Enuresis has been shown to be heritable, with a child being at least twice as likely to have the diagnosis if either parent has had it.
B. Mode of toilet training or its neglect can affect rates of enuresis, as shown by high rates seen in orphanages.
C. In girls with enuresis, nocturnal enuresis is the more common form.
D. Rates of enuresis are much higher in European countries than in developing countries.

Correct Answer: B. Mode of toilet training or its neglect can affect rates of enuresis, as shown by high rates seen in orphanages.

Explanation: Enuresis has etiological sources in both genetics and learned behaviors. There are very high rates of enuresis in orphanages and other residential institutions, likely related to the mode and environment in which toilet training occurs. Heritability has been shown in family, twin, and segregation analyses. The relative risk of having a child who develops enuresis is greater for previously enuretic fathers (odds ratio of 10.1) than for previously enuretic mothers (odds ratio of 3.6). Nocturnal enuresis is more common in males; diurnal incontinence is more common in females. Enuresis has been reported in a variety of European, African, and Asian countries as well as in the United States. At a national level, prevalence rates are remarkably similar, and there is great similarity in the developmental trajectories found in different countries.

11.5—Enuresis / Risk and Prognostic Factors; Culture-Related Diagnostic Issues; Sex- and Gender-Related Diagnostic Issues (p. 401)

11.6   A 4-year-old boy with moderate developmental delay presents with a history of accidentally passing feces into his underwear during the day about once every 2 weeks, even during school. He is now refusing to go to school for fear of soiling his pants and being ridiculed by classmates. Which of the following statements accurately describes the diagnostic options regarding encopresis in this case?

A. Encopresis diagnosis is incorrect because the frequency is less than twice per week.
B. Encopresis diagnosis is incorrect because the incontinence is unintentional.
C. Encopresis diagnosis is incorrect because the patient's mental age is likely less than 4 years old.
D. Encopresis diagnosis is correct.

Correct Answer: C. Encopresis diagnosis is incorrect because the patient's mental age is likely less than 4 years old.

Explanation: Criterion C requires that an individual be of an age in which consistent continence can be reasonably expected. Although this ordinarily occurs at age 4, in the case of developmental delay, one goes by the child's mental age. In this vignette it is likely that the child has not yet attained a mental age of 4 years and is ineligible for the diagnosis even though he has clinically significant distress. Criterion B requires that the incontinence be clinically significant, and this condition can be met by the frequency/duration requirement of once monthly for 3 months. In this vignette the child has sufficient frequency, so Criterion B is met and would not be a reason to withhold the diagnosis. The passage of feces may be voluntary or involuntary under Criterion A.

11.6—Encopresis / diagnostic criteria (p. 402)

11.7   Which of the following statements about encopresis is *true*?

A. When oppositional defiant disorder or conduct disorder is present, one cannot diagnose encopresis.

B. When constipation is present, one cannot diagnose encopresis.

C. Urinary tract infections can be comorbid with encopresis.

D. Although it is embarrassing, encopresis has no effect on children's self-esteem.

Correct Answer: C. Urinary tract infections can be comorbid with encopresis.

Explanation: Urinary tract infections are more common in children with encopresis. Children with encopresis often present with significant self-esteem issues. When the passage of feces is involuntary rather than intentional, it is often related to constipation, impaction, and retention with subsequent overflow. Smearing feces may be deliberate or accidental, resulting from the child's attempt to clean or hide feces that were passed involuntarily. When the incontinence is clearly deliberate, features of oppositional defiant disorder or conduct disorder may also be present.

11.7—Encopresis / Diagnostic Features and Associated Features (p. 403)

11.8 Which of the following statements about the encopresis specifier *with constipation and overflow incontinence* is accurate?

A. Encopresis with constipation and overflow incontinence is often involuntary.

B. Encopresis with constipation and overflow incontinence usually involves well-formed stool.

C. Encopresis with constipation and overflow incontinence cannot be diagnosed if the behavior results from psychologically motivated avoidance of defecation.

D. Encopresis with constipation and overflow incontinence rarely resolves after treatment of the constipation.

Correct Answer: A. Encopresis with constipation and overflow incontinence is often involuntary.

Explanation: When the passage of feces is involuntary rather than intentional, it is often related to constipation, impaction, and retention with subsequent overflow. The constipation may develop for psychological reasons (e.g., anxiety about defecating in a particular place or a more general pattern of anxious or oppositional behavior), leading to avoidance of defecation.

Feces in the *with constipation and overflow incontinence* subtype are characteristically (but not invariably) poorly formed, and leakage can be infrequent to continuous, occurring mostly during the day and rarely during slee11

p. Only part of the feces is passed during toileting, and the incontinence resolves after treatment of the constipation. In the *without constipation and overflow incontinence* subtype, feces are likely to be of normal form and consistency, and soiling is intermittent. Feces may be deposited in a prominent location. This is usually associated with the presence of oppositional defiant disorder or conduct disorder or may be the consequence of anal masturbation. Soiling without constipation appears to be less common than soiling with constipation.

11.8—Encopresis / Subtypes; Diagnostic Features; Associated Features (pp. 402–403)

11.9   When enuresis persists into late childhood or adolescence, the incontinence may resolve. What else is known about enuresis for this population?

A. Urinary frequency generally persists over time.
B. The diurnal form is more likely to persist into adolescence.
C. Incontinence is highly unlikely to recur later in adulthood in women.
D. Cognitive and behavioral problems are less likely.

Correct Answer: A. Urinary frequency generally persists over time.

Explanation: Although occasional diurnal incontinence is not uncommon in middle childhood, it is substantially more common in those who also have other co-occurring mental health problems, including cognitive and behavioral problems. When enuresis persists into late childhood or adolescence, the incontinence may resolve, but urinary frequency generally persists, and incontinence can recur later in adulthood in women. Diurnal enuresis is uncommon after age 9 years.

11.9—Enuresis / Development and Course (p. 400)

11.10   What are comorbidities associated with nocturnal enuresis?

A. Gastrointestinal infections.
B. Restless legs syndrome.
C. Depression.
D. Insomnia.

Correct Answer: B. Restless legs syndrome.

Explanation: Developmental delays, including speech, language, learning, and motor skills delays, are present in a portion of children with enuresis. Restless legs syndrome and parasomnias such as non–rapid eye movement sleep arousal disorders (sleepwalking and sleep terror types) are associated with nocturnal enuresis. Additionally, there is a link between nocturnal enuresis and heavy snoring or sleep apneas.

11.10—Enuresis / Comorbidity (p. 402)

CHAPTER 12

Sleep-Wake Disorders

12.1   Which of the following is a diagnostic criterion for insomnia disorder?

A. The sleep difficulty occurs at least 1 night per week.
B. A prominent complaint of dissatisfaction with sleep quantity or quality.
C. The sleep difficulty is present for at least 6 months.
D. The sleep difficulty may be related to inadequate opportunity to sleep.

Correct Answer: B. A prominent complaint of dissatisfaction with sleep quantity or quality.

Explanation: The diagnostic criteria for insomnia disorder include a predominant complaint of dissatisfaction with sleep quantity or quality (option B is correct). Criterion C requires that the sleep difficulty occurs at least 3 nights per week (option A is incorrect). Criterion D requires that the sleep difficulty is present for at least 3 months (option C is incorrect). Criterion E requires that the sleep difficulty occurs despite adequate opportunity for sleep (option D is incorrect).

12.1—Insomnia Disorder / diagnostic criteria (pp. 409–410)

12.2   Which of the following is necessary to make a diagnosis of insomnia disorder?

A. Absence of a coexisting medical condition.
B. Difficulty with initiating or maintaining sleep or early morning awakening with inability to return to sleep.
C. Absence of a coexisting mental disorder.
D. Absence of a coexisting sleep disorder.

Correct Answer: B. Difficulty with initiating or maintaining sleep or early morning awakening with inability to return to sleep.

Explanation: Criterion A for the diagnosis of insomnia disorder requires the presence of dissatisfaction with sleep quantity or quality, associated with one (or more) of the following symptoms: 1) difficulty initiating sleep; 2) difficulty maintaining sleep, characterized by frequent awakenings or problems returning to sleep after awakenings; or 3) early morning awakening with inability to return to sleep (option B is correct). The diagnosis of insomnia disorder is given whether it occurs as an independent condition or is comorbid with another mental disorder, a medical condition, or another sleep disorder (options A, C, and D are incorrect).

12.2—Insomnia Disorder / diagnostic criteria (pp. 409–410)

12.3 An 80-year-old man has a history of myocardial infarction and had coronary artery bypass graft surgery 8 years ago. He plays tennis three times a week, takes care of his grandchildren two afternoons each week, generally enjoys life, and manages all of his activities of daily living independently; however, he complains of excessively early morning awakening. He goes to sleep at 9:00 P.M. and sleeps well, with nocturia once nightly, but wakes at 3:30 A.M. although he would like to rise at 5:00 A.M. He does not endorse daytime sleepiness as a problem. His physical examination, mental status, and cognitive function are normal. What is the most likely sleep-wake disorder diagnosis?

A. Insomnia disorder.
B. Circadian rhythm sleep-wake disorder.
C. Situational/acute insomnia.
D. Normal sleep variations (no sleep-wake disorder diagnosis).

Correct Answer: D. Normal sleep variations (no sleep-wake disorder diagnosis).

Explanation: Normal sleep duration varies considerably across persons. Some individuals who require little sleep ("short sleepers") may be concerned about their sleep duration (option D is correct). Short sleepers differ from individuals with insomnia disorder by the lack of difficulty falling or staying asleep and by the absence of characteristic daytime symptoms (e.g., fatigue, concentration problems, irritability); option A is incorrect. Individuals with the delayed sleep phase type of circadian rhythm sleep-wake disorder report sleep-onset insomnia only when they try to sleep at socially normal times, but they do not report difficulty falling asleep or staying asleep when their bed and rising times are delayed and coincide with their endogenous circadian rhythm. This pattern is observed particularly among adolescents and younger adults (option B is incorrect). Situational/acute insomnia is a condition lasting a few days to several weeks, often associated with acute stress due to life events or with changes in sleep schedules. These acute or short-term insomnia symptoms may also produce significant distress and interfere with social, personal, and occupational functioning (option C is incorrect).

12.3—Insomnia Disorder / Differential Diagnosis (pp. 415–416)

12.4 Which of the following symptoms is most likely to indicate the presence of hypersomnolence disorder?

A. Sleep inertia.
B. Nonrestorative sleep.

C. Chronic sleepiness.

D. Multiple sleep latency test with mean sleep latency <10 minutes.

Correct Answer: A. Sleep inertia.

Explanation: Hypersomnolence disorder includes symptoms of excessive quantity of sleep (e.g., extended nocturnal sleep, long naps), sleepiness, and *sleep inertia* (i.e., a period of impaired performance and reduced vigilance following awakening from the regular sleep episode or from a nap). About 40% of individuals with hypersomnolence disorder may have sleep inertia, and this symptom may help differentiate hypersomnolence disorder from other causes of sleepiness (option A is correct). Approximately 80% of individuals with hypersomnolence disorder report that their sleep is nonrestorative, but this symptom is nonspecific and can occur with disorders that disrupt sleep, such as obstructive sleep apnea (option B is incorrect). As in hypersomnolence disorder, individuals with narcolepsy have chronic sleepiness; chronic sleepiness is also common in breathing-related sleep disorders (option C is incorrect). The multiple sleep latency test documents sleep tendency, typically indicated by mean sleep latency values of <8 minutes. In hypersomnolence disorder, the mean sleep latency is typically <10 minutes and frequently 8 minutes or less. Unfortunately, the multiple sleep latency test has poor test-retest reliability, and it does not distinguish well between hypersomnolence disorder and narcolepsy type 2 (option D is incorrect).

12.4—Hypersomnolence Disorder / Diagnostic Features (p. 418); Associated Features (p. 419); Diagnostic Markers (pp. 419–420); Differential Diagnosis (pp. 420–421)

12.5 An obese 52-year-old man complains of daytime sleepiness, and his partner confirms snoring, snorting, and gasping during nighttime sleep. What polysomnographic finding is needed to confirm the diagnosis of obstructive sleep apnea hypopnea?

A. No polysomnography is necessary.

B. Apnea hypopnea index greater than 30.

C. Evidence by polysomnography of at least 5 obstructive apneas or hypopneas per hour of sleep.

D. Evidence by polysomnography of 15 or more obstructive apneas and/or hypopneas per hour of sleep.

Correct Answer: C. Evidence by polysomnography of at least 5 obstructive apneas or hypopneas per hour of sleep.

Explanation: Criterion A for obstructive sleep apnea hypopnea requires either 1) evidence by polysomnography (option A is incorrect) of at least five obstructive apneas or hypopneas per hour of sleep with either a) nocturnal breathing disturbances (snoring, snorting/gasping, or breathing pauses during sleep) (option C is correct) or b) daytime sleepiness, fatigue, or unrefreshing sleep despite sufficient opportunities to sleep that is not better explained by another mental disorder (including a sleep disorder) and is not attributable to another medical condition or 2) evidence by polysomnography of 15 or more obstructive apneas and/or hypopneas per hour of sleep regardless of accompanying symptoms (option D is incorrect).

Disease severity is measured by a count of the number of apneas plus hypopneas per hour of sleep (apnea hypopnea index) using polysomnography or other overnight monitoring. The disorder is considered to be more severe when the apnea hypopnea index is greater than 30 (option B is incorrect).

12.5—Obstructive Sleep Apnea Hypopnea / diagnostic criteria (p. 429); Specifiers (pp. 429–430)

12.6 Diagnostic Criterion B for narcolepsy requires the presence of cataplexy, hypocretin deficiency, *or* characteristic abnormalities on sleep polysomnography or multiple sleep latency testing. Which of the following is a defining characteristic of cataplexy?

A. It is sudden.
B. It occurs unilaterally.
C. It persists for hours.
D. It is accompanied by hypertonia.

Correct Answer: A. It is sudden.

Explanation: In individuals with long-standing narcolepsy, cataplexy is defined as brief (seconds to minutes; option C is incorrect) episodes of sudden (option A is correct) bilateral (option B is incorrect) loss of muscle tone (option D is incorrect) with maintained consciousness that are precipitated by laughter or joking. In children or in individuals within 6 months of onset, cataplexy is defined as spontaneous grimaces or jaw-opening episodes with tongue thrusting or a global hypotonia, without any obvious emotional triggers.

12.6—Narcolepsy / diagnostic criteria (pp. 422–423)

12.7 A 68-year-old female patient complains of excessive daytime sleepiness. Nocturnal polysomnography demonstrates 10 episodes of apneas and hypopneas during sleep caused by variability in respiratory effort. Periods of breathing cessation last longer than 10 seconds. There are no nocturnal breathing disturbances and no sustained periods of oxygen desaturation. What is the appropriate DSM-5-TR diagnosis for this individual?

A. Insomnia due to substance use.
B. Sleep-related hypoventilation.
C. Obstructive sleep apnea hypopnea.
D. Central sleep apnea.

Correct Answer: D. Central sleep apnea.

Explanation: The diagnostic criteria for central sleep apnea is evidence by polysomnograpy of five or more central apnea episodes per hour, not explained by another current sleep disorder. Idiopathic central sleep apnea is characterized by repeated episodes of apneas and hypopneas during sleep caused by variability in respiratory effort but without evidence of airway obstruction (option D is correct). Central sleep apnea can be distinguished from obstructive sleep apnea hypopnea by the presence of at least five central apneas per hour of sleep. Central sleep apneas are recorded when periods of breathing cessation for longer than 10 seconds occur. Central sleep apnea may co-occur with obstructive sleep apnea hypopnea, but central sleep apnea is considered to predominate when central respiratory events are >50% of the total number of respiratory events. If there is no evidence of nocturnal breathing disturbance, there must be at least 15 or more obstructive apneas and/or hypopneas per hour of sleep, regardless of accompanying symptoms, in order to make a diagnosis of obstructive sleep apnea hypopnea (option C is incorrect). Central sleep apnea comorbid with opioid use is attributed to the effects of opioids on the respiratory rhythm generators in the medulla as well as the differential effects on hypoxic versus hypercapnic respiratory drive. It can be distinguished from insomnia due to drug or substance use on the basis of polysomnographic evidence of central sleep apnea (option A is incorrect). Sleep-related hypoventilation typically shows more sustained periods of oxygen desaturation rather than the periodic episodes seen in obstructive sleep apnea hypopnea and central sleep apnea (option B is incorrect).

12.7—Central Sleep Apnea / diagnostic criteria (pp. 435–436); Diagnostic Markers (p. 438); Differential Diagnosis (p. 438); Obstructive Sleep Apnea Hypopnea / diagnostic criteria (p. 429); Sleep-Related Hypoventilation / Differential Diagnosis (p. 442)

12.8 Which of the following metabolic changes is the cardinal feature of sleep-related hypoventilation?

A. Hypocretin deficiency.
B. Hypoxemia.
C. Hypercapnia.
D. Diabetes.

Correct Answer: C. Hypercapnia.

Explanation: Sleep-related hypoventilation is diagnosed using polysomnography, which shows sleep-related hypoxemia and hypercapnia that are not better explained by another breathing-related sleep disorder. The documentation of 1) increased arterial pCO_2 levels to >55 mm Hg during sleep or 2) a ≥ 10 mm Hg increase in pCO_2 levels (to a level that also exceeds 50 mm Hg) during sleep in comparison with awake supine values, in each case exceeding 10 minutes' duration, is the gold standard for diagnosis (option C is correct). Prolonged and sustained decreases in oxygen saturation in the absence of evidence of upper airway obstruction are often used as an indication of sleep-related hypoventilation. However, this finding is not specific; there are other potential causes of hypoxemia (option B is incorrect). Hypocretin (orexin) is a neuropeptide; deficiency of hypocretin is a feature of narcolepsy type 1 (option A is incorrect). Diabetes is consistently associated with obstructive sleep apnea (option D is incorrect).

12.8—Sleep-Related Hypoventilation / Diagnostic Markers (pp. 441–442); Narcolepsy / diagnostic criteria (pp. 422–423); Subtypes (p. 423); Diagnostic Features (pp. 423–424)

12.9   A 51-year-old man presents with symptoms of chronic fatigue. On weekday nights, it takes him several hours to fall asleep, with subsequent difficulty getting up to go to work in the morning and sleepiness for the first few hours of awake time. On weekends, he awakens later in the morning and feels less fatigue and sleepiness. Which of the following is the correct diagnosis?

A. Circadian rhythm sleep-wake disorder, advanced sleep phase type.
B. Circadian rhythm sleep-wake disorder, irregular sleep-wake type.
C. Circadian rhythm sleep-wake disorder, non-24-hour sleep-wake type.
D. Circadian rhythm sleep-wake disorder, delayed sleep phase type.

Correct Answer: D. Circadian rhythm sleep-wake disorder, delayed sleep phase type.

Explanation: Circadian rhythm sleep-wake disorder, delayed sleep phase type, is characterized by delay in the timing of the major sleep period (usually more than 2 hours) in relation to the desired sleep and wake-up time, resulting in symptoms of insomnia and excessive sleepiness. When allowed to set their own schedule, individuals with delayed sleep phase type exhibit normal sleep quality and duration for age. Symptoms of sleep-onset insomnia, difficulty waking in the morning, and excessive sleepiness early in the day are prominent (option D is correct). Circadian rhythm sleep-wake disorder, advanced sleep phase type, is a pattern of advanced sleep onset and awakening times, with an inability to remain awake or asleep until the desired or conventionally acceptable later sleep or wake times (option A is incorrect). Circadian rhythm sleep-wake disorder, irregular sleep-wake type, is characterized by a temporally disorganized sleep-wake pattern, such that the timing of sleep and wake periods is variable through the 24-hour period (option B is incorrect). Circadian rhythm sleep-wake disorder, non-24-hour sleep-wake type, is characterized by a pattern of sleep-wake cycles that is not synchronized to the 24-hour environment, with a consistent daily drift (usually to later and later times) of sleep onset and wake times (option C is incorrect).

12.9—Circadian Rhythm Sleep-Wake Disorders / diagnostic criteria (pp. 443–444); Delayed Sleep Phase Type / Diagnostic Features (p. 444)

12.10 A 67-year-old woman complains of insomnia. She does not have trouble falling asleep between 10 and 11 P.M., but after 1–2 hours she awakens for several hours in the middle of the night, sleeps again for 2–4 hours in the early morning, and then naps three or four times during the day for 1–3 hours at a time. She has a family history of dementia. On examination, she appears fatigued and exhibits deficits in short-term memory, calculation, and abstraction. What is the most likely diagnosis?

    A. Major neurocognitive disorder.
    B. Circadian rhythm sleep-wake disorder, irregular sleep-wake type.
    C. Insomnia disorder.
    D. Major depressive disorder.

Correct Answer: B. Circadian rhythm sleep-wake disorder, irregular sleep-wake type.

Explanation: Irregular sleep-wake type circadian rhythm sleep-wake disorder is characterized by a lack of discernible sleep-wake circadian rhythm. The diagnosis of irregular sleep-wake type is based primarily on a history of symptoms of insomnia at night (during the usual sleep period) and excessive sleepiness (napping) during the day. There is no major sleep period, and sleep and wake periods across 24 hours are fragmented, with sleep fragmented into at least three periods during the 24-hour day. The longest sleep period tends to occur between 2:00 A.M. and 6:00 A.M. and is usually <4 hours (option B is correct). Irregular sleep-wake type is often comorbid with neurodegenerative and neurodevelopmental disorders, such as major neurocognitive disorder, intellectual developmental disorder (intellectual disability), and traumatic brain injury (option A is incorrect). Careful attention should be taken to rule out other sleep-wake disorders (e.g., insomnia disorder), other mental disorders (e.g., depressive disorders, bipolar disorders), and medical conditions that can cause early morning awakening (options C and D are incorrect).

12.10—Circadian Rhythm Sleep-Wake Disorders / Irregular Sleep-Wake Type / Diagnostic Features (p. 447), Comorbidity (p. 448); Advanced Sleep Phase Type / Differential Diagnosis (p. 447)

12.11 Following a traumatic brain injury resulting in blindness, a 50-year-old man develops waxing and waning daytime sleepiness interfering with daytime activity. Serial actigraphy (a method of measuring human activity/rest cycles) demonstrates that the time of onset of the major sleep period occurs progressively later day after day, with a normal duration of the major sleep period. What is the most likely diagnosis?

    A. Major depressive disorder.
    B. Circadian rhythm sleep-wake disorder, delayed sleep phase type.

C. Circadian rhythm sleep-wake disorder, non-24-hour sleep-wake type.

D. Neurodegenerative disorder.

Correct Answer: C. Circadian rhythm sleep-wake disorder, non-24-hour sleep-wake type.

Explanation: Non-24-hour sleep-wake type circadian rhythm sleep disorder is most common among individuals who are blind or visually impaired and have decreased light perception. The pattern of sleep-wake cycles is not synchronized to the 24-hour environment, with a consistent daily drift (usually to later and later times) of sleep onset and wake times (option C is correct). In sighted individuals, non-24-hour sleep-wake type should be differentiated from delayed sleep phase type because individuals with delayed sleep phase type may display a similar progressive delay in sleep period for several days (option B is incorrect). Depressive disorders may result in similar circadian dysregulation and symptoms (option A is incorrect). Irregular sleep-wake type is often comorbid with neurodegenerative and neurodevelopmental disorders (option D is incorrect).

12.11—Circadian Rhythm Sleep-Wake Disorders / diagnostic criteria (pp. 443–444); Non-24-Hour Sleep-Wake Type / Diagnostic Features (pp. 448–449), Differential Diagnosis (p. 450)

12.12 A 50-year-old emergency department nurse complains of sleepiness at work interfering with her ability to function. History is notable for a recent switch from the 7 A.M. to 4 P.M. day shift to the 11 P.M. to 8 A.M. night shift. Symptoms include finding it difficult to sleep in the mornings at home, having little energy for recreational activities or household chores in the afternoon, and feeling exhausted by the middle of the overnight shift. What is the most likely diagnosis?

A. Normal variation in sleep with shift work.

B. Circadian rhythm sleep-wake disorder, shift work type.

C. Insomnia disorder.

D. Narcolepsy.

Correct Answer: B. Circadian rhythm sleep-wake disorder, shift work type.

Explanation: Diagnosis of circadian rhythm sleep-wake disorder, shift work type, is based primarily on a history of the individual working outside the normal 8:00 A.M. to 6:00 P.M. daytime window (particularly at night) on a regularly scheduled (i.e., non-overtime) basis. Symptoms of excessive sleepiness at work and impaired sleep at home on a persistent basis are prominent. Presence of both symptoms is usually required for a diagnosis of shift work type (option B is correct). The diagnosis of shift work type, as opposed to the normal difficulties of shift work, depends to some extent on the severity of symptoms and/or level of distress experienced by the individual (option A is incorrect). The presence of shift work type symptoms even when the individual is able to live on a day-oriented routine for several weeks at a time may suggest the presence of other sleep disorders, such as sleep apnea, insomnia, and narcolepsy, which should be ruled out (options C and D are incorrect).

12.12—Circadian Rhythm Sleep-Wake Disorders / Shift Work Type; Diagnostic Features (p. 450); Differential Diagnosis (p. 451)

12.13 A 14-year-old adolescent wakes in the morning with clear recollection of very frightening dreams. Once awake, she is normally alert and oriented, but the dreams are a persistent source of distress. Her parents report occasional murmurs or groans but no talking or moving during the period before waking. Other pertinent positives include a history of having been homeless in a series of temporary shelter accommodations for 1 year during childhood. What is the most likely diagnosis?

A. Sleep terror disorder.
B. Rapid eye movement (REM) sleep behavior disorder.
C. Nightmare disorder.
D. Posttraumatic stress disorder (PTSD).

Correct Answer: C. Nightmare disorder.

Explanation: Nightmare disorder is characterized by repeated occurrences of extended, extremely dysphoric, and well-remembered dreams that usually involve efforts to avoid threats to survival, security, or physical integrity and that generally occur during the second half of the major sleep episode. On awakening from the dysphoric dreams, the affected individual rapidly becomes oriented and alert (option C is correct). Both nightmare disorder and sleep terror disorder include awakenings or partial awakenings with fearfulness and autonomic activation, but the two disorders can be readily differentiated. Nightmares typically occur later in the night, during REM sleep, and produce vivid, story-like, and clearly recalled dreams; mild autonomic arousal; and complete awakenings. Sleep terrors typically arise in the first third of the night during deep non-REM sleep (especially during stage 3 sleep, now called N3 sleep) and produce either no dream recall or images without an elaborate story-like quality (option A is incorrect). The presence of complex vocal and motor activity during frightening dreams should prompt further evaluation for REM sleep behavior disorder, which occurs more typically among late middle- and older-age men but may also affect women. Although nightmares are typically characteristic of REM sleep behavior disorder, unlike nightmare disorder, REM sleep behavior disorder is associated with dream enactment that may cause nocturnal injuries. If the nightmares precede REM sleep behavior disorder and warrant independent clinical attention, an additional diagnosis of nightmare disorder may be given (option B is incorrect). Nightmares in which the content or affect of the dream is related to a traumatic event may be a component of PTSD or acute stress disorder (option D is incorrect).

12.13—Nightmare Disorder / diagnostic criteria (p. 457); Differential Diagnosis (pp. 460–461)

12.14　Which of the following is a type of rapid eye movement (REM) sleep arousal disorder?

A. Sleepwalking.
B. Sleep terrors.
C. Nightmare disorder.
D. Confusional arousals.

Correct Answer: C. Nightmare disorder.

Explanation: Both nightmare disorder and sleep terror disorder include awakenings or partial awakenings with fearfulness and autonomic activation, but the two disorders can be readily differentiated. Nightmares typically occur later in the night, during REM sleep, and produce vivid, story-like, and clearly recalled dreams; mild autonomic arousal; and complete awakenings. Sleep terrors typically arise in the first third of the night during deep non-REM (NREM) sleep (especially during stage 3 sleep, now called N3 sleep) and produce either no dream recall or images without an elaborate story-like quality (option C is correct and option B is incorrect). Confusional arousals, sleepwalking, and sleep terrors can easily be confused with REM sleep behavior disorder. They arise from NREM sleep and therefore tend to occur in the early portion of the sleep period (options A and D are incorrect).

12.14—Nightmare Disorder / Differential Diagnosis (pp. 460–461); Rapid Eye Movement Sleep Behavior Disorder / Differential Diagnosis (p. 463)

12.15　Which of the following is a specific subtype of non–rapid eye movement sleep arousal disorder, sleepwalking type?

A. Sleep terrors.
B. Sleep-related sexual behavior (sexsomnia).
C. Parasomnia overlap syndrome.
D. Night eating syndrome.

Correct Answer: B. Sleep-related sexual behavior (sexsomnia).

Explanation: Diagnostic criteria for non–rapid eye movement sleep arousal disorders specify two types: sleepwalking and sleep terrors. The sleepwalking type is further specified as having sleep-related eating or sleep-related sexual behavior (sexsomnia) (option B is correct and option A is incorrect). Parasomnia overlap syndrome consists of clinical and polysomnographic features of both sleepwalking and rapid eye movement sleep behavior disorder (option C is incorrect). In contrast to the sleep-related eating form of sleepwalking, which is characterized by recurrent episodes of eating during incomplete arousals from sleep, night eating syndrome is considered to be an abnormality in the circadian rhythm of meal timing, with a normal circadian timing of sleep onset in which the individual wakes up in the middle of the night and overeats (option D is incorrect).

12.15—Non–Rapid Eye Movement Sleep Arousal Disorders / diagnostic criteria (p. 452)

12.16   What is the key abnormality in sleep physiology in rapid eye movement (REM) sleep behavior disorder?

   A. Infrequent periodic extremity electromyography active during non-REM (NREM) sleep.
   B. Increased muscle activity uniformly across all muscle groups.
   C. Sleep paralysis.
   D. REM sleep without atonia.

Correct Answer: D. REM sleep without atonia.

Explanation: Rapid eye movement sleep disorder is characterized by repeated episodes of arousal during sleep associated with vocalization and/or complex motor behaviors. The presence of REM sleep without atonia during a polysomnogram is typically required for the diagnosis of REM sleep behavior disorder. Associated laboratory findings from polysomnography indicated increased tonic and/or phasic electromyographic activity during REM sleep, which is normally associated with muscle atonia. The increased muscle activity variably affects different muscle groups (option B is incorrect). Other polysomnographic findings may include very frequent periodic and aperiodic extremity electromyography activity during NREM sleep (option A is incorrect). In nightmare disorder, if nightmares occur during sleep-onset REM periods (hypnagogic), the dysphoric emotion is frequently accompanied by an awakening and being unable to move voluntarily (*sleep paralysis*; option C is incorrect).

12.16—Rapid Eye Movement Sleep Behavior Disorder / Diagnostic Features (pp. 461–462); Diagnostic Markers (p. 463); Nightmare Disorder / Diagnostic Features (p. 458)

12.17   Which of the following conditions is commonly associated with rapid eye movement (REM) sleep behavior disorder?

   A. Narcolepsy.
   B. Synucleinopathies.

C. Seizure disorder.
D. Dissociative disorders.

Correct Answer: B. Synucleinopathies.

Explanation: In individuals with idiopathic REM sleep behavior disorder, the risk of developing a defined neurodegenerative disease, most often a synucleinopathy (i.e., Parkinson's disease, major or mild neurocognitive disorder with Lewy bodies, or multiple system atrophy), is approximately 75% within 10–15 years following diagnosis, with an annualized risk of approximately 6%–7% per year (option B is correct). REM sleep behavior disorder is present concurrently in approximately 30% of patients with narcolepsy (option A is incorrect). Nocturnal seizures may mimic REM sleep behavior disorder, but the behaviors characteristic of nocturnal seizures are generally stereotyped (option C is incorrect). Unlike virtually all other parasomnias, which arise precipitously from non-REM or REM sleep, psychogenic dissociative behaviors arise from a period of well-defined wakefulness during the sleep period (option D is incorrect).

12.17—Rapid Eye Movement Sleep Behavior Disorder / Development and Course (p. 462); Differential Diagnosis (pp. 463–464); Comorbidity (p. 464)

12.18 Which of the following classes of psychotropic drugs may result in rapid eye movement (REM) sleep without atonia and REM sleep behavior disorder?

A. Selective serotonin reuptake inhibitors (SSRIs).
B. Opioids.
C. Benzodiazepines.
D. Stimulants.

Correct Answer: A. Selective serotonin reuptake inhibitors (SSRIs).

Explanation: Many widely prescribed medications, including tricyclic antidepressants, SSRIs, and serotonin-norepinephrine reuptake inhibitors, may result in polysomnographic evidence of REM sleep without atonia and in frank REM sleep behavior disorder (option A is correct). During acute short-term use, opioids may produce an increase in sleepiness and in subjective depth of sleep and reduced REM and slow-wave sleep (option B is incorrect). Sedatives, hypnotics, and anxiolytics (e.g., benzodiazepine receptor agonists) have similar effects as opioids on sleep (option C is incorrect). During acute intoxication, stimulants reduce the total amount of sleep, increase sleep latency and sleep continuity disturbances, and decrease REM sleep (option D is incorrect).

12.18—Rapid Eye Movement Sleep Behavior Disorder / Differential Diagnosis (p. 463); Substance/Medication-Induced Sleep Disorder / Associated Features (p. 471)

12.19 A 10-year-old boy is referred for evaluation of difficulty sitting still in school, which is interfering with his academic performance. He complains of an unpleasant "creepy-crawly" sensation in his legs for the past 3 months and an urge to move his legs when sitting still that is relieved by movement. This symptom is present most of the day but less so when he is playing sports after school or watching television in the evening, and it generally does not occur in bed at night. What aspect of this clinical presentation rules out a diagnosis of restless legs syndrome (RLS)?

A. The urge to move the legs is partially or totally relieved by movement.
B. The urge to move the legs begins or worsens during periods of rest or inactivity.
C. The symptoms have persisted for only 3 months.
D. The urge to move the legs is worse during the day than at night.

Correct Answer: D. The urge to move the legs is worse during the day than at night.

Explanation: Criterion A for RLS specifies that all of the following must be present: 1) the urge to move the legs begins or worsens during periods of rest or inactivity (option B is incorrect); 2) the urge to move the legs is partially or totally relieved by movement (option A is incorrect); 3) the urge to move the legs is worse in the evening or at night than during the day or occurs only in the evening or at night (option D is correct). Criterion B specifies that the symptoms in Criterion A must occur at least three times per week and have persisted for at least 3 months (option C is incorrect).

12.19—Restless Legs Syndrome / diagnostic criteria (pp. 464–465)

12.20 A 28-year-old pregnant patient reports restlessness and difficulty falling asleep at the onset of the sleep period, as well as daytime fatigue. There have been no changes in her sleep-work schedule. What sleep disorder is suggested by the onset of these symptoms in the third trimester of pregnancy?

A. Nocturnal leg cramps.
B. Narcolepsy.
C. Restless legs syndrome (RLS).
D. Obstructive sleep apnea.

Correct Answer: C. Restless legs syndrome (RLS).

Explanation: The prevalence of RLS during pregnancy is two to three times greater than in the general population. RLS associated with pregnancy peaks during the third trimester and improves or resolves in most cases soon after delivery (option C is correct). Unlike RLS, nocturnal leg cramps do not typically manifest with the desire to move the limbs, nor are there frequent limb movements (option A is incorrect). There may be an association between RLS and other sleep disorders, including narcolepsy and obstructive sleep apnea (options B and D are incorrect).

12.20—Restless Legs Syndrome / Sex- and Gender-Related Diagnostic Issues (pp. 466–467); Differential Diagnosis (p. 467)

12.21 Which of the following sleep disturbances is associated with *chronic* opioid use?

A. Increase in sleepiness.
B. Insomnia.
C. Increased total sleep time.
D. Increased rapid eye movement (REM) and slow-wave sleep.

Correct Answer: B. Insomnia.

Explanation: Opioids may produce an increase in sleepiness and in subjective depth of sleep and reduced REM and slow-wave sleep during *acute* short-term use. With continued administration, tolerance to the sedative effects of opioids develops and there are complaints of insomnia (option B is correct). Polysomnographic studies demonstrate reduced sleep efficiency and total sleep time (option C is incorrect), with reduction of slow-wave sleep and possibly REM sleep (option D is incorrect). Consistent with their respiratory depressant effects, opioids exacerbate obstructive sleep apnea. Emergence of central sleep apnea is also observed, especially with chronic use of longer-acting opioids.

12.21—Substance/Medication-Induced Sleep Disorder / Associated Features (pp. 471–472)

12.22 Which of the following substances is associated with parasomnias?

A. Amphetamines.
B. Zolpidem.
C. Cannabis.
D. Caffeine.

Correct Answer: B. Zolpidem.

Explanation: Parasomnias (sleepwalking and sleep-related eating) have been associated with use of benzodiazepine receptor agonists, especially when these drugs are taken at high doses and when they are combined with other sedative drugs. Zolpidem is a newer benzodiazepine receptor agonist (option B is correct). Sleep disorders induced by amphetamine-type substances and other stimulants are characterized by insomnia during intoxication and excessive sleepiness during withdrawal (option A is incorrect). Acute administration of cannabis may shorten sleep latency, although arousing effects with increments in sleep latency also occur. In chronic users, tolerance of the sleep-inducing and slow-wave sleep-enhancing effects develops (option C is incorrect). Caffeine consumed in low to moderate doses during the morning hours typically produces no significant effect on nighttime sleep in normal sleepers or those with insomnia. Caffeine may produce insomnia in a dose- and timing-dependent manner, particularly when larger doses are consumed later in the day or during evening hours. Prolongation of sleep latency, reduction of slow-wave sleep, increased nocturnal awakening, and reduced sleep duration are reported. Some individuals, particularly high consumers, may present with daytime sleepiness and performance impairments related to withdrawal (option D is incorrect).

12.22—Substance/Medication-Induced Sleep Disorder / Associated Features (pp. 471–472)

12.23 A 56-year-old college professor complains of having difficulty sleeping for more than 5 hours per night over the past few weeks, with associated daytime sleepiness. Awakening occurs an hour or two before her intended waking time in the morning, with associated restless sleep with frequent awakenings until it is time to get up. There is no initial insomnia or depressed mood. She attributes the sleep trouble to intrusive thoughts that arise, after an initially momentary awakening, about the need to complete an overdue academic project. What is the most appropriate diagnosis?

A. Unspecified insomnia disorder.
B. Other specified insomnia disorder (restricted to nonrestorative sleep).
C. Insomnia disorder.
D. Other specified insomnia disorder (short-term insomnia disorder).

Correct Answer: D. Other specified insomnia disorder (short-term insomnia disorder).

Explanation: The *other specified insomnia disorder* category applies to presentations in which symptoms characteristic of insomnia disorder that cause clinically significant distress or impairment in social, occupational, or other important areas of functioning predominate but do not meet the full criteria for insomnia disorder or any of the disorders in the sleep-wake disorders diagnostic class. The *other specified insomnia disorder* category is used in situations in which the clinician chooses to communicate the specific reason that the presentation does not meet the criteria for insomnia disorder or any specific sleep-wake disorder. This particular case is an example of a short-term insomnia disorder (duration less than 3 months; option D is correct). In the "restricted to nonrestorative sleep" example of the *other specified* category, the predominant complaint is nonrestorative sleep unaccompanied by other sleep symptoms such as difficulty falling asleep or remaining asleep (option B is incorrect). The *unspecified insomnia disorder* category is used in situations in which the clinician chooses *not* to specify the reason that the criteria are not met for insomnia disorder or a specific sleep-wake disorder and includes presentations in which there is insufficient information to make a more specific diagnosis (option A is incorrect). Sleep difficulty must be present for at least 3 months for a diagnosis of insomnia disorder (option C is incorrect).

12.23—Other Specified Insomnia Disorder (p. 475); Unspecified Insomnia Disorder (p. 475); Insomnia Disorder / diagnostic criteria (pp. 409–410)

CHAPTER 13

Sexual Dysfunctions

13.1 Which of the following is required for a diagnosis of female sexual interest/arousal disorder?

A. The disturbance has been present since the individual became sexually active.
B. At least three manifestations of lack of, or significantly reduced, sexual interest/arousal.
C. The symptoms are not limited to certain types of stimulation, situations, or partners.
D. The symptoms have persisted for a minimum duration of approximately 6 weeks.

Correct Answer: B. At least three manifestations of lack of, or significantly reduced, sexual interest/arousal.

Explanation: For the criteria for female sexual interest/arousal disorder to be met, there must be lack of, or significantly reduced, sexual interest/arousal, as manifested by at least three of the following: 1) absent or reduced interest in sexual activity; 2) absent or reduced sexual/erotic thoughts or fantasies; 3) no or reduced initiation of sexual activity and typically unreceptive to a partner's attempts to initiate; 4) absent or reduced sexual excitement/pleasure during sexual activity in almost all or all (approximately 75%–100%) sexual encounters (in identified situational contexts or, if generalized, in all contexts); 5) absent or reduced sexual interest/arousal in response to any internal or external sexual/erotic cues (e.g., written, verbal, visual); 6) absent or reduced genital or nongenital sensations during sexual activity in almost all or all (approximately 75%–100%) sexual encounters (in identified situational contexts or, if generalized, in all contexts) (option B is correct).

Diagnosis of a female sexual interest/arousal disorder requires a minimum duration of symptoms of approximately 6 months as a reflection that the symptoms must be a persistent problem (option D is incorrect).

Specifiers exist for *lifelong* (the disturbance has been present since the individual became sexually active) versus *acquired* (the disturbance began after a period of relatively normal sexual function (option A is incorrect). Specifiers also exist for *generalized* (not limited to certain types of stimulation, situations, or partners) versus *situational* (occurs only with certain types of stimulation, situations, or partners (option C is incorrect).

13.1—Female Sexual Interest/Arousal Disorder / diagnostic criteria (p. 489) / Diagnostic Features (pp. 489–490)

13.2   Which of the following is a subtype of sexual dysfunction in DSM-5-TR?

    A. Lifelong.
    B. Secondary to a medical condition.
    C. Due to partner violence.
    D. Due to an anxiety disorder.

Correct Answer: A. Lifelong.

Explanation: Subtypes are used to designate the onset of the difficulty. *Lifelong* refers to a sexual problem that has been present from first sexual experiences (option A is correct), and *acquired* applies to sexual disorders that develop after a period of relatively normal sexual function. If the sexual dysfunction is attributable to another medical condition (e.g., peripheral neuropathy), the person would not receive a psychiatric diagnosis (option B is incorrect). If severe relationship distress, partner violence, or significant stressors better explain the sexual difficulties, then a sexual dysfunction diagnosis is not made, but an appropriate Z code for the relationship problem or stressor may be listed (option C is incorrect). If the sexual dysfunction is mostly explainable by another nonsexual mental disorder (e.g., depressive or bipolar disorder, anxiety disorder, posttraumatic stress disorder, psychotic disorder), then only the other mental disorder diagnosis should be made (option D is incorrect).

13.2—chapter introduction (pp. 477–478)

13.3   A 65-year-old man presents with difficulty in obtaining an erection due to diabetes and severe vascular disease (previously diagnosed in DSM-IV as sexual dysfunction due to…[indicate the general medical condition] [coded as *607.84 male erectile disorder due to diabetes mellitus*]). What is the correct DSM-5-TR diagnosis for this presentation?

    A. Sexual dysfunction due to a general medical condition.
    B. Erectile disorder.
    C. Erectile dysfunction.
    D. No psychiatric diagnosis.

Correct Answer: D. No psychiatric diagnosis.

Explanation: A sexual dysfunction diagnosis requires ruling out problems that are better explained by a medical condition. If sexual dysfunction is attributable to another medical condition (e.g., peripheral neuropathy), the person would not receive a psychiatric diagnosis (option A is incorrect and option D is correct). Criterion D for erectile disorder specifies that the sexual dysfunction is not better explained by a nonsexual mental disorder or as a consequence of severe relationship distress or other significant stressors and is not attributable to the effects of a substance/medication or another medical condition (option B is incorrect). *Erectile dysfunction* is a widely used descriptive term (including in ICD-10) that refers to difficulty getting and maintaining an erection (option C is incorrect).

13.3—chapter introduction (pp. 477–478); Erectile Disorder / diagnostic criteria (pp. 481–482); Diagnostic Features (p. 482)

13.4 A 35-year-old man with new-onset diabetes presents with a 6-month history of inability to maintain an erection. The erectile dysfunction began suddenly 1 month after he was fired from his job. Serum glucose is well controlled with oral hypoglycemic medication. What is the appropriate DSM-5-TR diagnosis?

A. No psychiatric diagnosis.
B. Erectile disorder.
C. Substance/medication-induced sexual dysfunction.
D. Major depressive disorder.

Correct Answer: B. Erectile disorder.

Explanation: The essential feature of erectile disorder is a marked difficulty in obtaining or maintaining an erection or a marked decrease in erectile rigidity in all or almost all occasions of sexual activity (Criterion A) that has persisted for at least 6 months (Criterion B) and that causes clinically significant distress in the individual (Criterion C) (option B is correct). The most difficult aspect of the differential diagnosis of erectile disorder is ruling out erectile problems that are fully explained by medical factors. Such cases would not receive a diagnosis of a mental disorder (option A is incorrect). The distinction between erectile disorder as a mental disorder and erectile dysfunction as the result of another medical condition is usually unclear, and many cases will have complex, interactive biological and psychiatric etiologies. If the individual is older than 40–50 years and/or has concomitant medical problems, the differential diagnosis should include medical etiologies, especially vascular disease. The presence of an organic disease known to cause erectile problems does not confirm a causal relationship. For example, an individual with diabetes mellitus can develop erectile disorder in response to psychological stress. In general, erectile dysfunction due to organic factors is generalized and gradual in onset. An exception would be erectile problems after traumatic injury to the nervous innervation of the genital organs (e.g., spinal cord injury). Erectile problems that are situational and inconsistent and that have an acute onset after a stressful life event are most often due to psychological reasons.

An onset of erectile dysfunction that coincides with the beginning of substance/medication use and dissipates with discontinuation of the substance/medication or dose reduction is suggestive of a substance/medication-induced sexual dysfunction, which should be diagnosed instead of erectile disorder (option C is incorrect). Major depressive disorder and erectile disorder are closely associated, and erectile disorder accompanying severe depressive disorder may occur. If the erectile difficulties are better explained by another mental disorder, such as major depression, then a diagnosis of erectile disorder would not be made (option D is incorrect).

13.4—Erectile Disorder / Diagnostic Features (p. 482) / Differential Diagnosis (pp. 484–485)

13.5   Which of the following factors should be considered during assessment and diagnosis of a sexual dysfunction?

A. Biological factors only.
B. Factors related to the patient only and not their partner.
C. Cultural or religious factors.
D. The individual's specific sex assigned at birth.

Correct Answer: C. Cultural or religious factors.

Explanation: Several factors must be considered during assessment and diagnosis of a sexual dysfunction because they may be relevant to etiology or treatment and may contribute, to varying degrees, across individuals: 1) partner factors (e.g., partner's sexual problems, partner's health status; option B is incorrect); 2) relationship factors (e.g., poor communication; discrepancies in desire for sexual activity); 3) individual vulnerability factors (e.g., poor body image, history of sexual or emotional abuse), psychiatric comorbidity (e.g., depression, anxiety), or stressors (e.g., job loss, bereavement); 4) cultural/religious factors (e.g., inhibitions related to prohibitions against sexual activity or pleasure, attitudes toward sexuality; option C is correct); and 5) medical factors relevant to prognosis, course, or treatment.

Sexual response has a requisite biological underpinning, yet it is usually experienced in an intrapersonal, interpersonal, and cultural context. Thus, sexual function involves a complex interaction among biological, sociocultural, and psychological factors (option A is incorrect).

13.5—chapter introduction (pp. 477–478)

13.6   A 30-year-old woman comes to your office and reports that she is there only because her mother pleaded with her to see you. She tells you that although she has a good social network with friends of both sexes, she has never had any feelings of sexual arousal in response to men or women, does not have any erotic fantasies, and has little interest in sexual activity. She has found other like-minded individuals, and she and her friends accept themselves as asexual. What is the appropriate diagnosis, if any?

A. Female sexual interest/arousal disorder.
B. Other specified sexual dysfunction.

C. No diagnosis because she does not have the minimum number of symptoms required for female sexual interest/arousal disorder.
D. No diagnosis because she does not have clinically significant distress or impairment.

Correct Answer: D. No diagnosis because she does not have clinically significant distress or impairment.

Explanation: This patient has three of the six possible indicators in Criterion A, which is the minimum number needed (option C is incorrect): 1) absent or reduced interest in sexual activity, 2) absent or reduced sexual/erotic thoughts or fantasies, 3) no or reduced initiation of sexual activity and typically unreceptive to a partner's attempts to initiate, 4) absent or reduced sexual excitement or pleasure during sexual activity in almost all or all (approximately 75%–100%) sexual encounters (in identified situational contexts or, if generalized, in all contexts), 5) absent or reduced sexual interest/arousal in response to any internal or external sexual/erotic cues (e.g., written verbal, visual), and 6) absent or reduced genital or nongenital sensations during sexual activity in almost all or all (approximately 75%–100%) sexual encounters (in identified situational contexts or, if generalized, in all contexts). However, Criterion C specifies that the symptoms in Criterion A cause clinically significant distress in the individual (option D is correct). *Other specified sexual dysfunction* applies to presentations in which symptoms characteristic of a sexual dysfunction that cause clinically significant distress in the individual predominate but do not meet the full criteria for any of the disorders in the sexual dysfunctions diagnostic class (option B is incorrect).

13.6—Female Sexual Interest/Arousal Disorder / diagnostic criteria (p. 489) / Other Specified Sexual Dysfunction (p. 509)

13.7   Which of the following symptoms or conditions would rule out a diagnosis of erectile disorder?

A. Presence of diabetes mellitus.
B. Marked decrease in erectile rigidity.
C. Presence of alcohol use disorder.
D. Presence of symptoms for less than 3 months.

Correct Answer: D. Presence of symptoms for less than 3 months.

Explanation: A marked decrease in erectile rigidity is one of the three symptoms from Criterion A (at least one is required) that must be experienced on almost all or all (approximately 75%–100%) occasions of sexual activity (option B is incorrect). Criterion B specifies that the symptoms in Criterion A have persisted for a minimum duration of approximately 6 months (option D is correct). The presence of diabetes mellitus does not *in itself* rule out erectile disorder; erectile problems that are *fully* explained by medical factors would not receive a diagnosis of a mental disorder (option A is incorrect). Similarly, the mere presence of alcohol use disorder does not rule out the possibility of a separate, concurrent erectile disorder. However, an onset of erectile dysfunction that coincides with the beginning of substance/medication use and that dissipates with discontinuation of the substance/medication or dose reduction is suggestive of a substance/medication-induced sexual dysfunction, which should be diagnosed instead of erectile disorder (option C is incorrect).

13.7—Erectile Disorder / diagnostic criteria (pp. 481–482); Differential Diagnosis (pp. 484–485)

13.8   Which of the following is a distinctive feature of premature (early) ejaculation versus delayed ejaculation?

A. Symptoms have been present for at least 6 months.
B. Symptoms must be experienced during partnered sexual activity.
C. Symptoms cause clinically significant distress in the individual.
D. Severity is based on the level of distress experienced by the individual.

Correct Answer: D. Severity is based on the level of distress experienced by the individual.

Explanation: Criterion A for both premature (early) ejaculation and delayed ejaculation specifies that symptoms occur during partnered sexual activity (option B is incorrect). Both diagnoses require the presence of clinically significant distress (Criterion C). Similarly, Criterion B for both diagnoses requires that symptoms have been present for at least 6 months (option A is incorrect). For delayed ejaculation, current severity is based on the level of distress over the symptoms. For premature (early) ejaculation, current severity is based on how soon ejaculation occurs following initiation of sexual activity (option D is correct).

13.8—Delayed Ejaculation / diagnostic criteria (pp. 478–479); Premature (Early) Ejaculation / diagnostic criteria (pp. 501–502)

13.9   Which of the following medications is most likely to cause sexual dysfunction?

A. Bupropion.
B. Lamotrigine.
C. Citalopram.
D. Nefazodone.

Correct Answer: C. Citalopram.

Explanation: The most commonly reported side effect of antidepressant drugs is difficulty with orgasms or ejaculation in men and with arousal in women.

Certain agents (i.e., bupropion, mirtazapine, nefazodone, and vilazodone) appear to have lower rates of sexual side effects than other antidepressants (options A and D are incorrect). There are differences in the incidence of sexual side effects between some serotonergic and combined adrenergic-serotonergic antidepressants, with medications such as citalopram, fluoxetine, fluvoxamine, paroxetine, sertraline, and venlafaxine having the highest rates of sexual dysfunction (option C is correct). Although the effects of mood stabilizers on sexual function are unclear, it is possible that lithium and anticonvulsants, with the possible exception of lamotrigine, have adverse effects on sexual desire (option B is incorrect).

13.9—Substance/Medication-Induced Sexual Dysfunction / Associated Features (p. 507) / Prevalence (pp. 507–508)

13.10 Which of the following conditions would be appropriately diagnosed as *other specified sexual dysfunction*?

A. Substance/medication-induced sexual dysfunction.
B. Sexual aversion.
C. Delayed ejaculation.
D. Female sexual interest/arousal disorder.

Correct Answer: B. Sexual aversion.

Explanation: Options A, C, and D are diagnosable sexual dysfunctions, each with its own specific set of criteria. *Other specified sexual dysfunction* applies to presentations in which symptoms characteristic of a sexual dysfunction that cause clinically significant distress in the individual predominate but do not meet the full criteria for any of the disorders in the sexual dysfunctions diagnostic class. The *other specified sexual dysfunction* category is used in situations in which the clinician chooses to communicate the specific reason that the presentation does not meet the criteria for any specific sexual dysfunction. This is done by recording "other specified sexual dysfunction" followed by the specific reason (e.g., "sexual aversion"; option B is correct).

13.10—Other Specified Sexual Dysfunction (p. 509)

CHAPTER 14

Gender Dysphoria

14.1   In order for a child to meet criteria for a diagnosis of gender dysphoria, which of the following *must* be present?

    A. A co-occurring disorder of sex development.
    B. A strong desire to be of the other gender or an insistence that one *is* the other gender (or some alternative gender different from one's assigned gender).
    C. A strong dislike of one's sexual anatomy.
    D. A strong desire for the primary and/or secondary sex characteristics that match one's experienced gender.

Correct Answer: B. A strong desire to be of the other gender or an insistence that one *is* the other gender (or some other alternative gender different from one's assigned gender).

Explanation: For gender dysphoria in children, Criterion A is a marked incongruence between one's experienced/expressed gender and assigned gender, of at least 6 months' duration, as manifested by at least six of the following (one of which must be criterion A1): 1) a strong desire to be of the other gender or an insistence that one *is* the other gender (or some alternative gender different from one's assigned gender; option B is correct); 2) in boys (assigned gender), a strong preference for cross-dressing or simulating female attire, or in girls (assigned gender), a strong preference for wearing only typical masculine clothing and a strong resistance to the wearing of typical feminine clothing; 3) a strong preference for cross-gender roles in make-believe play or fantasy play; 4) a strong preference for the toys, games, or activities stereotypically used or engaged in by the other gender; 5) a strong preference for playmates of the other gender; 6) in boys (assigned gender), a strong rejection of typically masculine toys, games, and activities and a strong avoidance of rough-and-tumble play, or in girls (assigned gender), a strong rejection of typically feminine toys, games, and activities; 7) a strong dislike of one's sexual anatomy (option C is incorrect); 8) a strong desire for the primary and/or secondary sex characteristics that match one's experienced gender (option D is incorrect). A specifier exists if there is also a disorder/difference of sex development (option A is incorrect).

14.1—Gender Dysphoria / diagnostic criteria (pp. 512–513)

14.2   Which of the following statements about the diagnosis of gender dysphoria in adolescents and adults is *true*?

   A. The *posttransition* specifier is used to indicate that the individual has undergone (or is preparing to have) at least one gender-affirming medical procedure or treatment regimen.
   B. To qualify for the diagnosis, the individual must be pursuing some kind of sex reassignment treatment.
   C. To qualify for the diagnosis, the individual must have a strong desire to be of a different gender or must insist that they *are* the other gender.
   D. To qualify for the diagnosis, the individual must have an associated disorder of sex development.

Correct Answer: A. The *posttransition* specifier is used to indicate that the individual has undergone (or is preparing to have) at least one gender-affirming medical procedure or treatment regimen.

Explanation: In the diagnostic criteria for gender dysphoria in adolescents and adults, the *posttransition* specifier is used to identify individuals who have undergone (or are preparing to have) at least one gender-affirming medical procedure or treatment regimen—namely, regular gender-affirming hormone treatment or gender reassignment surgery confirming the experienced gender (option A is correct).

   Unlike the case for a child, an adolescent or adult need not have a strong desire to be of a different gender or insist that they are another gender to qualify for the diagnosis of gender dysphoria.

14.2—Gender Dysphoria / diagnostic criteria (pp. 512–513); Specifiers (p. 513)

14.3   Match each of the following terms (A–D) to its correct definition (i–iv).

   A. Transgender.
   B. Gender.
   C. Sex.
   D. Transsexual.

   i.   The biological indicators of male or female.
   ii. An individual's public, sociocultural (and usually legally recognized) lived role as boy or girl, man or woman.
   iii. An individual whose gender identity is different from their birth-assigned gender.
   iv. A term historically denoting an individual who seeks, or has undergone, a social transition from male to female or female to male.

Correct Answer: A: iii, B: ii, C: i, D: iv.

Explanation: The area of sex and gender is highly controversial and has led to a proliferation of terms whose meanings vary over time and within and between disciplines. In DSM-5-TR, *sex* refers to the biological indicators of male and female (understood in the context of reproductive capacity), such as in sex chromosomes, gonads, sex hormones, and nonambiguous internal and external genitalia (option C=i); *gender* is used to denote the public, sociocultural (and usually legally recognized) lived role as boy or girl, man or woman, or other gender (option B=ii). *Transgender* refers to the broad spectrum of individuals whose gender identity is different from their birth-assigned gender (option A=iii). *Transsexual* historically was used to denote an individual who seeks, is undergoing, or has undergone a social transition from male to female or female to male, which in many, but not all, cases also involves a somatic transition by gender-affirming hormone treatment and genital, breast, or other gender-affirming surgery (historically referred to as *sex reassignment surgery*).

14.3—chapter introduction (pp. 511–512)

14.4   How is a person's gender determined?

   A. Biological factors contribute, in interaction with social and psychological factors, to gender development.
   B. Gender is determined at birth.
   C. Gender is determined officially (and sometimes legally) when an individual changes gender.
   D. Gender is determined by medical procedures that align an individual's physical characteristics with their experienced gender.

Correct Answer: A. Biological factors contribute, in interaction with social and psychological factors, to gender development.

Explanation: *Gender* is used to denote the public, sociocultural (and usually legally recognized) lived role as boy or girl, man or woman, or other gender. Biological factors are seen as contributing, in interaction with social and psychological factors, to gender development (option A is correct).

Gender assignment refers to the assignment as male or female. This usually occurs at birth on the basis of phenotypic sex and, thereby, yields the *birth-assigned gender*, historically referred to as *biological sex* or, more recently, *natal gender* (option B is incorrect). *Gender reassignment* denotes an official (and sometimes legal) change of gender (option C is incorrect). *Gender-affirming treatments* are medical procedures (hormones or surgeries or both) that aim to align an individual's physical characteristics with their *experienced gender* (option D is incorrect).

14.4—chapter introduction (pp. 511–512)

14.5   What DSM-5-TR diagnosis has replaced the former DSM-IV diagnosis of gender identity disorder?

   A. Gender atypical.
   B. Transvestic disorder.

C. Gender dysphoria.
D. Nonconformity to gender roles.

Correct Answer: C. Gender dysphoria.

Explanation: *Gender dysphoria* as a general descriptive term refers to the distress that may accompany the incongruence between one's experienced or expressed gender and one's assigned gender. Although not all individuals will experience distress from incongruence, many are distressed if the desired physical interventions using hormones and/or surgery are not available. The current term is more descriptive than the previous DSM-IV term *gender identity disorder* and focuses on dysphoria, not identity per se, as the clinical problem (option C is correct).

Gender atypical refers to somatic features or behaviors that are not typical (in a statistical sense) of individuals with the same assigned gender in a given society and historical era; *gender-nonconforming*, *gender variant*, and *gender diverse* are alternative nondiagnostic terms (options A and D are incorrect).

Gender dysphoria should be distinguished from simple nonconformity to stereotypical gender role behavior by the strong desire to be of a gender other than the assigned one and by the extent and pervasiveness of gender-variant activities and interests (option D is incorrect).

Transvestic disorder is diagnosed in heterosexual (or bisexual) adolescent and adult males (rarely in females) for whom wearing women's clothing generates sexual excitement and causes distress and/or impairment without drawing their assigned gender into question. It is occasionally accompanied by gender dysphoria (option B is incorrect). An individual with transvestic disorder who also has clinically significant gender dysphoria can be given both diagnoses. In some cases of postpubertal-onset gender dysphoria in individuals assigned male at birth who are attracted to women, cross-dressing with sexual excitement is a precursor to the diagnosis of gender dysphoria.

14.5—chapter introduction (pp. 511–512); Gender Dysphoria / Differential Diagnosis (pp. 519–520)

CHAPTER 15

Disruptive, Impulse-Control, and Conduct Disorders

15.1 A 7-year-old boy has shown extreme stubbornness and defiance for the past year. This behavior is seen primarily at home and does not typically involve significant mood instability or anger, although he occasionally can be spiteful and vindictive. These symptoms have affected his sibling relationships in an extremely negative fashion, and more recently this behavior has been seen with peers and has begun to affect his friendships. His parents demonstrate a somewhat hostile parenting style. Which of the following statements about the diagnosis of oppositional defiant disorder (ODD) for this patient is correct?

   A. The child does not qualify for a diagnosis of ODD because his symptoms lack a significant mood component.
   B. The child may qualify for a diagnosis of ODD, despite lacking a persistently negative mood, if he meets the other symptom criteria.
   C. The child does not qualify for a diagnosis of ODD because his symptoms are confined primarily to the home setting.
   D. The child does not qualify for a diagnosis of ODD because his symptoms have not been present for a sufficient period of time.

Correct Answer: B. The child may qualify for a diagnosis of ODD, despite lacking a persistently negative mood, if he meets the other symptom criteria.

Explanation: According to DSM-5-TR, it is not unusual for individuals with ODD to show the behavioral features of the disorder without problems of negative mood. The symptoms of ODD may be confined to only one setting, and this is most frequently the home. Individuals who show enough symptoms to meet the diagnostic threshold, even if it is only at home, may be significantly impaired in their social functioning. Because these behaviors are common among siblings, they must be observed during interactions with persons other than siblings. Also, because symptoms of the disorder are typically more evident in interactions with adults or peers whom the individual knows well, they may not be apparent during a clinical examination. For children younger than

5 years, the behavior should occur on most days for a period of at least 6 months. For individuals 5 years or older, the behavior should occur at least once per week for at least 6 months, unless otherwise noted.

15.1—Oppositional Defiant Disorder / diagnostic criteria (pp. 522–523)

15.2   A 3-year-old boy has had severe temper tantrums occurring approximately weekly for a 6-month period. The tantrums are characterized by anger and defiant behavior, with the boy arguing back against his parents' instructions. The tantrums are usually preceded by a change in routine, fatigue, or hunger and rarely include any aggression or property destruction. The boy is generally well behaved in nursery school and during periods between his tantrums. Which of the following is the most appropriate diagnosis?

A. Oppositional defiant disorder (ODD).
B. Intermittent explosive disorder (IED).
C. Disruptive mood dysregulation disorder (DMDD).
D. None of the above.

Correct Answer: D. None of the above.

Explanation: Criterion A for ODD requires a pattern of angry/irritable mood, argumentative/defiant behavior, or vindictiveness lasting at least 6 months as evidenced by at least four symptoms from any of the following categories and exhibited during interaction with at least one individual who is not a sibling:

Angry/Irritable Mood

1. Loses temper.
2. Is touchy or easily annoyed by others.
3. Is angry and resentful.

Argumentative/Defiant Behavior

4. Argues with authority figures or adults.
5. Actively defies or refuses to comply with requests from authority figures or adults or with rules.
6. Deliberately annoys people.
7. Blames others for their mistakes or misbehavior.

Vindictiveness

8. Has been spiteful or vindictive at least twice within the past 6 months.

Temper outbursts for a preschool child would be considered a symptom of ODD only if they occurred on most days for the preceding 6 months, if they occurred with at least three other symptoms of the disorder, and if the temper outbursts contributed to the significant impairment associated with the disorder (e.g., led to destruction of property during outbursts, resulted in the child being asked to leave a preschool). In this vignette, the child's tantrums are the sole symptom; therefore, they would not meet Criterion A. Although the boy's tantrums have occurred at least weekly for a 6-month period, DSM-5-TR specifically notes that for a child younger than 5 years, behavior meeting Criterion A can be considered a symptom of ODD only if it occurs *on most days* for the preceding 6 months. Finally, the tantrums do not appear to cause significant distress or impairment in functioning (Criterion B) and could be developmental in nature.

A diagnosis of IED should not be given to individuals younger than 6 years, or the equivalent developmental level. The diagnosis of DMDD should not be made for the first time before age 6 years or after age 18 years. In DMDD, tantrums must occur frequently (i.e., on average, three or more times per week; Criterion C) over at least 1 year, and they must be developmentally inappropriate (Criterion B). The severe irritability of DMDD consists of chronic, persistently irritable or angry mood that is present between the severe temper outbursts. This irritable or angry mood must be characteristic of the child; be present most of the day, nearly every day; and be noticeable by others in the child's environment (Criterion D).

15.2—Oppositional Defiant Disorder / diagnostic criteria (pp. 522–523) and Differential Diagnosis (pp. 525–526)

15.3 The diagnostic criteria for oppositional defiant disorder (ODD) include specifiers for indicating severity of the disorder as manifested by pervasiveness of symptoms across settings and relationships. Which of the following specifiers would be appropriate for an 11-year-old child who meets Criterion A symptoms at home and at school?

A. Mild.
B. Moderate.
C. Severe.
D. Insufficient information.

Correct Answer: B. Moderate.

Explanation: The *mild* specifier requires symptoms to be confined to one setting, the *moderate* specifier requires symptoms to be present in at least two settings, and the *severe* specifier requires symptoms to be present in at least three settings.

15.3—Oppositional Defiant Disorder / diagnostic criteria; Specifiers (pp. 522–523)

15.4 A previously well-behaved 13-year-old begins to display extremely defiant and oppositional behavior, with vindictiveness, for the past 8 months. They are angry and argumentative and refuse to accept responsibility for their behavior, which is significantly affecting their life at home and in school. Which aspect of this presentation fits poorly with a diagnosis of oppositional defiant disorder (ODD)?

A. Lack of remorse.
B. Duration of symptoms.
C. Age at onset.
D. Symptoms in multiple settings.

Correct Answer: C. Age at onset.

Explanation: The first symptoms of ODD usually appear during the preschool years and rarely later than early adolescence. ODD is an unlikely diagnosis if the onset is in adolescence after a childhood marked by compliant behavior. Environmental and family stressors may be associated with externalizing manifestations of emotion dysregulation. These may manifest as tantrums and oppositional behavior in children and as aggressive behaviors in adolescents. Temporal association with a stressor and symptom duration of less than 6 months after the resolution of the stressor may help distinguish adjustment disorder from ODD. In this case, the relatively late onset suggests a mood disorder, an adjustment disorder (to a stressor not described in the vignette), or a substance use disorder. To count toward a diagnosis of a major depressive episode, a symptom must either be newly present or have clearly worsened compared with the individual's pre-episode status. Many individuals report or exhibit increased irritability (e.g., persistent anger, a tendency to respond to events with angry outbursts or blaming others, an exaggerated sense of frustration over minor matters). In children and adolescents, an irritable or cranky mood may develop rather than a sad or dejected mood.

15.4—Oppositional Defiant Disorder / Development and Course (p. 524)

15.5   What is an associated risk factor with oppositional defiant disorder (ODD)?

A. Heightened cortisol reactivity.
B. Being bullied.
C. Permissive parenting.
D. Low emotional reactivity.

Correct Answer: B. Being bullied.

Explanation: Children with ODD are at greater risk for both bullying peers and being bullied by peers. Although a number of neurobiological markers (e.g., lower heart rate and skin conductance reactivity; reduced basal cortisol reactivity; abnormalities in the prefrontal cortex and amygdala) have been identified in association with ODD, they cannot be used diagnostically because the vast majority of studies have not separated children with ODD from those with conduct disorder. Thus, it is unclear whether there are markers specific to ODD. Harsh, inconsistent, or neglectful child-rearing practices predict increases in symptoms, and manifestations of the disorder across development appear to be consistent. Temperamental factors related to problems in emotion regulation (e.g., high levels of emotional reactivity, poor frustration tolerance) have been predictive of the disorder.

15.5—Oppositional Defiant Disorder / Development and Course; Risk and Prognostic Factors (pp. 524–525)

15.6   A 16-year-old boy with a long history of defiant behavior toward authority figures also has a history of aggression toward peers (gets into fights at school), his parents, and objects (punching holes in walls, breaking doors). He lies frequently. Recently, he began to steal merchandise from local stores and money and jewelry from his parents. He does not seem pervasively irritable or depressed, has no sleep disturbance, and denies any history of psychotic symptoms. What is the most likely diagnosis?

A. Oppositional defiant disorder (ODD).
B. Conduct disorder.
C. Attention-deficit/hyperactivity disorder (ADHD).
D. Disruptive mood dysregulation disorder (DMDD).

Correct Answer: B. Conduct disorder.

Explanation: This boy displays aggression toward people, destruction of property, and deceitfulness or theft—all part of Criterion A for conduct disorder in DSM-5-TR. Individuals with ODD are not typically aggressive toward people or animals, and they do not generally destroy property or exhibit patterns of behavior involving theft or deceit. In addition, individuals with ODD have problems with emotion dysregulation as a more prominent and pervasive feature of their presentation. There is not enough information from the vignette to establish a diagnosis of ADHD. Although children with ADHD often exhibit hyperactive and impulsive behavior that may be disruptive, this behavior does not by itself violate societal norms or the rights of others. The lack of a pervasive mood disturbance argues against a diagnosis of DMDD.

15.6—Conduct Disorder / diagnostic criteria (pp. 530–531)

15.7   A 15-year-old boy has a history of episodic violent behavior that is out of proportion to the precipitant. During a typical episode, which escalates rapidly, he becomes extremely angry, punching holes in walls or destroying furniture in the home. There seems to be no specific purpose or gain associated with the outbursts, and within 30 minutes he is calm and "back to normal," a state that is not associated with any predominant mood disturbance. What diagnosis best fits this clinical picture?

A. Bipolar disorder.
B. Disruptive mood dysregulation disorder (DMDD).

C. Intermittent explosive disorder (IED).
D. Attention-deficit/hyperactivity disorder (ADHD).

Correct Answer: C. Intermittent explosive disorder (IED).

Explanation: This teenager's presentation is characteristic of IED. The fact that there is no mood disturbance between episodes argues against bipolar disorder or DMDD. In contrast to IED, DMDD is characterized by a persistently negative mood state most of the day, nearly every day, between impulsive aggressive outbursts. The aggression in IED is impulsive and ADHD can be comorbid with IED, but ADHD symptoms other than impulsivity (inattention and restlessness) are not described in this vignette.

15.7—Intermittent Explosive Disorder / diagnostic criteria (p. 527)

15.8   Which of the following is *not* a risk factor for intermittent explosive disorder (IED)?

A. First-degree relatives with IED.
B. Separation from family members in refugee populations.
C. Schizotypal personality disorder.
D. Borderline personality disorder.

Correct Answer: C. Schizotypal personality disorder.

Explanation: According to DSM-5-TR, first-degree relatives of individuals with IED are at higher risk of also having the disorder, which has a strong genetic component to the impulsive aggression. Individuals with antisocial personality disorder or borderline personality disorder and those who have a history of disorders with disruptive behaviors (e.g., ADHD, conduct disorder, oppositional defiant disorder) are at greater risk of comorbid IED. Long-term displacement from home and separation from family members are risk factors in some refugee population settings.

15.8—Intermittent Explosive Disorder / Risk and Prognostic Factors; Comorbidity (p. 529)

15.9   Which of the following biological markers is associated with intermittent explosive disorder (IED)?

A. Serotonergic abnormalities in the limbic system and orbitofrontal cortex.
B. Reduced amygdala responses to anger stimuli during functional MRI (fMRI) scanning.
C. Abnormalities in adrenal function.
D. Increased urinary catecholamines.

Correct Answer: A. Serotonergic abnormalities in the limbic system and orbitofrontal cortex.

Explanation: Research provides neurobiological support for the presence of serotonergic abnormalities, globally and in the brain, specifically in areas of the limbic system (anterior cingulate) and orbitofrontal cortex in individuals with IED. Amygdala responses to anger stimuli during fMRI scanning are *greater* in individuals with IED compared with healthy individuals. There is no current evidence for the abnormalities in adrenal function or changes in urinary catecholamines.

15.9—Intermittent Explosive Disorder / Associated Features (p. 528)

15.10 Which of the following statements about the differential diagnosis of intermittent explosive disorder (IED) is *false*?

A. In children, the diagnosis of IED can be made in the context of an adjustment disorder.
B. In contrast to IED, disruptive mood dysregulation disorder is characterized by a persistently negative mood state (i.e., irritability, anger) most of the day, nearly every day, between impulsive aggressive outbursts.
C. The level of impulsive aggression in individuals with antisocial personality disorder or borderline personality disorder is lower than that in individuals with IED.
D. Aggression in oppositional defiant disorder is typically characterized by temper tantrums and verbal arguments with authority figures, whereas impulsive aggressive outbursts in IED are in response to a broader array of provocation and include physical assault.

Correct Answer: A. In children, the diagnosis of IED can be made in the context of an adjustment disorder.

Explanation: DSM-5-TR stipulates that for children ages 6–18 years, aggressive behavior that occurs as part of an adjustment disorder should not be considered for the diagnosis of IED.

15.10—Intermittent Explosive Disorder / diagnostic criteria; Diagnostic Features (pp. 527–528)

15.11 A 17-year-old adolescent with a history of bullying and initiating fights using bats and knives has also stolen from others, set fires, destroyed property, broken into homes, and "conned" others. Which conduct disorder Criterion A category is not met in this vignette?

A. Aggression to people and animals.
B. Destruction of property.
C. Deceitfulness or theft.
D. Serious violations of rules.

Correct Answer: D. Serious violations of rules.

Explanation: The essential feature of conduct disorder is a repetitive and persistent pattern of behavior in which the basic rights of others or major age-appropriate societal norms or rules are violated (Criterion A). These behaviors fall into four main groupings: aggressive conduct that causes or threatens physical harm to other people or animals (Criteria A1–A7); nonaggressive conduct that causes property loss or damage (Criteria A8–A9); deceitfulness or theft (Criteria A10–A12); and serious violations of rules (Criteria A13–A15). According to DSM-5-TR, *serious violations of rules* include the following: often stays out at night despite parental prohibitions, beginning before age 13 years; has run away from home overnight at least twice while living in the parental or parental surrogate home, or once without returning for a lengthy period; and is often truant from school, beginning before age 13 years.

15.11—Conduct Disorder / Diagnostic Features (pp. 533)

15.12 A 15-year-old adolescent with a history of cruelty to animals, stealing, school truancy, and running away from home shows no remorse when caught or when confronted with how these behaviors affect her family. She disregards the feelings of others and seems to not care that her conduct is compromising her school performance. The behavior has been present for more than a year and in multiple relationships and settings. Which of the following components of the *with limited prosocial emotions* specifier is absent in this clinical picture?

A. Lack of remorse or guilt.
B. Callous—lack of empathy.
C. Unconcerned about performance.
D. Shallow or deficient affect.

Correct Answer: D. Shallow or deficient affect.

Explanation: *Shallow or deficient affect* is defined in DSM-5-TR as "does not express feelings or show emotions to others, except in ways that seem shallow, insincere, or superficial (e.g., actions contradict the emotion displayed; can turn emotions 'on' or 'off' quickly) or when emotional expressions are used for gain (e.g., emotions displayed to manipulate or intimidate others)." Not enough information is given in this vignette to indicate whether this patient has shallow or deficient affect.

15.12—Conduct Disorder / diagnostic criteria (pp. 530–532)

15.13 Which of the following does *not* qualify as aggressive behavior under Criterion A definitions for the diagnosis of conduct disorder?

A. Cyberbullying.
B. Forcing someone into sexual activity.
C. Stealing while confronting a victim.
D. Aggression in the context of a mood disorder.

Correct Answer: D. Aggression in the context of a mood disorder.

Explanation: Irritability, aggression, and conduct problems can occur in children or adolescents with a major depressive disorder, a bipolar disorder, or disruptive mood dysregulation disorder. On the basis of their course, the behavioral problems associated with these mood disorders can usually be distinguished from the pattern of conduct problems seen in conduct disorder. Specifically, persons with conduct disorder will display substantial levels of aggressive or nonaggressive conduct problems during periods in which there is no mood disturbance, either historically (i.e., a history of conduct problems predating the onset of the mood disturbance) or concurrently (i.e., display of some conduct problems that are premeditated and do not occur during periods of intense emotional arousal). In those cases in which criteria for conduct disorder and a mood disorder are met, both diagnoses can be given.

Criterion A in conduct disorder, aggression to people and animals, includes the following: 1) often bullies, threatens, or intimidates others; 2) often initiates physical fights; 3) has used a weapon that can cause serious physical harm to others (e.g., a bat, brick, broken bottle, knife, gun); 4) has been physically cruel to people; 5) has been physically cruel to animals; 6) has stolen while confronting a victim (e.g., mugging, purse snatching, extortion, armed robbery); and 7) has forced someone into sexual activity.

15.13—Conduct Disorder / diagnostic criteria (pp. 530–532); Differential Diagnosis (p. 536)

15.14 A 16-year-old adolescent who has started to miss school at least three times a week this year is argumentative with her teachers and parents. Her parents recall many tantrums due to not getting her way when she was preschool age. Recently, she has been breaking curfew and returning home intoxicated around 2 A.M. There was a time last year where she was missing for 2 weeks. Which of this patient's symptoms is a symptom of conduct disorder?

A. School truancy.
B. Tantrums during preschool age.
C. Running away for a lengthy period.
D. Breaking curfew.

Correct Answer: C. Running away for a lengthy period.

Explanation: DSM-5-TR Criterion A14 for conduct disorder specifies running away once if it is for a lengthy period or overnight at least twice. The patient's school truancy and breaking of curfew started this year; DSM-5-TR specifies that for conduct disorder this behavior needs to start before age 13 years. For a preschool-age child, temper outbursts and their frequency are considered in the diagnosis of oppositional defiant disorder but not in conduct disorder.

15.14—Conduct Disorder / Diagnostic Features (p. 533)

15.15   Compared with individuals with childhood-onset conduct disorder, what are patients with adolescent-onset conduct disorder more likely to have?

A. Oppositional defiant disorder (ODD).
B. Attention-deficit/hyperactivity disorder (ADHD).
C. Persistent symptoms into adulthood.
D. Normative peer relationships.

Correct Answer: D. Normative peer relationships.

Explanation: In childhood-onset conduct disorder, individuals are usually male, frequently display physical aggression toward others, have disturbed peer relationships, may have had ODD during early childhood, and usually have symptoms that meet full criteria for conduct disorder prior to puberty. Many children with this subtype also have concurrent ADHD or other neurodevelopmental difficulties. Individuals with childhood-onset type are more likely to have persistent conduct disorder into adulthood than are those with adolescent-onset conduct disorder. Compared with individuals with childhood-onset conduct disorder, individuals with adolescent-onset conduct disorder are less likely to display aggressive behaviors and tend to have more normative peer relationships (although they often display conduct problems in the company of others). These individuals are less likely to have conduct disorder that persists into adulthood.

15.15—Conduct Disorder / Subtypes (p. 532)

15.16   What is more common in individuals who qualify for the *with limited prosocial emotions* specifier for conduct disorder?

A. Personality features such as risk avoidance, fearfulness, and extreme sensitivity to punishment.
B. Engaging in aggression that is impulsive.
C. A *mild severity* specifier rating.
D. Childhood-onset subtype of conduct disorder.

Correct Answer: D. Childhood-onset subtype of conduct disorder.

Explanation: To qualify for the *with limited prosocial emotions* specifier, an individual must have displayed at least two of the listed characteristics—lack of remorse or guilt, callousness/lack of empathy, unconcern about performance, and shallow or deficient affect—persistently over at least 12 months and in multiple relationships and settings. These characteristics must reflect the individual's typical pattern of interpersonal and emotional functioning over this period and not just occasional occurrences in some situations.

A minority of individuals with conduct disorder exhibit characteristics that qualify for this specifier. The indicators of this specifier are those that have often been labeled as callous and unemotional traits in research. Other personality features, such as thrill seeking, fearlessness, and insensitivity to punishment, may also distinguish individuals with characteristics described in the specifier. These individuals may be more likely than others with conduct disorder to engage in aggression that is planned for instrumental gain. Individuals with conduct disorder of any subtype or any level of severity can have characteristics that qualify for the specifier with limited prosocial emotions, although individuals with the specifier are more likely to have childhood-onset type and a severity specifier rating of severe.

15.16—Conduct Disorder / diagnostic criteria; Specifiers (pp. 531–533)

15.17 When comparing populations, which population is associated with a higher prevalence of conduct disorder?

A. United States compared with other Western countries.
B. Socially oppressed adolescents compared with socially advantaged adolescents.
C. Females compared with males.
D. Children compared with adolescents.

Correct Answer: B. Socially oppressed adolescents compared with socially advantaged adolescents.

Explanation: One-year population prevalence rates range from 2% to more than 10%, with a median of 4%, in the United States and other largely high-income countries. The prevalence of conduct disorder in largely Western samples appears to be fairly consistent across various countries. Prevalence of adolescent-onset conduct disorder is more frequently associated with psychosocial stressors (e.g., being a member of a socially oppressed ethnic group facing discrimination). Prevalence rates rise from childhood to adolescence and are higher among males than among females.

15.17—Conduct Disorder / Specifiers (pp. 532–533); Prevalence (p. 534)

15.18 Which of the following statements about the onset and developmental course of conduct disorder is *true*?

A. Onset may occur as early as the preschool years.
B. Age at onset has no bearing on the developmental course of the disorder.
C. Oppositional defiant disorder is generally not a precursor to the childhood-onset type of conduct disorder.
D. Onset is common after age 16.

Correct Answer: A. Onset may occur as early as the preschool years.

Explanation: The onset of conduct disorder typically occurs in the period from middle childhood through middle adolescence, although symptoms may appear in the preschool years. Individuals with adolescent-onset type and those with fewer and milder symptoms tend to have a greater likelihood of being successful (from a social and occupational standpoint) as adults. Oppositional defiant disorder is a common precursor to the childhood-onset type of conduct disorder.

15.18—Conduct Disorder / Development and Course (p. 534)

15.19 Which of the following is a risk factor for the development of conduct disorder?

A. Higher-than-average verbal IQ.
B. Small family size.
C. Refugee status.
D. Parental history of attention-deficit/hyperactivity disorder (ADHD).

Correct Answer: D. Parental history of attention-deficit/hyperactivity disorder (ADHD).

Explanation: Conduct disorder appears to be more common in children of biological parents with severe alcohol use disorder, depressive and bipolar disorders, or schizophrenia or biological parents who have a history of ADHD or conduct disorder. Temperamental risk factors include a difficult undercontrolled infant temperament and lower-than-average intelligence, particularly with regard to verbal IQ. Family-level risk factors include parental rejection and neglect, inconsistent child-rearing practices, harsh discipline, physical or sexual abuse, lack of supervision, early institutional living, frequent changes of caregivers, large family size, parental criminality, and certain kinds of familial psychopathology (e.g., substance-related disorders). Community-level risk factors include peer rejection, association with a delinquent peer group, neighborhood disadvantage, and exposure to violence. Parental migration is a risk factor for children who are left in the country of origin as well as for those who migrated with their parents, with conduct problems being attributable to acculturation processes. However, first-generation immigrants and refugees often have fewer conduct problems than their peers do.

15.19—Conduct Disorder / Risk and Prognostic Factors (pp. 534–535)

15.20 What is *not* a risk or prognostic factor associated with conduct disorder?

A. Biological sibling with conduct disorder.
B. Low skin conductance.
C. Adoptive parent with conduct disorder.
D. Increased autonomic fear conditioning

Correct Answer: D. Increased autonomic fear conditioning.

Explanation: *Reduced* autonomic fear conditioning, particularly *low* skin conductance, is well documented in individuals with conduct disorder; however, this finding is not diagnostic of the disorder. The risk of conduct disorder is increased in children with a biological or an adoptive parent or a sibling with conduct disorder. Structural and functional differences in brain areas associated with affect regulation and affect processing, particularly frontotemporal-limbic connections involving the brain's ventral prefrontal cortex and amygdala, have been consistently noted in individuals with conduct disorder. Persistence is more likely for individuals with behaviors that meet criteria for the childhood-onset subtype and qualify for the specifier *with limited prosocial emotions*. The risk that conduct disorder will persist is also increased by co-occurring attention-deficit/hyperactivity disorder and by substance abuse.

15.20—Conduct Disorder / Risk and Prognostic Factors (pp. 534–535)

15.21 Which of the following helps distinguish conduct disorder from oppositional defiant disorder (ODD)?

A. Conduct disorder is more likely to involve aggression toward other people.
B. ODD is more likely to involve conflict with parents.
C. Conduct disorder is more likely to involve an angry or irritable mood.
D. A diagnosis of conduct disorder supersedes and precludes the diagnosis of ODD.

Correct Answer: A. Conduct disorder is more likely to involve aggression toward other people.

Explanation: Conduct disorder and ODD are both related to symptoms that bring the individual in conflict with adults and other authority figures (e.g., parents, teachers, work supervisors). The behaviors of ODD are typically of a less severe nature than those of individuals with conduct disorder and do not include aggression toward people or animals, destruction of property, or a pattern of theft or deceit. Furthermore, ODD includes problems of emotion dysregulation (i.e., angry and irritable mood) that are not included in the definition of conduct disorder. When criteria are met for both ODD and conduct disorder, both diagnoses can be given.

15.21—Conduct Disorder / Differential Diagnosis (pp. 536–537)

15.22 Which of the following comorbid disorders is *not* associated with pyromania?

A. Antisocial personality disorder.
B. Substance use disorders.
C. Obsessive-compulsive disorder
D. Gambling disorder.

Correct Answer: C. Obsessive-compulsive disorder.

Explanation: There appears to be a high co-occurrence of substance use disorders; gambling disorder; depressive and bipolar disorders; and other disruptive, impulse-control, and conduct disorders with pyromania. Juvenile fire setting may also be associated with conduct disorders or attention-deficit/hyperactivity disorder. Although fire setting in the United States among children and adolescents is a major problem, the actual diagnosis of pyromania is rare.

15.22—Pyromania / Differential Diagnosis (p. 539)

15.23 A 15-year-old student in private school, without known psychiatric history, has been caught stealing other students' laptops and cell phones, even though he comes from a wealthy family and his parents continue to purchase the newest electronics for him in an effort to deter him from stealing. Which of the following would raise your clinical suspicion that the patient may have kleptomania?

   A. He demonstrates recurrent failure to resist impulses to steal objects that are not needed for personal use or for their monetary value.
   B. He demonstrates recurrent failure to resist impulses to steal objects during periods of detachment or boredom.
   C. He experiences increased tension before committing the theft but does not experience relief, pleasure, or gratification while committing the theft.
   D. He has a strong family history for antisocial personality disorder and conduct disorder.

Correct Answer: A. He demonstrates recurrent failure to resist impulses to steal objects that are not needed for personal use or for their monetary value.

Explanation: Kleptomania is defined by the recurrent failure to resist impulses to steal items even though the items are not needed for personal use or for monetary value (Criterion A). The individual experiences a rising sense of tension before the act (Criterion B) and then derives pleasure or gratification when committing the theft (Criterion C). The act is not done in response to anger or vengeance, and the stealing that occurs in kleptomania is not better explained by conduct disorder, a manic episode, or antisocial personality disorder (Criterion E). There appears to be a higher rate of alcohol use disorders in first-degree relatives of individuals with kleptomania than in the general population.

15.23—Kleptomania / diagnostic criteria (p. 539), Risk and Prognostic Factors (p. 540)

15.24 Which of the following statements about kleptomania is *false*?

   A. The prevalence of kleptomania in the general population is generally very low, and the disorder is more frequent among females.

B. First-degree relatives of individuals with kleptomania may have higher rates of obsessive-compulsive disorder and/or substance use disorders than the general population.

C. Kleptomania can occur in a manic episode as a response to a delusion or hallucination.

D. Individuals with kleptomania generally do not preplan their thefts.

Correct Answer: C. Kleptomania can occur in a manic episode as a response to a delusion or hallucination.

Explanation: Kleptomania should be distinguished from intentional or inadvertent stealing that may occur during a manic episode, in response to delusions or hallucinations (e.g., in schizophrenia), or as a result of a major neurocognitive disorder. The key feature of kleptomania is recurrent failure to resist impulses to steal items even though they are not needed and the individual is aware that the act is senseless.

15.24—Kleptomania / Diagnostic Features (p. 539), Prevalence (p. 540), Differential Diagnosis (pp. 540–541)

15.25 Which diagnosis is associated with higher risk for suicidal ideation and behavior?

A. Intermittent explosive disorder (IED).

B. Kleptomania.

C. Oppositional defiant disorder (ODD).

D. All of the above.

Correct Answer: D. All of the above.

Explanation: A study of 1,460 research volunteers found that IED comorbid with posttraumatic stress disorder was associated with a markedly elevated rate of lifetime suicide attempt. ODD has been associated with increased risk for suicide attempts, even after comorbid disorders are controlled for. Kleptomania has been associated with an increased risk for suicide attempts.

15.25—Oppositional Defiant Disorder / Associated Features (p. 524), Intermittent Explosive Disorder / Association With Suicidal Thoughts or Behavior (p. 529); Kleptomania / Association With Suicidal Thoughts or Behavior (p. 540)

15.26 A 12-year-old boy with a history of verbal arguments with his parents and teachers was physically cruel to the family's pet hamster 3 months ago. Last month he stole his mother's credit card to purchase video games and clothes. He is brought to the emergency department after the police pick him up for setting a fire in one of the alleys near his parents' apartment building. What piece of information would indicate this could be due to pyromania rather than conduct disorder?

A. He burned the clothes he had stolen to avoid getting caught.
B. He is intoxicated and voices were commanding him to set the fire.
C. He practiced setting smaller fires at school and home and saved the ashes.
D. He set the fire on purpose.

Correct Answer: C. He practiced setting smaller fires at school and home and saved the ashes.

Explanation: The essential feature of pyromania is the presence of multiple episodes of deliberate and purposeful fire setting (Criterion A). There is a fascination with, interest in, curiosity about, or attraction to fire and its situational contexts (e.g., paraphernalia, uses, consequences) (Criterion C). The fire setting is not done to conceal criminal activity, to express anger or vengeance, or in response to a delusion or a hallucination (Criterion E). The fire setting does not result from impaired judgment. Fire setting can be deliberate in both conduct disorder and pyromania.

15.25—Pyromania / diagnostic criteria and Diagnostic Features (pp. 537–538)

CHAPTER 16

Substance-Related and Addictive Disorders

16.1 The diagnostic criteria for substance abuse, substance dependence, substance intoxication, and substance withdrawal were not equally applicable to all substances in DSM-IV and were changed in DSM-5. This remains the case in DSM-5-TR, with *substance use disorder* replacing the DSM-IV diagnoses of *substance abuse* and *substance dependence*. For which of the following substance classes is there adequate evidence to support diagnostic criteria in DSM-5 for the three major categories of *use disorder, intoxication,* and *withdrawal?*

A. Caffeine.
B. Cannabis.
C. Tobacco.
D. Hallucinogen.

Correct Answer: B. Cannabis.

Explanation: The essential feature of a substance use disorder is a cluster of cognitive, behavioral, and physiological symptoms indicating that the individual continues using the substance despite significant substance-related problems. As seen in Table 1, "Diagnoses associated with substance class" (p. 545), the diagnosis of a substance use disorder can be applied to all 10 substance classes included in this chapter except caffeine. For certain classes, some symptoms are less salient, and in a few instances not all symptoms apply (e.g., withdrawal symptoms are not specified for phencyclidine use disorder, other hallucinogen use disorder, or inhalant use disorder).

Marked and generally easily measured physiological signs of withdrawal are common with alcohol; opioids; and sedatives, hypnotics, and anxiolytics. Withdrawal signs and symptoms with stimulants (amphetamine-type substances, cocaine, other or unspecified stimulants), as well as tobacco and cannabis, are often present but may be less apparent. Significant withdrawal has *not* been documented in humans after repeated use of phencyclidine, other hallucinogens, and inhalants; therefore, this criterion is not included for these substances. Cannabis withdrawal and caffeine withdrawal are included in DSM-5-TR. However, only cannabis has sufficient evidence to support all three categories of substance-related disorders.

16.1—chapter introduction (pp. 543–544)

16.2 Which of the following pairs of drugs falls into a single class in DSM-5-TR?

A. Cocaine and phencyclidine (PCP).
B. Cocaine and methylphenidate.
C. 3,4-Methylenedioxymethamphetamine (MDMA [ecstasy]) and metham-phetamine.
D. Lorazepam and alcohol.

Correct Answer: B. Cocaine and methylphenidate.

Explanation: Stimulants covered in this chapter include amphetamine and prescription stimulants with similar effects (e.g., methylphenidate) and cocaine. Substance-related disorders involving certain other substances with stimulant properties are classified in other sections of this chapter. These include caffeine (in caffeine-related disorders); nicotine (in tobacco-related disorders); and MDMA (in other hallucinogen-related disorders), which has both stimulant and hallucinogenic effects.

16.2—Stimulant Use Disorder / Diagnostic Features (pp. 635–636)

16.3 Which of the following statements about tolerance and withdrawal in the DSM-5-TR diagnosis of substance use disorder is *true*?

A. Tolerance and withdrawal are no longer considered to be valid diagnostic symptoms of substance use disorder.
B. The definitions of tolerance and withdrawal have been updated because the previous definitions had poor interrater reliability.
C. The presence of either tolerance or withdrawal is now required to make a substance use disorder diagnosis for some but not all classes of substances.
D. Tolerance and withdrawal are still listed as criteria, but if they occur during appropriate medically supervised treatment, they are not counted toward the diagnosis of a substance use disorder.

Correct Answer: D. Tolerance and withdrawal are still listed as criteria, but if they occur during appropriate medically supervised treatment, they are not counted toward the diagnosis of a substance use disorder.

Explanation: Symptoms of tolerance and withdrawal occurring during appropriate use of prescribed medications given as part of medical treatment (e.g., opioid analgesics, sedatives, stimulants) are specifically not counted when diagnosing a substance use disorder. The appearance of normal, expected pharmacological tolerance and withdrawal during the course of medical treatment have been known to lead to an erroneous diagnosis of addiction even when they were the only symptoms present. Individuals whose only symptoms are those that occur as a result of medical treatment (i.e., tolerance and withdrawal as part of medical care when the medications are taken as prescribed) should not receive a diagnosis solely on the basis of these symptoms.

16.3—chapter introduction; Substance Use Disorders / Diagnostic Features (p. 547)

16.4   Which of the following differentiates alcohol use disorder from the other alcohol-related disorders?

A. Alcohol use disorder involves impaired control over alcohol use.
B. Alcohol use disorder requires a high quantity of alcohol to be consumed.
C. Alcohol use disorder is an intractable condition.
D. The majority of people who use heavy doses of alcohol develop the disorder.

Correct Answer: A. Alcohol use disorder involves impaired control over alcohol use.

Explanation: Alcohol use disorder is often erroneously perceived as an intractable condition, perhaps on the basis of the fact that individuals who present for treatment typically have a history of many years of severe alcohol-related problems. However, these most severe cases represent only a minority of individuals with this disorder, and the typical individual with the disorder has a much more promising prognosis.

The key element of alcohol use disorder is the use of heavy doses of alcohol with resulting repeated and significant distress or impaired functioning. Although most drinkers sometimes consume enough alcohol to feel intoxicated, only a minority (<20%) ever develop alcohol use disorder. Therefore, drinking, even daily, in low doses and occasional intoxication do not by themselves make this diagnosis.

Alcohol use disorder is differentiated from alcohol intoxication, alcohol withdrawal, and alcohol-induced mental disorders (e.g., alcohol-induced depressive disorder) in that alcohol use disorder describes a problematic pattern of alcohol use that involves impaired control over alcohol use, social impairment due to alcohol use, risky alcohol use (e.g., driving while intoxicated), and pharmacological symptoms (the development of tolerance or withdrawal), whereas alcohol intoxication, alcohol withdrawal, and alcohol-induced mental disorders describe psychiatric syndromes that develop in the context of heavy use. Alcohol intoxication, alcohol withdrawal, and alcohol-induced mental disorders occur frequently in individuals with alcohol use disorder. In such cases, a diagnosis of alcohol intoxication, alcohol withdrawal, or an alcohol-induced mental disorder should be given in addition to a diagnosis of alcohol use disorder, the presence of which is indicated in the diagnostic code.

16.4—Alcohol Use Disorder/ Development and Course (pp. 556–557); Differential Diagnosis (pp. 560–561)

16.5   Which of the following is *not* a recognized alcohol-related disorder in DSM-5-TR?

A. Alcohol dependence.
B. Alcohol use disorder.
C. Alcohol intoxication.
D. Alcohol withdrawal.

Correct Answer: A. Alcohol dependence.

Explanation: The alcohol-related disorders are alcohol use disorder, alcohol intoxication, alcohol withdrawal, and alcohol-induced mental disorders. The following alcohol-induced mental disorders are described in other DSM-5-TR chapters with disorders with which they share phenomenology (see the substance/medication-induced mental disorders in these chapters): alcohol-induced psychotic disorder ("Schizophrenia Spectrum and Other Psychotic Disorders"); alcohol-induced bipolar and related disorder ("Bipolar and Related Disorders"); alcohol-induced depressive disorder ("Depressive Disorders"); alcohol-induced anxiety disorder ("Anxiety Disorders"); alcohol-induced sleep disorder ("Sleep-Wake Disorders"); alcohol-induced sexual dysfunction ("Sexual Dysfunctions"); and alcohol-induced major or mild neurocognitive disorder ("Neurocognitive Disorders").

16.5—Alcohol-Related Disorders/ Alcohol-Induced Mental Disorders (pp. 567–568)

16.6   Which of the following statements is correct about the diagnosis of a caffeine-related disorder?

A. The individual must be aware of consuming caffeine.
B. In order to diagnose caffeine intoxication, the amount consumed must exceed 200 mg.
C. The diagnosis of caffeine withdrawal requires the preceding use of caffeine on a daily basis.
D. Caffeine withdrawal may be diagnosed even in the absence of clinically significant distress or impairment in social, occupational, or other important areas of functioning.

Correct Answer: C. The diagnosis of caffeine withdrawal requires the preceding use of caffeine on a daily basis.

Explanation: The essential feature of caffeine intoxication is recent consumption of caffeine and five or more signs or symptoms that develop during or shortly after caffeine use (Criteria A and B). Symptoms include restlessness, nervousness, excitement, insomnia, flushed face, diuresis, and gastrointestinal complaints, which can occur with low doses (e.g., 200 mg) in vulnerable individuals such as children, the elderly, or individuals who have not been exposed to caffeine previously.

Caffeine can be consumed from a number of different sources, including coffee, tea, caffeinated soda, "energy" drinks, over-the-counter analgesics and cold remedies, weight-loss aids, and chocolate. Caffeine is also increasingly being used as an additive to vitamins and to food products.

More than 85% of adults and children in the United States regularly consume caffeine, with adult caffeine consumers ingesting about 280 mg/day on average. The incidence and prevalence of the caffeine withdrawal syndrome in the general population are unclear.

The essential feature of caffeine withdrawal is the presence of a characteristic withdrawal syndrome that develops after the abrupt cessation of (or substantial reduction in) prolonged daily caffeine ingestion (Criterion B). Because individuals may be unaware of the wide array of sources of caffeine beyond coffee, colas, and energy drinks (e.g., over-the-counter analgesics and cold remedies, weight loss aids, chocolate), they may not connect ingestion of these substances with symptoms of caffeine withdrawal. The caffeine withdrawal syndrome is indicated by three or more of the following (Criterion B): headache; marked fatigue or drowsiness; dysphoric mood, depressed mood, or irritability; difficulty concentrating; and flu-like symptoms (nausea, vomiting, or muscle pain/stiffness). The withdrawal syndrome causes clinically significant distress or impairment in social, occupational, or other important areas of functioning (Criterion C).

16.6—Caffeine-Related Disorders (pp. 569–574)

16.7 Which of the following symptoms is more common in women than men as a consequence of the abrupt termination of daily or near-daily cannabis use?

A. Less severe withdrawal symptoms.
B. Suicide.
C. Hunger.
D. Irritability.

Correct Answer: D. Irritability.

Explanation: Common cannabis withdrawal symptoms include irritability, depressed mood, anxiety, restlessness, sleep difficulty, and decreased appetite or weight loss. Compared with men, women report more severe cannabis withdrawal symptoms, especially mood symptoms such as irritability, restlessness, and anger, and gastrointestinal symptoms such as stomachache and nausea, which may contribute to potential telescoping (faster transition from first cannabis use to cannabis use disorder). In particular, men with cannabis use disorder have a suicide rate of 79 per 100,000 person-years, and women with cannabis use disorder have a suicide rate of 47 per 100,000 person-years.

16.7—Cannabis Withdrawal (pp. 584–586)

16.8   Which of the following is *not* a recognized symptom associated with hallucinogen use?

A. Withdrawal.
B. Tolerance.
C. A persistent desire or unsuccessful efforts to cut down or control use of the substance.
D. Recurrent use of the substance in situations in which it is physically hazardous.

Correct Answer: A. Withdrawal.

Explanation: The essential feature of a substance use disorder is a cluster of cognitive, behavioral, and physiological symptoms indicating that the individual continues using the substance despite significant substance-related problems. For certain classes, some symptoms are less salient, and in a few instances not all symptoms apply (e.g., withdrawal symptoms are not specified for phencyclidine use disorder, other hallucinogen use disorder, or inhalant use disorder).

Withdrawal (Criterion A11) is a syndrome that occurs when blood or tissue concentrations of a substance decline in an individual who had maintained prolonged, heavy use of the substance. After developing withdrawal symptoms, the individual is likely to consume the substance to relieve the symptoms. Withdrawal symptoms vary greatly across the classes of substances, and separate criteria sets for withdrawal are provided for the drug classes. Marked and generally easily measured physiological signs of withdrawal are common with alcohol; opioids; and sedatives, hypnotics, and anxiolytics. Withdrawal signs and symptoms with stimulants (amphetamine-type substances, cocaine, other or unspecified stimulants), as well as tobacco and cannabis, are often present but may be less apparent. Significant withdrawal has not been documented in humans after repeated use of phencyclidine, other hallucinogens, and inhalants; therefore, this criterion is not included for these substances.

16.8—Substance Use Disorders / Diagnostic Features (pp. 544–547)

16.9   To meet proposed criteria for *neurobehavioral disorder associated with prenatal alcohol exposure,* an individual's prenatal alcohol exposure must have been "more than minimal." How is "more than minimal" exposure defined, in terms of how much alcohol was used by the mother during gestation?

A. Any exposure to alcohol during the pregnancy.
B. Fewer than 10 drinks per month and no more than 1 drink per drinking occasion.
C. Fewer than 7 drinks per month and no more than 3 drinks per drinking occasion.
D. Fewer than 13 drinks per month and no more than 2 drinks per drinking occasion.

Correct Answer: D. Fewer than 13 drinks per month and no more than 2 drinks per drinking occasion.

Explanation: A clinical diagnosis of fetal alcohol syndrome, including specific prenatal alcohol-related facial dysmorphology and growth retardation, can be used as evidence of significant levels of prenatal alcohol exposure; specific guidelines for facial dysmorphology have been developed for diverse ethnoracial physiognomies. Although both animal and human studies have documented adverse effects of lower levels of drinking, identifying how much prenatal exposure is needed to significantly impact neurodevelopmental outcome remains challenging. Data suggest that a history of more than minimal gestational exposure prior to pregnancy recognition and/or following pregnancy recognition may be required. More than minimal exposure is defined as greater than 13 drinks per month during pregnancy or more than 2 drinks on any one occasion. Identifying a minimal threshold of drinking during pregnancy will require consideration of a variety of factors known to affect exposure and/or interact to influence developmental outcomes, including stage of prenatal development, gestational smoking, maternal and fetal genetics, and maternal physical status (i.e., age, health, and certain obstetric problems).

16.9—Conditions for Further Study / Neurobehavioral Disorder Associated With Prenatal Alcohol Exposure / proposed criteria / Diagnostic Features (pp. 916–918)

16.10   Which of the following is the only non-substance-related disorder to be included in the DSM-5-TR chapter "Substance-Related and Addictive Disorders"?

A. Gambling disorder.
B. Internet gaming disorder.
C. Electronic communication addiction disorder.
D. Compulsive computer use disorder.

Correct Answer: A. Gambling disorder.

Explanation: In addition to the substance-related disorders, this chapter also includes gambling disorder, reflecting evidence that gambling behaviors activate reward systems similar to those activated by drugs of abuse and produce some behavioral symptoms that appear comparable to those produced by the substance use disorders.

16.10—chapter introduction (p. 543)

16.11   In most substance/medication-induced mental disorders (with the exception of substance/medication-induced major or mild neurocognitive disorder and hallucinogen persisting perception disorder), if the person abstains from substance use, the disorder will eventually disappear or no longer be clinically relevant even without formal treatment. In what time frame is this likely to happen?

A. One hour.
B. One month.
C. Three months.
D. One year.

Correct Answer: B. One month.

Explanation: Most substance/medication-induced mental disorders, regardless of the severity of the symptoms, are likely to improve relatively quickly with abstinence and unlikely to remain clinically relevant for more than 1 month after complete cessation of use.

16.11—chapter introduction; Substance-Induced Disorders / Substance/Medication-Induced Mental Disorders / Development and Course (pp. 551–552)

16.12 Because opioid withdrawal and sedative, hypnotic, or anxiolytic withdrawal can involve very similar symptoms, distinguishing between the two can be difficult. Which of the following presenting symptoms would aid in differentiating opioid withdrawal from sedative, hypnotic, or anxiolytic withdrawal?

A. Nausea or vomiting.
B. Anxiety.
C. Yawning.
D. Restlessness or agitation.

Correct Answer: C. Yawning.

Explanation: The anxiety and restlessness associated with opioid withdrawal resemble symptoms seen in sedative-hypnotic withdrawal. However, opioid withdrawal is also accompanied by rhinorrhea, lacrimation, and pupillary dilation, which are not seen in sedative-type withdrawal. Dilated pupils are also seen in hallucinogen intoxication and stimulant intoxication. However, other signs or symptoms of opioid withdrawal, such as nausea, vomiting, diarrhea, abdominal cramps, rhinorrhea, or lacrimation, are not present.

16.12—Opioid Use Disorder / Differential Diagnosis (pp. 614–615); Opioid Withdrawal / diagnostic criteria (pp. 617–618)

16.13 In DSM-5-TR, the sedative, hypnotic, or anxiolytic class contains all prescription sleeping medications and almost all prescription antianxiety medications. What is the reason that nonbenzodiazepine antianxiety agents (e.g., buspirone, gepirone) are *not* included in this class?

A. They are not generally available in nonparenteral (intravenous or intramuscular) formulations.

B. They do not appear to be associated with significant misuse.

C. They are not associated with illicit manufacturing or diversion (e.g., Schedule I–V drugs in the United States, list of psychotropic substances recognized by the International Narcotics Control Board and the United Nations).

D. They are not respiratory depressants.

Correct Answer: B. They do not appear to be associated with significant misuse.

Explanation: Sedative, hypnotic, or anxiolytic substances include benzodiazepines, benzodiazepine-like drugs (e.g., zolpidem, zaleplon), carbamates (e.g., glutethimide, meprobamate), barbiturates (e.g., secobarbital), and barbiturate-like hypnotics (e.g., glutethimide, methaqualone, propofol). This class of substances includes most prescription sleeping medications and most prescription antianxiety medications. Nonbenzodiazepine antianxiety agents (e.g., buspirone, gepirone) are not included in this class because they do not appear to be associated with significant misuse.

16.13—Sedative, Hypnotic, or Anxiolytic Use Disorder / Diagnostic Features (p. 622)

16.14 Which of the following criteria was *not* one of the criteria for either substance abuse or substance dependence in DSM-IV but was included in DSM-5 and has been continued in DSM-5-TR?

A. Important social, occupational, or recreational activities are given up or reduced because of substance use.

B. The substance is often taken in larger amounts or over a longer period than was intended.

C. Craving, or a strong desire or urge to use the substance, is present.

D. Recurrent substance use results in a failure to fulfill major role obligations at work, school, or home.

Correct Answer: C. Craving, or a strong desire or urge to use the substance, is present.

Explanation: Overall, the diagnosis of a substance use disorder is based on a pathological pattern of behaviors related to use of the substance. To assist with organization, the diagnostic items making up Criterion A can be considered to fit within overall groupings of impaired control, social impairment, risky use, and pharmacological criteria. Impaired control over substance use is the first criteria grouping (Criteria A1–A4). The individual may take the substance in larger amounts or over a longer period than was originally intended (Criterion A1). The individual may express a persistent desire to cut down or regulate substance use and may report multiple unsuccessful efforts to decrease or discontinue use (Criterion A2). The individual may spend a great deal of time obtaining the substance, using the substance, or recovering from its effects

(Criterion A3). In some instances of more severe substance use disorders, virtually all of the individual's daily activities revolve around the substance. Craving (Criterion A4) is manifested by an intense desire or urge for the drug that may occur at any time but is more likely when the individual is in an environment where the drug previously was obtained or used. Craving has also been shown to involve classical conditioning and is associated with activation of specific reward structures in the brain. Craving might be queried by asking if there has ever been a time when there were such strong urges to take the drug that the individual could not think of anything else. Current craving is often used as a treatment outcome measure because it may be a signal of impending relapse.

16.14—chapter introduction; Substance Use Disorders / Diagnostic Features (pp. 545–546)

16.15 A 27-year-old woman presents for psychiatric evaluation after almost hitting someone with her car while driving under the influence of marijuana. She reports that her husband pushed her to seek treatment. He has told her that her ongoing marijuana use is a serious stress in the marriage. Nevertheless, she continues to smoke two joints daily and drive while under the influence of marijuana. What is the appropriate diagnosis?

A. Cannabis abuse.
B. Cannabis dependence.
C. Cannabis intoxication.
D. Cannabis use disorder.

Correct Answer: D. Cannabis use disorder.

Explanation: Cannabis use disorder is defined by the same 11 criteria that define the other substance use disorders, as supported by considerable empirical evidence. The cluster of behavioral and physical symptoms that make up these criteria leads to clinically significant impairment or distress and can include withdrawal, tolerance, craving, spending a great deal of time in activities related to the substance, and hazardous use (e.g., driving while under its influence).

16.15—Cannabis Use Disorder / Diagnostic Features (p. 576–577)

16.16 A 35-year-old man with a long-standing history of heavy alcohol use is referred for psychiatric evaluation after his recent admission to the hospital for acute hepatitis. The patient reports that he drank 2–3 drinks daily in college. Over the past 10 years, he has gradually increased his nightly alcohol intake from a single 6-pack to two 12-packs of beer. He frequently oversleeps and does not get to work. He has tried to moderate his alcohol use on numerous occasions with little success, particularly after developing complications associated with alcoholic cirrhosis. The patient admits that he becomes anxious and gets hand tremors when he doesn't drink. This patient meets the criteria for which of the following diagnoses?

A. Alcohol abuse.
B. Alcohol dependence.
C. Alcohol use disorder, severe.
D. Alcohol use disorder, moderate.

Correct Answer: C. Alcohol use disorder, severe.

Explanation: Alcohol use disorder is defined by a cluster of behavioral and physical symptoms, such as withdrawal, tolerance, and craving. Alcohol withdrawal is characterized by withdrawal symptoms that develop approximately 4–12 hours after the reduction of intake following prolonged, heavy alcohol ingestion. Because withdrawal from alcohol can be unpleasant and intense, individuals may continue to consume alcohol despite adverse consequences, often to avoid or to relieve withdrawal symptoms. Some withdrawal symptoms (e.g., sleep problems) can persist at lower intensities for months and can contribute to relapse. Once a pattern of repetitive and intense use develops, individuals with alcohol use disorder may devote substantial periods of their time to obtaining and consuming alcoholic beverages.

Severity of the disorder is based on the number of diagnostic criteria endorsed. For a given individual, changes in severity of alcohol use disorder across time are also reflected by reductions in the frequency (e.g., days of use per month) or dose (e.g., number of standard drinks consumed per day) of alcohol used, as assessed by the individual's self-report, report of knowledgeable others, clinician observations, and, when practical, biological testing (e.g., elevations in blood tests as described in the section "Diagnostic Markers" for this disorder).

16.16—Alcohol Use Disorder / Diagnostic Features (p. 555); Specifiers (p. 555)

16.17 Which of the following is the most accurate statement about predicting alcohol withdrawal or its consequences?

A. Fewer than 10% of individuals undergoing alcohol withdrawal experience dramatic symptoms such as severe autonomic hyperactivity, tremors, or alcohol withdrawal delirium.
B. All of the symptoms of alcohol withdrawal cease after 7 days.
C. Alcohol withdrawal varies widely across U.S. ethnoracial groups.
D. Tonic-clonic seizures occur in approximately 25% of individuals who meet criteria for alcohol withdrawal.

Correct Answer: A. Fewer than 10% of individuals undergoing alcohol withdrawal experience dramatic symptoms such as severe autonomic hyperactivity, tremors, or alcohol withdrawal delirium.

Explanation: Alcohol withdrawal is characterized by withdrawal symptoms that develop approximately 4–12 hours after the reduction of intake following prolonged, heavy alcohol ingestion. Because withdrawal from alcohol can be unpleasant and intense, individuals may continue to consume alcohol despite adverse consequences, often to avoid or to relieve withdrawal symptoms. Some withdrawal symptoms (e.g., sleep problems) can persist at lower intensities for months and can contribute to relapse.

Less than 10% of individuals who develop alcohol withdrawal will ever develop dramatic symptoms (e.g., severe autonomic hyperactivity, tremors, alcohol withdrawal delirium). Tonic-clonic seizures occur in less than 3% of individuals.

It is estimated that approximately 50% of middle-class, highly functional individuals with alcohol use disorder in the United States have ever experienced a full alcohol withdrawal syndrome. Among individuals with alcohol use disorder who are hospitalized or homeless, the rate of alcohol withdrawal may be greater than 80%. Less than 10% of individuals in withdrawal ever demonstrate alcohol withdrawal delirium or withdrawal seizures. The prevalence of alcohol withdrawal symptoms does not seem to vary across U.S. ethnoracial groups.

16.17—Alcohol Use Disorder / Diagnostic Features (p. 555); Prevalence (p. 556); Alcohol Withdrawal / diagnostic criteria (p. 553–554)

16.18 How many remission specifiers are included in the DSM-5-TR diagnostic criteria for alcohol use disorder?

A. One.
B. Two.
C. Three.
D. Four.

Correct Answer: B. Two.

Explanation: There are two remission specifiers:

In early remission: After full criteria for alcohol use disorder were previously met, none of the criteria for alcohol use disorder have been met for at least 3 months but for less than 12 months (with the exception that Criterion A4, "craving, or a strong desire or urge to use alcohol," may be met).

In sustained remission: After full criteria for alcohol use disorder were previously met, none of the criteria for alcohol use disorder have been met at any time during a period of 12 months or longer (with the exception that Criterion A4, "craving, or a strong desire or urge to use alcohol," may be met).

16.18—Alcohol Use Disorder / diagnostic criteria (pp. 553–554)

16.19 In which of the following situations would the specifier for a patient in remission be considered to be in a controlled environment?

A. Enlisted in the U.S. armed services.
B. Working on a cargo ship out at sea.

C. Imprisoned in a city jail.

D. Inpatient on a locked hospital unit.

Correct Answer: D. Inpatient on a locked hospital unit.

Explanation: *In a controlled environment* applies as a further specifier of remission if the individual is both in remission and in a controlled environment (i.e., in early remission in a controlled environment or in sustained remission in a controlled environment). Examples of these environments are closely supervised and substance-free jails, therapeutic communities, and locked hospital units.

16.19—Alcohol Use Disorder/ Specifiers (p. 555)

16.20 Which of the following substances is most likely to be associated with poly-drug use?

A. Alcohol.

B. Tobacco.

C. 3,4-Methylenedioxymethamphetamine (MDMA [ecstasy]).

D. Methamphetamine.

Correct Answer: C. 3,4-Methylenedioxymethamphetamine (MDMA [ecstasy]).

Explanation: Other hallucinogen use disorder is highly associated with cocaine use disorder, stimulant use disorder, other substance use disorder, tobacco (nicotine) use disorder, any personality disorder, posttraumatic stress disorder, and panic attacks.

16.20—Other Hallucinogen Use Disorder / Comorbidity (p. 594)

16.21 For which of the following substances might laboratory testing be unreliable?

A. Lysergic acid diethylamide (LSD).

B. Cocaine.

C. Alcohol.

D. Opioids.

Correct Answer: A. Lysergic acid diethylamide (LSD).

Explanation: Hallucinogens comprise a diverse group of substances that, despite having different chemical structures and possibly involving different molecular mechanisms, produce similar alterations of perception, mood, and cognition in users. Hallucinogens included are phenylalkylamines (e.g., mescaline, 2,5-dimethoxy-4-methylamphetamine [DOM], and 3,4-methylenedioxymethamphetamine [MDMA; also called ecstasy or molly]); the indoleamines, including psilocybin (and its metabolite psilocin, the compound primarily responsible for the psychedelic effects of hallucinogenic mushrooms) and dimethyltryptamine (DMT); and the ergolines, such as LSD and morning glory seeds. In addition, miscellaneous other ethnobotanical compounds are classified as hallucinogens, of which *Salvia divinorum* and jimsonweed are two examples.

Laboratory testing can be useful in distinguishing among the different hallucinogens. However, because some agents (e.g., LSD) are so potent that as little as 75 μg can produce severe reactions, typical toxicological examination will not always reveal which substance has been used.

Phencyclidine may be detected in urine for up to 8 days or even longer at very high doses.

Routine urine toxicology test results are often positive for opioid drugs in individuals with opioid use disorder. Urine test results remain positive for most opioids (e.g., heroin, morphine, codeine, oxycodone, propoxyphene) for 12–36 hours after administration.

Almost all sedative, hypnotic, or anxiolytic substances can be identified through laboratory evaluations of urine or blood (the latter of which can quantify the amounts of these agents in the body). Urine test results are likely to remain positive for up to approximately 1 week after the use of long-acting substances such as diazepam or flurazepam.

Benzoylecgonine, a metabolite of cocaine, typically remains in the urine for 1–3 days after a single dose and may be present for 7–12 days in individuals using repeated high doses.

The most direct test available to measure alcohol consumption cross-sectionally is blood alcohol concentration, which can also be used to judge tolerance to alcohol. For example, an individual with a concentration of 150 mg of ethanol per deciliter (dL) of blood who does not show signs of intoxication can be presumed to have acquired at least some degree of tolerance to alcohol. At 200 mg/dL, most nontolerant individuals demonstrate severe intoxication. Regarding laboratory tests, one sensitive laboratory indicator of heavy drinking is a modest elevation or high-normal levels (>35 units) of γ-glutamyltransferase (GGT). This may be the only laboratory finding. At least 70% of individuals with a high GGT level are persistent heavy drinkers (i.e., consuming eight or more drinks daily on a regular basis).

16.21—Alcohol Use Disorder / Diagnostic Markers (pp. 558–559); Phencyclidine Use Disorder / Diagnostic Markers (p. 589); Other Hallucinogen Use Disorder / Diagnostic Features (p. 592); Diagnostic Markers (p. 593); Opioid Use Disorder / Diagnostic Markers (p. 612); Sedative, Hypnotic, or Anxiolytic Use Disorder / Diagnostic Markers (p. 625); Stimulant Use Disorder / Diagnostic Markers (p. 638)

16.22 Alcohol intoxication, phencyclidine intoxication, cannabis intoxication, and inhalant intoxication have which Criterion C sign in common?

A. Depressed reflexes.
B. Generalized muscle weakness.

C. Nystagmus.

D. Impairment in attention or memory.

Correct Answer: C. Nystagmus.

Explanation: Nystagmus is the only one of these signs found in Criterion C of alcohol, cannabis, inhalant, and phencyclidine intoxication.

16.22—multiple: diagnostic criteria for Alcohol Intoxication (p. 561); Inhalant Intoxication (pp. 605–606); Cannabis (pp. 582–583); Phencyclidine Intoxication (pp. 594–595)

16.23 A 25-year-old medical student presents to the student health service at 7 A.M. complaining of having a "panic attack" and vomiting twice. He reports that he stayed up all night studying for his final exam in gross anatomy. The exam starts in an hour, but he feels too anxious to attend. The patient is restless and appears flushed, with visible muscle twitching. He is urinating excessively and has tachycardia, and his electrocardiogram shows premature ventricular complexes. His thoughts and speech appear to be rambling in nature. His urine toxicology screen is negative. What is the most likely diagnosis?

A. Panic disorder.

B. Amphetamine intoxication, amphetamine-like substance.

C. Caffeine intoxication.

D. Cocaine intoxication.

Correct Answer: C. Caffeine intoxication.

Explanation: This patient is exhibiting signs of restlessness, flushed face, gastrointestinal disturbance, muscle twitching, diuresis, rambling flow of speech, and cardiac abnormalities, all of which are consistent with caffeine intoxication. Although a panic episode might be associated with tachycardia or gastrointestinal distress, it would not cause muscle twitching or cardiac arrhythmias. Intoxication with stimulants such as amphetamine or cocaine would manifest very similarly with psychomotor agitation and cardiac arrhythmias, but these substances would not cause diuresis and would be expected to show up on a urine toxicology screen. Alcohol withdrawal could also manifest similarly but is typically characterized by tremor rather than muscle twitching, and it also does not cause diuresis.

16.23—Caffeine Intoxication / diagnostic criteria; Diagnostic Features (pp. 569–570)

16.24 The use of which illicit psychoactive substance is the most prevalent in the United States?

A. 3,4-Methylenedioxymethamphetamine (MDMA [ecstasy]).

B. Phencyclidine.

C. Cannabis.

D. Lysergic acid diethylamide (LSD).

Correct Answer: C. Cannabis.

Explanation: Cannabinoids, especially cannabis, are the most widely used illicit psychoactive substances in the United States. The following prevalence data are drawn from U.S.-based studies, unless otherwise noted. Among youth (ages 12–17 years), the past-year prevalence of DSM-IV cannabis use disorder is 2.7%–3.1%. Among adults age 18 years and older, the prevalence is 1.5%–2.9%. Among cannabis users, the prevalence of DSM-IV cannabis use disorder is 20.4% among youth and 30.6% among adults. For DSM-5 cannabis use disorder, 12-month prevalence is approximately 2.5% among adults (1.4%, 0.6%, and 0.6% at mild, moderate, and severe levels, respectively).

16.24—Cannabis Use Disorder / Prevalence (p. 578)

16.25 Which of the following laboratory tests can be used in combination with γ-glutamyltransferase (GGT) to monitor abstinence from alcohol?

A. Alanine aminotransferase (ALT).

B. Alkaline phosphatase.

C. Carbohydrate-deficient transferrin (CDT).

D. Mean corpuscular volume (MCV).

Correct Answer: C. Carbohydrate-deficient transferrin (CDT).

Explanation: Regarding laboratory tests, one sensitive laboratory indicator of heavy drinking is a modest elevation or high-normal levels (>35 units) of GGT. This may be the only laboratory finding. At least 70% of individuals with a high GGT level are persistent heavy drinkers (i.e., consuming eight or more drinks daily on a regular basis). A second test with comparable or even higher levels of sensitivity and specificity is CDT, with levels of 20 units or higher useful in identifying individuals who regularly consume eight or more drinks daily. Given that both GGT and CDT levels return toward normal within days to weeks of stopping drinking, both state markers may be useful in monitoring abstinence, especially when the clinician observes increases, rather than decreases, in these values over time—a finding indicating that the individual is likely to have returned to heavy drinking. The combination of tests for CDT and GGT may have even higher levels of sensitivity and specificity than either test used alone.

16.25—Alcohol Use Disorder / Diagnostic Markers (p. 559)

16.26 A patient presents to the student health clinic after a week of drinking several cans of cola eight times a day for a week to complete a bet he lost. The last soda was consumed yesterday. The patient is complaining of the sudden onset of extreme fatigue. With which of the following symptoms is he most likely to present?

A. Vomiting.
B. Drowsiness.
C. Flu-like symptoms.
D. Headache.

Correct Answer: D. Headache.

Explanation: The essential feature of caffeine withdrawal is the presence of a characteristic withdrawal syndrome that develops after the abrupt cessation of (or substantial reduction in) prolonged daily caffeine ingestion (Criterion B). Because individuals may be unaware of the wide array of sources of caffeine beyond coffee, colas, and energy drinks (e.g., over-the counter analgesics and cold remedies, weight loss aids, chocolate), they may not connect ingestion of these substances with symptoms of caffeine withdrawal. Caffeine withdrawal syndrome is indicated by three or more of the following (Criterion B): headache; marked fatigue or drowsiness; dysphoric mood, depressed mood, or irritability; difficulty concentrating; and flu-like symptoms (nausea, vomiting, or muscle pain/stiffness). The withdrawal syndrome causes clinically significant distress or impairment in social, occupational, or other important areas of functioning (Criterion C). The symptoms must not be associated with the physiological effects of another medical condition and are not better explained by another mental disorder (Criterion D).

Headache is the hallmark feature of caffeine withdrawal and may be diffuse, gradual in development, throbbing, severe, and sensitive to movement. However, other symptoms of caffeine withdrawal can occur in the absence of headache.

16.26—Caffeine Withdrawal / Diagnostic Features (p. 572)

16.27 How much does cannabis use disorder increase the risk of an adult having any other substance disorder?

A. One time.
B. Five times.
C. Nine times.
D. Twenty times.

Correct Answer: C. Nine times.

Explanation: Cannabis use disorder is highly comorbid with other substance use disorders (e.g., alcohol, cocaine, opioids). For example, compared with adults without cannabis use disorder, having a cannabis use disorder multiplies the risk for any other substance disorder by a factor of about nine. Cannabis has been commonly considered as a "gateway" drug because individuals who use cannabis have a substantially greater lifetime probability than nonusers of subsequently using other, riskier substances (e.g., opioids, cocaine). Among adults seeking treatment for a cannabis use disorder, many (63%) report problematic use of secondary or tertiary substances, including alcohol, cocaine, methamphetamine/amphetamine, and heroin or other opiates, and cannabis use disorder is often a secondary or tertiary problem among those with a primary diagnosis of other substance use disorders.

16.27—Cannabis Use Disorder / Comorbidity (p. 581)

16.28   A patient presents to the emergency department complaining of vomiting that "comes and goes." Which drug is the patient likely using regularly?

A. Tobacco.
B. Alcohol.
C. Cannabis.
D. Cocaine.

Correct Answer: C. Cannabis.

Explanation: Regarding medical conditions, cannabinoid hyperemesis syndrome is a syndrome of nausea and cyclic vomiting associated with regular cannabis use that is increasingly seen in emergency departments as the prevalence of cannabis use increases.

16.28—Cannabis Use Disorder / Comorbidity (p. 581–582)

16.29   Which adult ethnoracial group has the highest prevalence of cannabis use disorder?

A. Asians and Pacific Islanders.
B. American Indians/Alaska Natives.
C. African Americans.
D. Whites.

Correct Answer: B. American Indians/Alaska Natives.

Explanation: According to age, the prevalence of cannabis use disorder in the United States is highest among individuals ages 18–29 years (6.9%) and lowest among individuals ages 45 years and older (0.8%). Rates of cannabis use disorder are greater in men than in women (3.5% vs. 1.7%) and in boys than in girls ages 12–17 years (3.4% vs. 2.8%), although gender differences have been narrowing in recent birth cohorts across several countries. Regarding ethnoracial differences, for adolescents ages 12–17 years, rates are highest among Hispanics (3.8%), followed by whites (3.1%), African Americans (2.9%), and other ethnoracial groups (2.3%). Among adults, the prevalence of cannabis use disorder is 5.3% in American Indians and Alaska Natives, 4.5% in African Americans, 2.6% in Hispanics, 2.2% in whites, and 1.3% in Asians and Pacific Islanders.

16.29—Cannabis Use Disorder / Prevalence (p. 578)

16.30 Which of the following drugs that can have hallucinogenic effects is not considered in the DSM-5-TR chemical classes of hallucinogens?

A. Mescaline.
B. 3,4-Methylenedioxymethamphetamine (MDMA [ecstasy]).
C. Cannabis.
D. Psilocybin.

Correct Answer: C. Cannabis.

Explanation: Hallucinogens comprise a diverse group of substances that, despite having different chemical structures and possibly involving different molecular mechanisms, produce similar alterations of perception, mood, and cognition in users. Hallucinogens included are phenylalkylamines (e.g., mescaline, 2,5-dimethoxy-4-methylamphetamine [DOM], and MDMA [also called ecstasy or molly]); the indoleamines, including psilocybin (and its metabolite psilocin, the compound primarily responsible for the psychedelic effects of hallucinogenic mushrooms) and dimethyltryptamine; and the ergolines, such as lysergic acid diethylamide (LSD) and morning glory seeds. In addition, miscellaneous other ethnobotanical compounds are classified as hallucinogens, of which *Salvia divinorum* and jimsonweed are two examples. Excluded from the hallucinogen group are cannabis and its active compound, delta-9-tetrahydrocannabinol (THC; see the section "Cannabis-Related Disorders"). These substances can have hallucinogenic effects but are diagnosed separately.

16.30—Other Hallucinogen Use Disorder / Diagnostic Features (p. 592)

16.31 Use of which of the following drugs is most likely to result in the development of a hallucinogen use disorder?

A. Lysergic acid diethylamide (LSD).
B. Psilocybin.
C. Dimethyltryptamine .
D. 3,4-Methylenedioxymethamphetamine (MDMA [ecstasy]).

Correct Answer: D. 3,4-Methylenedioxymethamphetamine (MDMA [ecstasy]).

Explanation: MDMA/ecstasy as a hallucinogen may have distinctive effects attributable to both its hallucinogenic and its stimulant properties. Ecstasy users have a higher risk of developing a hallucinogen use disorder than those using other hallucinogens. Among both adolescent and adult ecstasy users and users of other hallucinogens, the most frequently reported hallucinogen use disorder criteria are tolerance; hazardous use, use despite emotional or health problems; giving up activities in favor of use; and spending a lot of time obtaining, using, or recovering from the effects of use. As found for other substances, diagnostic criteria for other hallucinogen use disorder are arrayed along a single continuum of severity.

16.31—Other Hallucinogen Use Disorder / Diagnostic Features (p. 592)

16.32 For which of the following hallucinogens is there evidence of a withdrawal syndrome?

    A. Lysergic acid diethylamide (LSD).
    B. 3,4-Methylenedioxymethamphetamine (MDMA [ecstasy]).
    C. Psilocybin.
    D. Phencylidine.

Correct Answer: B. 3,4-Methylenedioxymethamphetamine (MDMA [ecstasy]).

Explanation: Given that a clinically significant withdrawal syndrome has not been consistently documented in humans, the diagnosis of hallucinogen withdrawal syndrome is not included in DSM-5-TR and therefore is not part of the hallucinogen use disorder diagnostic criteria. However, there may be evidence of withdrawal from MDMA, with endorsement of any two or more withdrawal symptoms (e.g., malaise, appetite disturbance, mood changes [anxious, depressed, irritable], poor concentration, sleep disruption) or withdrawal avoidance observed in more than half of individuals in diverse samples of ecstasy users in the United States and internationally.

16.32—Other Hallucinogen Use Disorder / Diagnostic Features (p. 592)

16.33 What distinguishes substance/medication-induced mental disorders from substance use disorders?

    A. They occur only during periods of intoxication.
    B. Symptoms continue in spite of cessation of use of the substance.
    C. Cognitive and behavioral symptoms contribute to the continued use.
    D. They occur only if the medication is taken at higher than suggested doses.

Correct Answer: C. Cognitive and behavioral symptoms contribute to the continued use.

Explanation: The substance/medication-induced mental disorders are potentially severe, usually temporary, but sometimes persisting CNS syndromes that develop in the context of the effects of substances of abuse, medications, and some toxins. They are distinguished from the substance use disorders, in which a cluster of cognitive, behavioral, and physiological symptoms contribute to the continued use of a substance despite significant substance-related problems.

Substance-induced mental disorders develop in the context of intoxication with or withdrawal from substances of abuse, whereas medication-induced mental disorders can be seen with prescribed or over-the-counter medications that are taken at the suggested doses. Both conditions are usually temporary and likely to disappear within 1 month or so of cessation of acute withdrawal, severe intoxication, or use of the medication.

16.33—Substance/Medication-Induced Mental Disorders (p. 550); Development and Course (pp. 551–552)

16.34 Which two groups of inhalant agents are *not* among the recognized substances qualifying for the DSM-5 inhalant use disorder diagnosis?

A. Butane lighters and toluene.
B. Xylene and butane.
C. Trichloroethane and hexane.
D. Nitrous oxide and nitrite gases.

Correct Answer: D. Nitrous oxide and nitrite gases.

Explanation: Examples of inhalant substances include volatile hydrocarbons, which comprise toxic gases from glues, fuels, paints, and other volatile compounds. When possible, the particular substance involved should be named (e.g., *toluene use disorder*). However, most compounds that are inhaled are a mixture of several substances that can produce psychoactive effects, and it is often difficult to ascertain the exact substance responsible for the disorder. Unless there is clear evidence that a single, unmixed substance has been used, the general term *inhalant* should be used in recording the diagnosis. Disorders arising from inhalation of nitrous oxide or of amyl-, butyl-, or isobutylnitrite are diagnosed as other (or unknown) substance use disorder.

16.34—Inhalant Use Disorder / Diagnostic Features (pp. 602–603)

16.35 A 22-year-old university student presents to his primary care physician complaining of progressive worsening of numbness, tingling, and weakness in both of his legs over the past several weeks. His gait is unsteady, and he has difficulty grasping objects in his hands. He did not use any substances on the day of presentation but admits that over the past 3 months he has been consistently using one particular substance on a daily basis. Which substance use disorder most likely accounts for this patient's symptoms?

A. Other (or unknown) substance use disorder.
B. Other hallucinogen use disorder.
C. Inhalant use disorder.
D. Opioid use disorder.

Correct Answer: A. Other (or unknown) substance use disorder.

Explanation: The diagnostic class *other (or unknown) substance–related disorders* applies to substances that are not included within any of the nine substance classes presented earlier in this chapter (i.e., alcohol; caffeine; cannabis; halluci-nogens [phencyclidine and others]; inhalants; opioids; sedatives, hypnotics, or anxiolytics; stimulants; or tobacco). Such substances include anabolic steroids; nonsteroidal anti-inflammatory drugs; corticosteroids; antiparkinsonian med-ications; antihistamines; nitrous oxide ("laughing gas"); amyl-, butyl-, or isobutylnitrites; betel nut, which is chewed in many geographic regions to pro-duce mild euphoria and a floating sensation; and kava (from a South Pacific pepper plant), which produces mild euphoria, sedation, incoordination, and weight loss, as well as health effects (e.g., mild hepatitis, lung abnormalities). Note that gaseous substances are included with the *inhalant* category only if they are hydrocarbon agents; other gaseous substances (including nitrous ox-ide mentioned earlier) are included in the *other (or unknown) substance* category. Unknown substance–related disorders are associated with unidentified sub-stances, such as intoxications in which the individual cannot identify the in-gested drug, or substance use disorders involving either new black market drugs not yet identified or familiar drugs sold illegally under false names.

Membership in certain populations with access to nitrous oxide may be asso-ciated with frequent use of the substance and possibly with a diagnosis of nitrous oxide use disorder. The role of this gas as an anesthetic agent leads to misuse by some medical and dental professionals, and its use as a propellant for commercial products (e.g., whipped cream dispensers) contributes to misuse by food service workers. Nitrous oxide misuse by adolescents and young adults is significant, and some individuals with very frequent use may present with serious medical complications and mental conditions, including myeloneuropathy, spinal cord subacute combined degeneration, peripheral neuropathy, and psychosis.

16.35—Other Substance Use Disorder / Diagnostic and Associated Features (p. 654)

16.36 Which organ system or anatomical function is most commonly affected by chronic use of 3,4-methylenedioxymethamphetamine (MDMA [ecstasy])?

A. Neurological.
B. Respiratory.
C. Cardiopulmonary.
D. Oral cavity.

Correct Answer: A. Neurological.

Explanation: There is evidence for persisting neurotoxic effects of MDMA use, including impairments in memory, psychological function, and neuroendo-crine function; serotonin system dysfunction; and sleep disturbance; as well as adverse effects on brain microvasculature, white matter maturation, and damage to axons.

16.36—Other Hallucinogen Use Disorder / Functional Consequences of Other Hallucinogen Use Disorder (p. 594)

16.37 What percentage of individuals who undergo untreated sedative, hypnotic, or anxiolytic withdrawal experience a grand mal seizure?

A. 5%–10%.
B. 10%–20%.
C. 20%–30%.
D. 30%–40%.

Correct Answer: C. 20%–30%.

Explanation: The essential feature of sedative, hypnotic, or anxiolytic withdrawal is the presence of a characteristic syndrome that develops after a marked decrease in or cessation of intake after several weeks or more of regular use (Criteria A and B). This withdrawal syndrome is characterized by two or more symptoms (similar to alcohol withdrawal) that include autonomic hyperactivity (e.g., increases in heart rate, respiratory rate, blood pressure, or body temperature, along with sweating); a tremor of the hands; insomnia; nausea, sometimes accompanied by vomiting; anxiety; and psychomotor agitation. A grand mal seizure may occur in perhaps as many as 20%–30% of individuals undergoing untreated withdrawal from these substances. In severe withdrawal, visual, tactile, or auditory hallucinations or illusions can occur but are usually in the context of a withdrawal delirium.

16.37—Sedative, Hypnotic, or Anxiolytic Withdrawal / Diagnostic Features (p. 629)

16.38 Which route of stimulant use is most prevalent among individuals who are in treatment for a stimulant use disorder?

A. Oral.
B. Intranasal.
C. Smoking.
D. Intravenous.

Correct Answer: C. Smoking.

Explanation: Some persons begin stimulant use to control weight or to improve performance in school, work, or athletics. Initial use may include obtaining medications such as methylphenidate or amphetamine salts prescribed to others for the treatment of attention-deficit/hyperactivity disorder. Among primary treatment admissions for amphetamine-type substance use in the United States, 61% reported smoking, 26% reported injecting, and 9% reported snorting, suggesting that stimulant use disorder can develop from multiple modes of administration.

16.38—Stimulant Use Disorder / Development and Course (p. 637)

16.39 What is the most common co-occurring psychiatric diagnosis among individuals with a history of significant prenatal alcohol exposure?

A. Major depressive disorder.
B. Generalized anxiety disorder.
C. Attention-deficit/hyperactivity disorder (ADHD).
D. Oppositional defiant disorder.

Correct Answer: C. Attention-deficit/hyperactivity disorder (ADHD).

Explanation: Mental health problems have been identified in more than 90% of individuals with histories of significant prenatal alcohol exposure. The most common co-occurring diagnosis is ADHD, but research has shown that individuals with neurobehavioral disorder associated with prenatal alcohol exposure (ND-PAE) differ in neuropsychological characteristics and in their responsiveness to pharmacological interventions. Other high-probability co-occurring disorders include oppositional defiant disorder and conduct disorder, but the appropriateness of these diagnoses should be weighed in the context of the significant impairments in general intellectual and executive functioning that are often associated with prenatal alcohol exposure. Mood symptoms, including symptoms of bipolar disorder and depressive disorders, have been described. History of prenatal alcohol exposure is associated with an increased risk for later tobacco, alcohol, and other substance use disorders.

16.39—Conditions for Further Study / Neurobehavioral Disorder Associated With Prenatal Alcohol Exposure / Comorbidity (p. 920)

16.40 Which of the following has been included in DSM-5-TR as a potential diagnosis?

A. Sex addiction.
B. Exercise addiction.
C. Shopping addiction.
D. Gaming addiction.

Correct Answer: D. Gaming addiction.

Explanation: In addition to the substance-related disorders, this chapter also includes gambling disorder, reflecting evidence that gambling behaviors activate reward systems similar to those activated by drugs of abuse and that they produce some behavioral symptoms that appear comparable to those produced by the substance use disorders. Other excessive behavioral patterns, such as internet gaming (see "Conditions for Further Study"), have also been described, but the research on these and other behavioral syndromes is less clear. Thus, groups of repetitive behaviors, sometimes termed behavioral addictions (with subcategories such as sex addiction, exercise addiction, and shopping addiction), are not included because there is insufficient peer-reviewed evidence to establish the diagnostic criteria and course descriptions needed to identify these behaviors as mental disorders.

Gambling disorder is currently the only non-substance-related disorder included in the DSM-5-TR Section II chapter "Substance-Related and Addictive Disorders." However, there are other behavioral disorders that show some similarities to substance use disorders and gambling disorder for which the word *addiction* is commonly used in nonmedical settings, and the one condition with a considerable literature is the compulsive playing of internet games. Internet gaming has been reportedly defined as an "addiction" by the Chinese government and is considered a public health threat in South Korea, where treatment and prevention systems have been set up. Reports of treatment of this condition have appeared in medical journals, mostly from Asian countries, but also in the United States and other high-income countries.

Excessive use of the internet not involving playing of online games (e.g., excessive use of social media, such as Facebook or TikTok; viewing pornography online) is not considered analogous to internet gaming disorder, and future research on other excessive uses of the internet would need to follow similar guidelines as suggested in DSM-5-TR.

16.40—Substance-Related and Addictive Disorders / chapter introduction (p. 543); Conditions for Further Study/Internet Gaming Disorder (pp. 913–916)

16.41 Which of the following is one of the most common medical consequences of drinking in people with alcohol use disorder?

A. Cirrhosis.
B. Cardiomyopathy.
C. Hypertension.
D. Pancreatitis.

Correct Answer: C. Hypertension.

Explanation: Repeated intake of high doses of alcohol can affect nearly every organ system, especially the gastrointestinal tract, cardiovascular system, and the central and peripheral nervous systems. Gastrointestinal effects include gastritis, stomach or duodenal ulcers, and, in about 15% of individuals who use alcohol heavily, liver cirrhosis and/or pancreatitis. There is also an increased rate of cancer of the esophagus, stomach, and other parts of the gastrointestinal tract. One of the most commonly associated conditions is low-grade hypertension. Cardiomyopathy and other myopathies are less common but occur at an increased rate among those who drink very heavily. These factors, along with marked increases in levels of triglycerides and low-density lipoprotein cholesterol, contribute to an elevated risk of heart disease. Peripheral neuropathy may be evidenced by muscular weakness, paresthesias, and decreased peripheral sensation. More persistent central nervous system effects include cognitive deficits, such as severe memory impairment and degenerative changes in the cerebellum. These effects are related to the direct effects of alcohol, trauma, or vitamin deficiencies (particularly of the B vitamins, including thiamine). One devastating central nervous system effect is the relatively rare alcohol-induced persisting amnestic disorder, or Wernicke-Korsakoff syndrome, in which the ability to encode new memory is severely impaired. This condition is now described in the chapter "Neurocognitive Disorders" and would be termed a substance/medication-induced neurocognitive disorder.

16.41 Alcohol Use Disorder/Associated Features (pp. 555–556)

CHAPTER 17

Neurocognitive Disorders

17.1 The essential feature of the DSM-5-TR diagnosis of delirium is a disturbance in attention/awareness and in cognition that develops over a short period of time, represents a change from baseline, and tends to fluctuate in severity during the course of a day. Which of the following additional conditions must apply?

A. There must be laboratory evidence of an evolving dementia.
B. The disturbance must be associated with a disruption of the sleep-wake cycle.
C. The disturbance must not occur in the context of a severely reduced level of arousal, such as coma.
D. The disturbance must not be superimposed on a preexisting neurocognitive disorder.

Correct Answer: C. The disturbance must not occur in the context of a severely reduced level of arousal, such as coma.

Explanation: The essential feature of delirium is a disturbance of attention or awareness (Criterion A) that is accompanied by a change in baseline cognition (Criterion C) that cannot be better explained by a preexisting or evolving neurocognitive disorder (Criterion D). The ability to evaluate cognition to diagnose delirium depends on there being a level of arousal sufficient for response to verbal stimulation; hence, delirium should not be diagnosed in the context of coma (Criterion D). The disturbance develops over a short period of time, usually hours to a few days, and tends to fluctuate in severity during the course of the day (Criterion B). There is evidence from the history, physical examination, or laboratory findings that the disturbance is a physiological consequence of another underlying medical condition, substance intoxication or withdrawal, use of a medication, or a toxin exposure, or a combination of these factors (Criterion E).

Both major and mild neurocognitive disorders (NCDs) can increase the risk for delirium and complicate the course. The most common differential diagnostic issue when evaluating confusion in older adults is disentangling symptoms of delirium and dementia. The clinician must determine whether the individual has delirium; a delirium superimposed on a preexisting NCD, such as that due to Alzheimer's disease; or an NCD without delirium. The traditional distinction between delirium and dementia according to acuteness of onset and temporal course is particularly difficult in those elderly individuals who had a prior NCD that may not have been recognized or who develop persistent cognitive impairment following an episode of delirium.

17.1—Delirium / diagnostic criteria (p. 672); Diagnostic Features (p. 675); Differential Diagnosis (pp. 677–678)

17.2   Both major and mild neurocognitive disorders can increase the risk of delirium and complicate its course. Delirium is distinguished from dementia on the basis of the key features of acute onset, impairment in attention, and which of the following?

   A. Fluctuating course.
   B. Steady course.
   C. Presence of depression.
   D. Cogwheeling movements.

Correct Answer: A. Fluctuating course.

Explanation: According to Criterion B for delirium, the disturbance develops over a short period of time, usually hours to a few days, and tends to fluctuate during the course of the day, often with worsening in the evening and night when external orienting stimuli decrease.

17.2—Delirium / Diagnostic Features (p. 675)

17.3   A 79-year-old woman with a history of depression is being evaluated at a nursing home for a suspected urinary tract infection. She is easily distracted, perseverates on answers to questions, asks the same question repeatedly, is unable to focus, and cannot answer questions regarding orientation. The mental status changes evolved over a single day. Her family reports that they thought she "wasn't herself" when they saw her the previous evening, but the nursing report this morning indicates that the patient was cordial and appropriate. What is the most likely diagnosis?

   A. Major depressive disorder, recurrent episode.
   B. Depressive disorder due to another medical condition.
   C. Delirium.
   D. Major depressive disorder, with anxious distress.

Correct Answer: C. Delirium.

Explanation: This patient's symptoms are proximally related to the urinary tract infection: her mental status changes had a temporal, fluctuating course with disturbance in attention and cognition. These are the diagnostic features of delirium.

17.4   The diagnostic criteria for major or mild neurocognitive disorder with Lewy bodies (NCDLB) include fulfillment of criteria for major or mild neurocognitive disorder and presence of a combination of core diagnostic features and suggested diagnostic features for either probable or possible neurocognitive disorder with Lewy bodies. Another feature necessary for the diagnosis is that the disturbance is not better explained by cerebrovascular disease, another neurodegenerative disease, the effects of a substance, or another mental, neurological, or systemic disorder. Which of the following completes the list of features necessary for the diagnosis?

A. An acute onset and rapid progression.
B. An insidious onset and gradual progression.
C. An insidious onset and rapid progression.
D. A waxing and waning presentation.

Correct Answer: B. An insidious onset and gradual progression.

Explanation: NCDLB includes not only progressive cognitive impairment (with early changes in complex attention and executive function rather than learning and memory) but also recurrent complex visual hallucinations; concurrent symptoms of rapid eye movement sleep behavior disorder (which can be a very early manifestation); as well as hallucinations in other sensory modalities, depression, apathy, anxiety, and delusions. The symptoms fluctuate in a pattern that can resemble a delirium, but no adequate underlying cause can be found. The variable presentation of NCDLB symptoms reduces the likelihood of all symptoms being observed in a brief clinic visit and necessitates a thorough assessment of caregiver observations. The use of assessment scales specifically designed to assess fluctuation may aid in diagnosis. Another core feature is spontaneous parkinsonism, which must begin after the onset of cognitive decline; by convention, major cognitive deficits are observed *at least 1 year before* the motor symptoms. NCDLB is a gradually progressive disorder with insidious onset. However, there is often a prodromal history of confusional episodes (delirium) of acute onset, often precipitated by illness or surgery.

17.4—Major or Mild Neurocognitive Disorder With Lewy Bodies / diagnostic criteria (pp. 699–700); Development and Course (p. 701); Differential Diagnosis (p. 702)

17.5   Which of the following is *not* a diagnostic criterion, feature, or marker of major or mild neurocognitive disorder with Lewy bodies (NCDLB)?

A. Concurrent symptoms of rapid eye movement (REM) sleep behavior disorder.
B. High striatal dopamine transporter uptake in basal ganglia demonstrated by single-photon emission computed tomography (SPECT) or positron emission tomography (PET) imaging.

C. Low striatal dopamine transporter uptake in basal ganglia demonstrated by SPECT or PET imaging.

D. Severe neuroleptic sensitivity.

Correct Answer: B. High striatal dopamine transporter uptake in basal ganglia demonstrated by SPECT or PET imaging.

Explanation: The underlying neurodegenerative disease in NCDLB is primarily a synucleinopathy due to α-synuclein misfolding and aggregation. Cognitive testing beyond the use of a brief screening instrument may be necessary to define deficits clearly. Assessment scales developed to measure fluctuation can be useful. The associated condition REM sleep behavior disorder may be diagnosed through a formal sleep study or identified by questioning the patient or informant about relevant symptoms. Neuroleptic sensitivity (challenge) is not recommended as a diagnostic marker but raises suspicion of NCDLB if it occurs.

A diagnostically suggestive feature is *low* striatal dopamine transporter uptake on SPECT or PET scan. Biomarkers supportive of NCDLB but with more limited evidence of diagnostic value include the following: preservation of medial temporal volume relative to Alzheimer's disease on MRI, generalized low uptake on SPECT/PET perfusion scan with reduced occipital activity with or without the cingulate island sign (sparing of the posterior cingulate cortex relative to the precuneus plus cuneus on fluorodeoxyglucose-PET imaging), and prominent slow wave activity on electroencephalogram with periodic fluctuations in the pre-alpha/theta range.

17.5—Major or Mild Neurocognitive Disorder With Lewy Bodies / Diagnostic Markers (p. 701)

17.6   A 72-year-old man with no history of alcohol or other substance use disorders and no psychiatric history is brought to the emergency department (ED) because of transient episodes of unexplained loss of consciousness. His wife reports that he has experienced repeated falls and syncope over the past year, as well as auditory and visual hallucinations. A thorough workup for cardiac disease has found no evidence of structural heart disease or arrhythmias. In the ED, he is found to have severe autonomic dysfunction, including orthostatic hypotension and urinary incontinence. What is the best provisional diagnosis for this patient?

A. New-onset schizophrenia.

B. Possible major or mild neurocognitive disorder with Lewy bodies (NCDLB).

C. Possible major or mild neurocognitive disorder due to Alzheimer's disease.

D. New-onset seizure disorder.

Correct Answer: B. Possible major or mild neurocognitive disorder with Lewy bodies (NCDLB).

Explanation: Further information on cognition, time frame, and other etiologies must be ascertained, but the best working diagnosis with the limited information available is NCDLB. Individuals with NCDLB frequently experience repeated falls and syncope and transient episodes of unexplained loss of consciousness. Severe autonomic dysfunction, such as orthostatic hypotension and urinary incontinence, may also be observed. Auditory and other nonvisual hallucinations are common, as are systematized delusions, delusional misidentification, and depression.

The patient has auditory and visual hallucinations but no other feature of schizophrenia, and the age at onset, along with the associated neurological symptoms, suggests a neurodegenerative disorder rather than schizophrenia. Among neurocognitive disorders, the prominence of hallucinations, episodic loss of consciousness, and autonomic symptoms—rather than marked memory impairment—in the early course argue against a neurocognitive disorder due to Alzheimer's disease and in favor of NCDLB. The patient has one of the core diagnostic features of NCDLB, visual hallucinations, justifying a "possible" level of certainty for the diagnosis. A seizure disorder might cause episodic loss of consciousness but would not parsimoniously account for hallucinations and autonomic symptoms.

17.6—Major or Mild Neurocognitive Disorder With Lewy Bodies / Diagnostic Features and Associated Features (p. 700)

17.7 The diagnostic criteria for neurocognitive disorder (NCD) due to HIV infection include fulfillment of criteria for major or mild NCD and documented infection with HIV (as confirmed by established laboratory methods). Which of the following is a prominent feature of NCD due to HIV infection?

A. Impairment in executive functioning.
B. Significant delusions and hallucinations at onset of the disorder.
C. Marked difficulty with recall of learned information.
D. Rapid progression to profound neurocognitive impairment.

Correct Answer: A. Impairment in executive functioning.

Explanation: NCD associated with HIV infection generally shows a "subcortical pattern" with prominently impaired executive function, slowing of processing speed, problems with more demanding attentional tasks, and difficulty in learning new information but fewer problems with recall of learned information. In major NCD, slowing may be prominent. Language difficulties, such as aphasia, are uncommon, although reductions in fluency may be observed. HIV pathogenic processes can affect any part of the brain; therefore, other patterns are possible. An NCD due to HIV infection can resolve, improve, slowly worsen, or have a fluctuating course. Rapid progression to profound neurocognitive impairment is uncommon in the context of currently available combination antiviral treatment; consequently, an abrupt change in mental status in an individual with HIV may prompt an evaluation of other medical sources for the cognitive change, including secondary infections.

17.7—Major or Mild Neurocognitive Disorder Due to HIV Infection / Diagnostic Features; Development and Course (pp. 718–719)

17.8   In addition to documented infection with HIV and fulfillment of criteria for major or mild neurocognitive disorder (NCD), what other requirement must be met to qualify for a diagnosis of major or mild NCD due to HIV infection?

A. Presence of HIV in the cerebrospinal fluid.
B. A pattern of cognitive impairment characterized by early predominance of aphasia and impaired memory for previously learned information.
C. Inability to attribute the NCD to non-HIV conditions (including secondary brain diseases), another medical condition, or a mental disorder.
D. Presence of Kayser-Fleischer rings.

Correct Answer: C. Inability to attribute the NCD to non-HIV conditions (including secondary brain diseases), another medical condition, or a mental disorder.

Explanation: In addition to requiring fulfillment of criteria for major or mild NCD and documented infection with HIV, the diagnostic criteria for NCD due to HIV infection stipulate that the NCD is not better explained by non-HIV conditions, including secondary brain diseases such as progressive multifocal leukoencephalopathy or cryptococcal meningitis, and that it is not attributable to another medical condition and is not better explained by a mental disorder.

An NCD due to HIV infection generally shows a "subcortical pattern" with prominently impaired executive function, slowing of processing speed, problems with more demanding attentional tasks, and difficulty in learning new information but fewer problems with recall of learned information. In major NCD, slowing may be prominent. Language difficulties, such as aphasia, are uncommon, although reductions in fluency may be observed. HIV pathogenic processes can affect any part of the brain; therefore, other patterns are possible. NCD due to HIV is more prevalent in individuals with high viral loads in the cerebrospinal fluid, but this is not a diagnostic criterion. Kayser-Fleischer rings are observed in Wilson's disease, not HIV.

17.8—Major or Mild Neurocognitive Disorder Due to HIV Infection / diagnostic criteria and Diagnostic Features (pp. 717–718); Associated Features (p. 718)

17.9   Which of the following features characterizes alcohol-induced major or mild neurocognitive disorder, amnestic-confabulatory type?

A. Amnesia for new information and confabulation.
B. Seizures.

C. Amnesia for previously learned information and downward gaze paralysis.

D. Anosognosia and apraxia.

Correct Answer: A. Amnesia for new information and confabulation.

Explanation: Neurocognitive disorder induced by alcohol frequently manifests with a combination of impairments in executive function and memory and learning domains. Features of alcohol-induced amnestic-confabulatory (Korsakoff's) neurocognitive disorder include prominent amnesia (severe difficulty learning new information, with rapid forgetting) and a tendency to confabulate. These manifestations may co-occur with signs of thiamine encephalopathy (Wernicke's encephalopathy) with associated features such as nystagmus and ataxia. Ophthalmoplegia of Wernicke's encephalopathy is typically characterized by a lateral gaze paralysis.

17.9—Substance/Medication-Induced Major or Mild Neurocognitive Disorder / Diagnostic Features (pp. 714–715)

17.10 Which of the following statements about the diagnosis of neurocognitive disorder due to Huntington's disease (NCDHD) is *true*?

A. NCDHD is a laboratory-based diagnosis/disorder.

B. NCDHD is a disorder that requires positive neuroimaging for diagnosis.

C. NCDHD is a clinical diagnosis based on abnormal physical findings and family history/genetic findings.

D. NCDHD is a diagnosis that is best defined as patients who have a pill-rolling tremor.

Correct Answer: C. NCDHD is a clinical diagnosis based on abnormal physical findings and family history/genetic findings.

Explanation: Genetic testing is the primary laboratory test for the determination of Huntington's disease, which is an autosomal dominant disorder with complete penetrance. A diagnosis of definite Huntington's disease is given in the presence of unequivocal extrapyramidal motor abnormalities in an individual with either a family history of Huntington's disease or genetic testing showing a CAG trinucleotide repeat expansion in the *HTT* gene, located on chromosome 4.

17.10—Major or Mild Neurocognitive Disorder Due to Huntington's Disease / Diagnostic Features (p. 727); Diagnostic Markers (p. 728)

17.11 Depression, irritability, anxiety, obsessive-compulsive symptoms, and apathy are frequently associated with Huntington's disease and often precede the onset of motor symptoms. Psychosis more rarely precedes the onset of motor symptoms. Which of the following is a core feature of major or mild neurocognitive disorder due to Huntington's disease?

A. Progressive cognitive impairment with early changes in executive function.
B. Prominent early memory impairment, mostly affecting short-term memory.
C. Psychosis in the early stages, with marked olfactory hallucinations.
D. Voluntary jerking movements.

Correct Answer: A. Progressive cognitive impairment with early changes in executive function.

Explanation: A core feature of Huntington's disease is progressive cognitive impairment with early changes in executive function (i.e., processing speed, organization, and planning) rather than learning and memory. Cognitive and associated behavioral changes often precede the emergence of the typical motor abnormalities of bradykinesia (i.e., slowing of voluntary movement) and chorea (i.e., involuntary jerking movements).

17.11—Major or Mild Neurocognitive Disorder Due to Huntington's Disease / Diagnostic Features; Associated Features (p. 727)

17.12 Genetic testing is the primary laboratory test for the determination of Huntington's disease. Which of the following best characterizes the genetic nature of Huntington's disease?

A. X-linked recessive inheritance with incomplete penetrance.
B. Autosomal recessive inheritance with complete penetrance.
C. Autosomal dominant inheritance with complete penetrance.
D. X-linked dominant inheritance.

Correct Answer: C. Autosomal dominant inheritance with complete penetrance.

Explanation: The genetic basis of Huntington's disease is a fully penetrant autosomal dominant expansion of the CAG trinucleotide, often called a CAG repeat, in the huntingtin gene. A CAG repeat length of 40 or more is invariably associated with Huntington's disease, with longer repeat lengths associated with early age at onset. A CAG repeat length in the 36–39 range is considered to be partially penetrant, which means that this length may or may not lead to Huntington's disease. If Huntington's disease does occur with repeat lengths in this range, it is more often associated with onset late in life (diagnosis after age 70).

17.12—Major or Mild Neurocognitive Disorder Due to Huntington's Disease / Risk and Prognostic Factors; Diagnostic Markers (p. 728)

17.13 Major or mild neurocognitive disorder (NCD) due to prion disease encompasses NCDs associated with a group of subacute spongiform encephalopathies caused by transmissible agents known as *prions*. What is the most common prion disease?

A. Creutzfeldt-Jakob disease.

B. Bovine spongiform encephalopathy.

C. Huntington's disease.

D. Neurosyphilis.

Correct Answer: A. Creutzfeldt-Jakob disease.

Explanation: Prion diseases include sporadic Creutzfeldt-Jakob disease, genetic Creutzfeldt-Jakob disease, iatrogenic Creutzfeldt- Jakob disease, variant Creutzfeldt-Jakob disease, variably protease-sensitive prionopathy, kuru, Gerstmann-Sträussler-Scheinker syndrome, and fatal insomnia. The most common type is sporadic Creutzfeldt-Jakob disease, typically referred to as Creutzfeldt-Jakob disease (CJD). (Variant CJD is much rarer and is associated with transmission of bovine spongiform encephalopathy, also called "mad cow disease.") Typically, individuals with CJD present with neurocognitive deficits, ataxia, and abnormal movements such as myoclonus, chorea, or dystonia; a startle reflex is also common. Typically, the history reveals rapid progression to major NCD over as little as 6 months, and thus the disorder is typically seen only at the major level. However, many individuals with the disorder may have atypical presentations, and the disease can be confirmed only by biopsy or at autopsy.

Wernicke-Korsakoff syndrome, neurosyphilis, and Huntington's disease are not prion diseases; rather, Wernicke-Korsakoff syndrome is secondary to thiamine deficiency, Huntington's disease is secondary to a genetic defect, and neurosyphilis is caused by a sexually transmitted infection.

17.13—Major or Mild Neurocognitive Disorder Due to Prion Disease / Diagnostic Features (pp. 721–722)

17.14 Prion disease has been reported to occur in individuals of all ages, from the teenage years to late life. Which of the following best characterizes the time frame of disease progression?

A. Over a few months.

B. Over several days.

C. Over several weeks.

D. Over 5 years.

Correct Answer: A. Over a few months.

Explanation: Prion disease may develop at any age in adults—the peak age for sporadic Creutzfeldt-Jakob disease is approximately 67 years, although it has been reported to occur in individuals spanning the teenage years to late life. Non-Latinx whites were found to have an older mean age at onset compared with other ethnic and racial populations in the United States. Prodromal symptoms of prion disease may include fatigue, anxiety, problems with appetite or sleeping, or difficulties with concentration. After several weeks, these symptoms may be followed by incoordination, altered vision, or abnormal gait or other movements that may be myoclonic, choreoathetoid, or ballistic, along with a rapidly progressive dementia. The disease typically progresses very rapidly to a major level of impairment over several months. More rarely, it can progress over 2 years and appear similar in its course to other neurocognitive disorders.

17.14—Major or Mild Neurocognitive Disorder Due to Prion Disease / Development and Course (p. 722)

17.15 Major and mild neurocognitive disorders (NCDs) exist on a spectrum of cognitive and functional impairment. Which of the following constitutes an important threshold differentiating the two diagnoses?

A. Whether the individual is concerned about the decline in cognitive function.
B. Whether there is impairment in cognitive performance as measured by standardized testing or clinical assessment.
C. Whether the cognitive impairment is sufficient to interfere with independent completion of activities of daily living.
D. Whether the cognitive deficits occur exclusively in the context of a delirium.

Correct Answer: C. Whether the cognitive impairment is sufficient to interfere with independent completion of activities of daily living.

Explanation: Criterion B (for major and mild NCD) relates to the individual's level of independence in everyday functioning. Individuals with *major* NCD will have impairment of sufficient severity to interfere with independence such that others will have to take over tasks that the individuals were previously able to complete on their own. Individuals with *mild* NCD will have preserved independence, although there may be subtle interference with function or a report that tasks require more effort or take more time than previously. The distinction between major and mild NCD is inherently arbitrary, and the disorders exist along a continuum. Precise thresholds are therefore difficult to determine. Careful history taking, observation, and integration with other findings are required, and the implications of diagnosis should be considered when an individual's clinical manifestations lie at a boundary.

The core feature of both mild and major NCD, Criterion A requires evidence of a cognitive decline based on 1) concern on the part of the patient, a knowledgeable informant, or a clinician that there has been such a decline and 2) impairment in cognitive performance as documented by standardized neurological testing or other objective assessment. For major NCD, *significant* decline and *substantial* impairment are specified; for mild NCD, the words *modest* and *mild* are used. Both a concern and objective evidence are required because they are complementary. Neuropsychological testing, with performance compared with norms appropriate to the individuals' age, sex, educational attainment, and cultural background, is part of the standardized evaluation of NCDs and is particularly critical in the evaluation of mild NCD.

Both disorders can occur with comorbid delirium, but they cannot be diagnosed if the cognitive impairment occurs only in the context of delirium (Criterion C). Both disorders can occur in patients with other significant disorders, but in order to make the diagnosis, the cognitive deficits must not be primarily attributable to another disorder (Criterion D).

17.15—Major and Mild Neurocognitive Disorders / diagnostic criteria (A and B) (pp. 679–680); Diagnostic Features (pp. 686–685)

17.16 Expressed as a percentile, what is the typical performance on neuropsychological testing of individuals with major neurocognitive disorder (NCD)?

A. Sixtieth percentile or below.
B. Fiftieth percentile or below.
C. Sixteenth percentile or below.
D. Third percentile or below.

Correct Answer: D. Third percentile or below.

Explanation: Neuropsychological testing, with performance compared with norms appropriate to the patient's age, educational attainment, and cultural background, is part of the standard evaluation of NCDs. For major NCD, performance is typically 2 or more standard deviations below appropriate norms (3rd percentile or below). For mild NCD, performance typically lies in the 1–2 standard deviation range (between the 3rd and 16th percentiles).

17.16—Major and Mild Neurocognitive Disorders / Diagnostic Features (p. 685)

17.17 A 68-year-old semiretired cardiologist with responsibility for electrocardiogram (ECG) interpretation at his community hospital is referred by the hospital's Employee Assistance Program for clinical evaluation because of concerns expressed by other clinicians that he has been making many mistakes in his ECG interpretations over the past few months. The patient discloses symptoms of persistent sadness since the death of his wife 6 months prior to the evaluation, with frequent thoughts of death, trouble sleeping, and escalating usage of sedative-hypnotics and alcohol. He has some trouble concentrating, but he has been able to maintain his household, pay his bills, shop, and prepare meals by himself without difficulty. He scores 28/30 on the Mini-Mental State Examination (MMSE). Which of the following would be the primary consideration in the differential diagnosis?

A. Mild neurocognitive disorder (NCD).
B. Adjustment disorder.
C. Major depressive disorder.
D. No diagnosis.

Correct Answer: C. Major depressive disorder.

Explanation: Not enough information has been provided to know for certain whether this patient meets criteria for a specific mood disorder diagnosis—or for a substance use disorder diagnosis—but a major NCD can be ruled out. Although the patient's test score on the MMSE is within the normal range, he does meet Criterion A for major NCD, in that concerns about a decline in cognitive function have been raised because of his increased error rate in interpreting ECGs. Regarding Criterion B for major NCD, the patient does not demonstrate loss of ability to perform activities of daily living independently and so does not qualify for a diagnosis of major NCD. He does meet Criterion C, in that he is not demonstrating signs of delirium. The fact that his problems have become evident only in the context of mood issues strongly suggests that a depressive disorder and/or substance use may account for his work performance deficits; therefore, he likely will not meet Criterion D for NCD. Although he could meet Criterion B for mild NCD, a mood disorder would be the most prominent consideration in the differential diagnosis.

17.17—Major and Mild Neurocognitive Disorders / diagnostic criteria (pp. 679–680)

17.18 A 69-year-old semiretired radiologist with responsibility for chest X-ray interpretation at his academic medical center has been referred by the hospital's Employee Assistance Program for clinical evaluation because of concerns expressed by other clinicians that he has been making many mistakes in his X-ray interpretations over the past few months. Evaluation discloses a remote history of alcohol dependence with sobriety for the past 20 years and a depressive episode following the death of his wife 9 years before the current problem, treated with cognitive-behavioral therapy with full resolution of symptoms after 6 months and no recurrence. He acknowledges some trouble concentrating but no other symptoms, and he minimizes the alleged X-ray interpretation problems. He cannot state the correct date or day of the week and cannot recall the previous day's news events, but he can describe highlights of his long career in medicine in great detail. Collateral history from his children reveals that on several occasions in the past year, neighbors in his apartment building had complained that he forgot to turn off his stove while cooking, resulting in a smoke-filled apartment. He scores 21/30 on the Mini-Mental State Examination. What diagnosis best fits this clinical picture?

A. Major neurocognitive disorder (NCD).
B. Mild NCD.
C. Major depressive disorder.
D. No diagnosis.

Correct Answer: A. Major neurocognitive disorder (NCD).

Explanation: Concern has been raised about cognitive decline affecting this patient's functioning, and his test performance is very abnormal, so he clearly meets Criterion A for major NCD. Forgetting to keep track of what is cooking on the stovetop, with the result that neighbors have to intervene because of the smoky conditions, is a good example of inability to perform activities of daily living independently, so he meets Criterion B for major NCD, as opposed to mild NCD. He is not delirious, so he meets Criterion C. Neither his remote history of alcohol dependence nor his remote history of depression accounts for his cognitive problems, and there is no evidence of another mental disorder, so he probably also meets Criterion D.

17.18—Major and Mild Neurocognitive Disorders / diagnostic criteria (pp. 679–680)

17.19 In a patient with *mild* neurocognitive disorder (NCD), which of the following would distinguish *probable* from *possible* Alzheimer's disease?

A. Evidence of a causative Alzheimer's disease genetic mutation from either genetic testing or family history.
B. Clear evidence of decline in memory and learning.
C. No evidence of mixed etiology.
D. Onset after age 80.

Correct Answer: A. Evidence of a causative Alzheimer's disease genetic mutation from either genetic testing or family history.

Explanation: The only way that mild NCD due to *probable* Alzheimer's disease can be diagnosed is if there is evidence of a causative Alzheimer's disease genetic mutation from either genetic testing or family history. Mild NCD due to *possible* Alzheimer's disease is diagnosed on the basis of the presence of *all* of the clinical criteria described in options B–D above. Age at onset is not a diagnostic criterion.

17.19—Major or Mild Neurocognitive Disorder Due to Alzheimer's Disease / diagnostic criteria (pp. 690–691)

17.20 In major or mild frontotemporal neurocognitive disorder, which of the following is a diagnostic feature of the language variant?

A. Severe semantic memory impairment.
B. Severe deficits in perceptual-motor function.
C. Grammar, word-finding, or word-generation difficulty.
D. Hyperorality.

Correct Answer: C. Grammar, word-finding, or word-generation difficulty.

Explanation: The language variant diagnosis specifically requires worsening in language function with at least relative sparing of learning and memory and perceptual-motor function. Hyperorality is a diagnostic feature of the behavioral deficit variant. Signs of either the language variant or behavior variant can also occur in patients in whom the other variant is predominant, but the diagnosis would be based on the predominant features.

17.20—Major or Mild Frontotemporal Neurocognitive Disorder / diagnostic criteria (pp. 695–696)

17.21 Which of the following neurocognitive disorders (NCDs) is especially characterized by deficits in domains such as speech production, word finding, object naming, or word comprehension, whereas episodic memory, perceptual-motor abilities, and executive function are relatively preserved?

A. Major or mild NCD due to Alzheimer's disease.
B. Major or mild NCD with Lewy bodies.
C. Behavioral-variant major or mild frontotemporal NCD.
D. Language-variant major or mild frontotemporal NCD.

Correct Answer: D. Language-variant major or mild frontotemporal NCD.

Explanation: Major or mild frontotemporal NCD comprises a number of syndromic variants characterized by the progressive development of behavioral and personality change and/or language impairment. The behavioral variant and two language variants (semantic and agrammatic/nonfluent) exhibit distinct patterns of brain atrophy and some distinctive neuropathology. To make the diagnosis, the criteria must be met for either the behavioral or the language variant, but many individuals present with features of both.

Individuals with language-variant major or mild frontotemporal NCD present with primary progressive aphasia with gradual onset, with two subtypes commonly described (semantic variant and agrammatic/nonfluent variant), and each variant has distinctive features and corresponding neuropathology. A third form of progressive language decline, called logopenic progressive aphasia, is associated with left temporoparietal dysfunction and is often caused by Alzheimer's disease pathology.

Individuals with behavioral-variant major or mild frontotemporal NCD present with varying degrees of apathy or disinhibition. They may lose interest in socialization, self-care, and personal responsibilities or display socially inappropriate behaviors. Insight is usually impaired, and this often delays medical consultation. The first referral is often to a psychiatrist. Individuals may develop changes in social style and in religious and political beliefs, with repetitive movements, hoarding, changes in eating behavior, and hyperorality. In later stages, loss of sphincter control may occur. Cognitive decline is less prominent, and formal testing may show relatively few deficits in the early stages. Common neurocognitive symptoms are lack of planning and organization, distractibility, and poor judgment. Deficits in executive function, such as poor performance on tests of mental flexibility, abstract reasoning, and response inhibition, are present, but learning and memory are relatively spared, and perceptual motor abilities are almost always preserved in the early stages.

17.21—Major or Mild Frontotemporal Neurocognitive Disorder / Diagnostic Features (pp. 696–697)

17.22 Which of the following is a core feature of major or mild neurocognitive disorder with Lewy bodies?

A. Fluctuating cognition with pronounced variations in attention and alertness.
B. Recurrent auditory hallucinations.
C. Fulfillment of criteria for rapid eye movement (REM) sleep behavior disorder.
D. Evidence of low striatal dopamine transporter uptake in basal ganglia as demonstrated by single photon emission computed tomography (SPECT) or positron emission tomography (PET) imaging.

Correct Answer: A. Fluctuating cognition with pronounced variations in attention and alertness.

Explanation: Recurrent well-formed *visual* hallucinations (not auditory hallucinations) and parkinsonism arising *after* (not earlier than) cognitive impairment are the other core features of major or mild neurocognitive disorder with Lewy bodies. REM sleep behavioral disorder and excessive sensitivity to neuroleptic agents are suggestive diagnostic features; low dopamine transporter uptake in basal ganglia is a diagnostic marker but is not included in the diagnostic criteria.

17.22—Major or Mild Neurocognitive Disorder With Lewy Bodies / diagnostic criteria; Diagnostic Markers (pp. 699–701)

17.23 A previously healthy 67-year-old man is brought to the emergency department by his family. He is experiencing an acute change in mental status. There is no evidence in the initial history, physical examination, and laboratory studies to indicate substance intoxication or withdrawal or to suggest another medical problem as the cause of his altered mental state. Over the course of 1 hour of observation, his level of alertness varies from alert but distractible, with apparent auditory and visual hallucinations, to somnolent; he has difficulty sustaining attention to an examiner, and he cannot perform simple tasks such as serial subtractions or spelling words backward. What is the most appropriate diagnosis?

A. Delirium.
B. Delirium due to another medical condition.
C. Delirium due to substance intoxication.
D. Unspecified delirium.

Correct Answer: D. Unspecified delirium.

Explanation: This man meets criteria for some sort of delirium, but at this point in the course of his illness it cannot be determined what the cause is. The *unspecified delirium* category can be used when the clinician chooses not to specify a specific cause, when the diagnostic criteria for delirium are not entirely fulfilled, or when the specific diagnostic subtype of delirium cannot be ascertained.

17.23—Unspecified Delirium (p. 678)

17.24 A 35-year-old man brings his 60-year-old father for evaluation of cognitive and functional decline, stating that he thinks his father has dementia; the son is also worried about the possibility of a hereditary illness. The physician notes to herself that the patient has substantial cognitive impairment and features suggestive of the diagnosis of major neurocognitive disorder due to Huntington's disease, but she is not sure about the cause of the neurocognitive disorder. She also notes that the patient's son appears extremely anxious. She has a tight schedule and cannot provide a counseling session for the patient's son until the next day. What is the most appropriate diagnosis to record on the insurance claim form that the patient's son will submit on his father's behalf?

A. Unspecified central nervous system (CNS) disorder.
B. Unspecified neurocognitive disorder.
C. Unspecified mild neurocognitive disorder.
D. Huntington's disease.

Correct Answer: B. Unspecified neurocognitive disorder.

Explanation: The category u*nspecified neurocognitive disorder* applies to presentations in which symptoms characteristic of a neurocognitive disorder that cause clinically significant distress or impairment in social, occupational, or other important areas of functioning predominate but do not meet the full criteria for any of the disorders in the neurocognitive disorders diagnostic class. The *unspecified neurocognitive disorder* category is also used in situations in which the precise etiology cannot be determined with sufficient certainty to make an etiological attribution.

In this case, Huntington's disease is suspected but not established. Unspecified CNS disorder is not a DSM-5 diagnosis and would be inadequately specific to the patient's condition. The apparent severity of the deficits precludes a diagnosis of mild neurocognitive disorder or a V code designation of problem related to living alone.

17.24—Unspecified Neurocognitive Disorder (p. 732)

CHAPTER 18

Personality Disorders

18.1   Which of the following DSM-IV personality disorder diagnoses is no longer present in DSM-5-TR?

A. Antisocial personality disorder.
B. Avoidant personality disorder.
C. Borderline personality disorder.
D. Personality disorder not otherwise specified (NOS).

Correct Answer: D. Personality disorder not otherwise specified (NOS).

Explanation: The following personality disorders are included in the "Personality Disorders" chapter of DSM-5-TR: paranoid personality disorder, schizoid personality disorder, schizotypal personality disorder, antisocial personality disorder (option A is incorrect), borderline personality disorder (option C is incorrect), histrionic personality disorder, narcissistic personality disorder, avoidant personality disorder (option B is incorrect), dependent personality disorder, obsessive-compulsive personality disorder, personality change due to another medical condition, other specified personality disorder, and unspecified personality disorder. Therefore, option D is correct.

18.1—chapter introduction (pp. 733–734)

18.2   While collaborating on a presentation to their customers, the members of a sales team become increasingly frustrated with their team leader. He insists that the members of the team adhere to strict rules for developing the project. This involves approaching the task in sequential manner such that no new task can be begun until the prior one is perfected. When other members suggest alternative approaches, the leader becomes frustrated and insists that the team stick to his approach. Although the results are inarguably of high quality, the team is convinced that they will not finish in time for the scheduled presentation. Which of the following disorders would best explain the behavior of this team leader?

A. Narcissistic personality disorder.
B. Obsessive-compulsive disorder (OCD).
C. Schizoid personality disorder.
D. Obsessive-compulsive personality disorder (OCPD).

Correct Answer: D. Obsessive-compulsive personality disorder (OCPD).

Explanation: The essential feature of OCPD is a preoccupation with orderliness, perfectionism, and mental and interpersonal control at the expense of flexibility, openness, and efficiency. Individuals with OCPD attempt to maintain a sense of control through painstaking attention to rules, trivial details, procedures, lists, schedules, or form to the extent that the major point of the activity is lost. They are excessively careful and prone to repetition, paying extraordinary attention to detail and repeatedly checking for possible mistakes, losing track of time in the process. They may force themselves and others to follow rigid moral principles and very strict standards of performance (option D is correct).

Despite the similarity in names, OCD is usually easily distinguished from OCPD by the presence of true obsessions and compulsions in OCD (option B is incorrect). Individuals with narcissistic personality disorder may also profess a commitment to perfectionism and believe that others cannot do things as well, but these individuals are more likely to believe that they have achieved perfection, whereas those with OCPD are usually self-critical (option A is incorrect). Both schizoid personality disorder and OCPD may be characterized by an apparent formality and social detachment. In OCPD, this stems from discomfort with emotions and excessive devotion to work, whereas in schizoid personality disorder there is a fundamental lack of capacity for intimacy (option C is incorrect).

18.2—Obsessive-Compulsive Personality Disorder / Diagnostic Features (pp. 772–773); Differential Diagnosis (pp. 774–775)

18.3   Individuals with obsessive-compulsive personality disorder (OCPD) are primarily motivated by a need for which of the following?

A. Efficiency.
B. Admiration.
C. Control.
D. Intimacy.

Correct Answer: C. Control.

Explanation: The essential feature of OCPD is a preoccupation with orderliness, perfectionism, and mental and personal control (option C is correct), at the expense of flexibility, openness, and efficiency (option A is incorrect). Narcissistic personality disorder is a pattern of grandiosity, need for admiration, and lack of empathy (option B is incorrect). Both schizoid personality disorder and OCPD may be characterized by an apparent formality and social detachment. In OCPD, this stems from discomfort with emotions and excessive devotion to work, whereas in schizoid personality disorder there is a fundamental lack of capacity for intimacy (option D is incorrect).

18.3—chapter introduction (pp. 733–734); Obsessive-Compulsive Personality Disorder / Diagnostic Features (pp. 772–773); Differential Diagnosis (pp. 774–775)

18.4 Which of the following findings would rule out the diagnosis of obsessive-compulsive personality disorder (OCPD)?

    A. A concurrent diagnosis of obsessive-compulsive disorder (OCD).
    B. A concurrent diagnosis of hoarding disorder.
    C. A concurrent diagnosis of narcissistic personality disorder.
    D. Evidence that the behavioral patterns reflect culturally sanctioned interpersonal styles.

Correct Answer: D. Evidence that the behavioral patterns reflect culturally sanctioned interpersonal styles.

Explanation: In assessing an individual for OCPD, the clinician should not include behaviors that reflect habits, customs, or interpersonal styles that are culturally sanctioned by the individual's reference group. Such behaviors should not on their own be considered indications of OCPD (option D is correct). When criteria for both OCPD and OCD are met, both diagnoses should be recorded (option A is incorrect). Similarly, when criteria for both OCPD and hoarding disorder are met, both diagnoses should be recorded (option B is incorrect). If an individual has personality features that meet criteria for one or more personality disorders in addition to OCPD, all can be diagnosed (option C is incorrect).

18.4—Obsessive-Compulsive Personality Disorder / Culture-Related Diagnostic Issues (p. 774); Differential Diagnosis (pp. 774–775)

18.5 Despite working for a company for many years, a 36-year-old employee has not advanced beyond an entry level position. She gets good reviews and works long hours but has not asked for a promotion because she feels she is not as good as other employees and thus unworthy of promotion. She explains her long hours by saying that she is not very smart and needs to check over all her work because she is afraid that people will ridicule any mistakes. Which of the following personality disorders would best explain this woman's lack of job advancement?

    A. Dependent personality disorder.
    B. Avoidant personality disorder.
    C. Paranoid disorder.
    D. Schizoid personality disorder.

Correct Answer: B. Avoidant personality disorder.

Explanation: The essential feature of avoidant personality disorder is a pervasive pattern of social inhibition, feelings of inadequacy, and hypersensitivity to negative evaluation that begins by early adulthood and is present in a variety of contexts. Offers of job promotions may be declined because failure to manage the new responsibilities might result in criticism from coworkers (option B is correct). Both avoidant personality disorder and dependent personality disorder are characterized by feelings of inadequacy, hypersensitivity to criticism, and a need for reassurance. Similar behaviors (e.g., unassertiveness) and attributes (e.g., low self-esteem and low self-confidence) may be observed in both dependent personality disorder and avoidant personality disorder, although other behaviors are notably divergent, such as avoidance of social proximity in avoidant personality disorder but proximity seeking in dependent personality disorder. The motivations behind similar behaviors may be quite different. For example, the unassertiveness in avoidant personality disorder is described as more closely related to fears of being rejected or humiliated, whereas in dependent personality disorder it is motivated by the desire to avoid being left to fend for oneself (option A is incorrect). Like avoidant personality disorder, schizoid and schizotypal personality disorders are characterized by social isolation. However, individuals with avoidant personality disorder want to have relationships with others and feel their loneliness deeply, whereas those with schizoid or schizotypal personality disorder may be content with and even prefer their social isolation (option D is incorrect). Paranoid personality disorder and avoidant personality disorder are both characterized by a reluctance to confide in others. However, in avoidant personality disorder, this reluctance is attributable more to a fear of humiliation or being found inadequate than to a fear of others' malicious intent (option C is incorrect).

18.5—Avoidant Personality Disorder / Diagnostic Features (p. 765) / Differential Diagnosis (p. 767)

18.6 A cardiologist requests a psychiatric consultation for her patient, a 46-year-old man, because of concern that he "seems crazy." On evaluation, the patient makes poor eye contact, tends to ramble, and makes unusual word choices. He is modestly disheveled and wears clothes with mismatched colors. He expresses odd beliefs about supernatural phenomena, but these beliefs do not seem to be of delusional intensity. Collateral information from a sibling elicits the observation that the patient "has always been like this—weird, a loner, and likes it that way." Which of the following conditions best explains this patient's odd behaviors and beliefs?

A. Schizoid personality disorder.
B. Schizotypal personality disorder.
C. Delusional disorder.
D. Schizophrenia.

Correct Answer: B. Schizotypal personality disorder.

Explanation: The essential feature of schizotypal personality disorder is pervasive social and interpersonal deficits marked by acute discomfort with, and reduced capacity for, close relationships as well as by cognitive or perceptual distortions and eccentricities of behavior. Individuals with schizotypal personality are often considered to be odd or eccentric because of unusual mannerisms, an often unkempt manner of dress that does not quite "fit together," and inattention to the usual social conventions. They experience interpersonal relatedness as problematic and are uncomfortable relating to other people (option B is correct). These individuals often have ideas of reference (i.e., incorrect interpretations of casual incidents and external events as having a particular and unusual meaning specifically for the person) (Criterion A1). Ideas of reference should be distinguished from delusions of reference, in which the beliefs are held with delusional conviction. Individuals with schizotypal personality disorder may be superstitious or preoccupied with paranormal phenomena that are outside the norms of their subculture (Criterion A2). Schizotypal personality disorder can be distinguished from delusional disorder, schizophrenia, and bipolar or depressive disorder with psychotic features because these disorders are all characterized by a period of persistent psychotic symptoms (e.g., delusions and hallucinations). To give a diagnosis of schizotypal personality disorder, the personality disorder must have been present before the onset of psychotic symptoms and persist when the psychotic symptoms are in remission (options C and D are incorrect). Although schizoid personality disorder may also be characterized by social detachment and restricted affect, schizotypal personality disorder can be distinguished from this diagnosis by the presence of cognitive or perceptual distortions and marked eccentricity or oddness (option A is incorrect).

18.6—Schizotypal Personality Disorder / Diagnostic Features (pp. 745–746) / Differential Diagnosis (pp. 747–748)

18.7   Which of the following statements most accurately describes the development, course, and prognosis of borderline personality disorder (BPD)?

A. Suicide attempts increase with age.
B. A childhood history of neglect, rather than abuse, is unusual.
C. Prospective follow-up studies have found that stable remissions of up to 8 years are very common.
D. Affective symptoms remit more rapidly than impulsive symptoms.

Correct Answer: C. Prospective follow-up studies have found that stable remissions of up to 8 years are very common.

Explanation: BPD has long been thought of as a disorder with a poor symptomatic course, which tends to lessen in severity as individuals with BPD enter their 30s and 40s. However, prospective follow-up studies have found that stable remissions of 1–8 years are very common (option C is correct). A study of individuals with BPD followed for 10 years found that recurrent suicidal behavior was a defining characteristic of BPD, associated with declining rates of suicide attempts from 79% to 13% over time (option A is incorrect). BPD has been found to be associated with high rates of various forms of reported childhood abuse and emotional neglect (option B is incorrect). Impulsive symptoms of BPD remit the most rapidly, whereas affective symptoms remit at a substantially slower rate (option D is incorrect).

18.7—Borderline Personality Disorder / Development and Course (p. 755); Risk and Prognostic Factors (p. 755); Association With Suicidal Thoughts or Behavior (p. 756)

18.8   Which of the following is a characteristic of narcissistic personality disorder (NPD)?

    A. A requirement for much attention of any kind.
    B. Impulsive aggressivity and deceitfulness.
    C. Immersion in perfectionism related to order and rigidity.
    D. A pervasive pattern of grandiosity.

Correct Answer: D. A pervasive pattern of grandiosity.

Explanation: The essential feature of NPD is a pervasive pattern of grandiosity, need for admiration, and lack of empathy that begins by early adulthood and is present in a variety of contexts (option D is correct). Although individuals with borderline, histrionic, and narcissistic personality disorders may require much attention, those with NPD specifically need that attention to be admiring (option A is incorrect). Individuals with antisocial and narcissistic personality disorders share a tendency to be tough-minded, glib, superficial, exploitative, and unempathic. However, NPD does not necessarily include characteristics of impulsive aggressivity and deceitfulness (option B is incorrect). In both NPD and obsessive-compulsive personality disorder, the individual may profess a commitment to perfectionism and believe that others cannot do things as well. However, whereas those with obsessive-compulsive personality disorder tend to be more immersed in perfectionism related to order and rigidity, individuals with NPD tend to set high perfectionistic standards, especially for appearance and performance, and to be critically concerned if they are not measuring up (option C is incorrect).

18.8—Narcissistic Personality Disorder / Diagnostic Features (pp. 761–762); Differential Diagnosis (pp. 763–764)

18.9   Which of the following cognitive or perceptual disturbances are most characteristic of borderline personality disorder (BPD)?

    A. Overly concrete or overly abstract responses.
    B. Ideas of reference.
    C. Superstitiousness or preoccupation with paranormal phenomena.
    D. Transient paranoid ideation during periods of stress.

Correct Answer: D. Transient paranoid ideation during periods of stress.

Explanation: During periods of extreme stress, transient paranoid ideation or dissociative symptoms (e.g., depersonalization) may occur (Criterion 9), but these are generally of insufficient severity or duration to warrant an additional diagnosis. Paranoid ideas or illusions may be present in both BPD and schizotypal personality disorder, but these symptoms are more transient, interpersonally reactive, and responsive to external structuring in BPD. Individuals with schizotypal personality disorder often have ideas of reference (option B is incorrect). These individuals may be superstitious or preoccupied with paranormal phenomena that are outside the norms of their subculture (option C is incorrect). Responses can be either overly concrete or overly abstract (option A is incorrect).

18.9—Borderline Personality Disorder / Diagnostic Features (pp. 753–754); Differential Diagnosis (pp. 756–757); Schizotypal Personality Disorder / Diagnostic Features (pp. 745–746)

18.10 A 43-year-old warehouse security guard comes to your office complaining of vague feelings of depression for the past few months, with no particular sense of fear or anxiety. He feels little desire for relationships but notes that his co-workers seem happier, and they have many relationships. He has never felt comfortable with other people, not even with family. He has lived alone since early adulthood and is self-sufficient. He almost always works night shifts to avoid interactions with others. He tries to remain low-key and undistinguished to discourage others from striking up conversations. Mental status examination is notable for significantly constricted, bland affect. No cognitive or perceptual disturbances are present. Which personality disorder would best fit with this presentation?

A. Paranoid.
B. Schizoid.
C. Schizotypal.
D. Avoidant.

Correct Answer: B. Schizoid.

Explanation: The essential feature of schizoid personality disorder is a pervasive pattern of detachment from social relationships and a restricted range of emotions in interpersonal settings. Individuals with schizoid personality disorder appear to lack a desire for intimacy, seem indifferent to opportunities to develop close relationships, and do not seem to derive much satisfaction from being part of a family or other social group (Criterion A1; option B is correct). Although characteristics of social isolation and restricted affectivity are common to schizoid, schizotypal, and paranoid personality disorders, schizoid personality disorder can be distinguished from schizotypal personality disorder by the lack of cognitive and perceptual distortions and from paranoid personality disorder by the lack of suspiciousness and paranoid ideation (options A and C are incorrect). The social isolation of schizoid personality disorder can be distinguished from that of avoidant personality disorder, which is attributable to fear of being embarrassed or found inadequate and excessive anticipation of rejection. In contrast, people with schizoid personality disorder have a more pervasive detachment and limited desire for social intimacy (option D is incorrect).

18.10—Schizoid Personality Disorder / Diagnostic Features (p. 742); Differential Diagnosis (pp. 743–744)

18.11   Which of the following behaviors or states would be least likely to occur in an individual with schizoid personality disorder?

A. An angry outburst at a colleague who criticizes their work.
B. Turning down an invitation to a party.
C. Lacking desire for sexual experiences.
D. Drifting with regard to life goals.

Correct Answer: A. An angry outburst at a colleague who criticizes their work.

Explanation: The essential feature of schizoid personality disorder is a pervasive pattern of detachment from social relationships and a restricted range of emotions in interpersonal settings. Individuals with schizoid personality disorder may have particular difficulty expressing anger, even in response to direct provocation, which contributes to the impression that they lack emotion (option A is correct). They prefer spending time by themselves rather than being with other people. They often appear to be socially isolated or "loners" and almost always choose solitary activities or hobbies that do not include interaction with others (Criterion A2; option B is incorrect). Criterion A3 states that individuals with schizoid personality disorder may have little, if any, interest in having sexual experiences with another person (option C is incorrect). Their lives sometimes seem directionless, and they may appear to "drift" in their goals (option D is incorrect).

18.11—Schizoid Personality Disorder / diagnostic criteria (pp. 741–742); Diagnostic Features (p. 742)

18.12   What is the relationship between a history of conduct disorder before age 15 and the diagnosis of antisocial personality after age 18?

A. A history of some conduct disorder symptoms before age 15 is one of the required criteria for a diagnosis of antisocial personality disorder in adulthood.
B. Childhood onset of conduct disorder has no relationship to the likelihood of developing antisocial personality disorder in adult life.

C. Both antisocial personality disorder and conduct disorder can be diagnosed before age 18 years.

D. Both antisocial personality disorder and conduct disorder can be diagnosed in individuals older than 18 years.

Correct Answer: A. A history of some conduct disorder symptoms before age 15 is one of the required criteria for a diagnosis of antisocial personality disorder in adulthood.

Explanation: The essential feature of antisocial personality disorder is a pervasive pattern of disregard for, and violation of, the rights of others that begins in childhood or early adolescence and continues into adulthood. Criterion C for the diagnosis of antisocial personality disorder specifically requires evidence of conduct disorder with onset before age 15 years (option A is correct). The likelihood of developing antisocial personality disorder in adult life is increased if the individual experienced childhood onset of conduct disorder (before age 10 years) and accompanying attention-deficit/hyperactivity disorder (option B is incorrect). By definition, antisocial personality disorder cannot be diagnosed before age 18 years (option C is incorrect). For individuals older than 18 years, a diagnosis of conduct disorder is given only if the criteria for antisocial personality disorder are not met (option D is incorrect).

18.12—Antisocial Personality Disorder / diagnostic criteria (p. 748); / Diagnostic Features (pp. 748–749); Development and Course (p. 750); Differential Diagnosis (pp. 751–752); Comorbidity (p. 752)

18.13 A 25-year-old patient has a childhood history of repeated instances of torturing animals, setting fires, stealing, running away from home, and school truancy, beginning at age 9 years. As an adult, he repeatedly lies to others; engages in petty thefts, con games, and frequent fights (including episodes involving the use of objects at hand—pipe wrenches, chairs, steak knives—to injure others); and uses aliases to avoid paying child support. There is no history of manic, depressive, or psychotic symptoms. The patient is dressed in expensive clothing and displays an expensive wristwatch for which he demands admiration. He expresses feelings of specialness and entitlement and endorses a sense of deserving exemption from ordinary rules, as well as feelings of anger that his special talents have not been adequately recognized by others. He shows devaluation of, contempt for, and lack of empathy for others and lack of remorse for his behavior. There is no sign of psychosis. What is the appropriate DSM-5-TR diagnosis?

A. Antisocial personality disorder.

B. Narcissistic personality disorder.

C. Antisocial personality disorder and narcissistic personality disorder.

D. Other specified personality disorder (mixed personality features).

Correct Answer: C. Antisocial personality disorder and narcissistic personality disorder.

Explanation: This individual meets diagnostic criteria for antisocial personality disorder. Criterion A specifies a pervasive pattern of disregard for and violation of the rights of others, occurring since age 15 years, as indicated by three (or more) of the following: 1) failure to conform to social norms with respect to lawful behaviors; 2) deceitfulness; 3) impulsivity or failure to plan ahead; 4) irritability and aggressiveness; 5) reckless disregard for safety of self or others; 6) consistent irresponsibility; and 7) lack of remorse. This antisocial behavior does not occur exclusively during the course of schizophrenia or bipolar disorder (Criterion D). The individual is at least age 18 years (Criterion B), and there is evidence of conduct disorder with onset before age 15 years (Criterion C).

The patient also meets diagnostic criteria for narcissistic personality disorder: a pervasive pattern of grandiosity (in fantasy or behavior), need for admiration, and lack of empathy, beginning by early adulthood and present in a variety of contexts (Criterion A), as indicated by five (or more) of the following: 1) a grandiose sense of self-importance; 2) preoccupation with fantasies of unlimited success, power, brilliance, beauty, or ideal love; 3) a belief that they are "special" and unique and can only be understood by, or should associate with, other special or high-status people (or institutions); 4) need for excessive admiration; 5) a sense of entitlement; 6) interpersonal exploitation of others; 7) lack of empathy; 8) envy of others or belief that others are envious of them; and 9) arrogant, haughty behaviors or attitudes.

Narcissistic personality disorder may be confused with antisocial personality disorder because both disorders have certain features in common. It is therefore important to distinguish between them on the basis of differences in their characteristic features. However, if an individual has personality features that meet criteria for one or more personality disorders in addition to antisocial personality disorder, all can be diagnosed. Individuals with antisocial personality disorder and narcissistic personality disorder share a tendency to be tough-minded, glib, superficial, and exploitative and to lack empathy. Because this patient meets diagnostic criteria for both personality disorders, option C is correct. The category *other specified personality disorder* applies to presentations in which symptoms characteristic of a personality disorder that cause clinically significant distress or impairment in social, occupational, or other important areas of functioning predominate but do not meet the full criteria for any of the disorders in the personality disorders diagnostic class. The *other specified personality disorder* category is used in situations in which the clinician chooses to communicate the specific reason that the presentation does not meet the criteria for any specific personality disorder. This is done by recording "other specified personality disorder" followed by the specific reason (e.g., "mixed personality features") (option D is incorrect).

18.13—Antisocial Personality Disorder / diagnostic criteria (p. 748); Differential Diagnosis (pp. 751–752); Narcissistic Personality Disorder / diagnostic criteria (p. 760); Other Specified Personality Disorder (p. 778)

18.14 Which of the following is one of the general criteria for a personality disorder in DSM-5-TR?

A. The pattern of inner experience deviates markedly from the expectations of the individual's culture.
B. The pattern of inner experience is flexible and confined to a single personal or social situation.
C. The pattern of inner experience is fluctuating and of short duration.
D. The pattern of inner experience is ego-syntonic and does not lead to distress.

Correct Answer: A. The pattern of inner experience deviates markedly from the expectations of the individual's culture.

Explanation: A personality disorder is an enduring pattern of inner experience and behavior that deviates markedly from the expectations of the individual's culture, is pervasive and inflexible (option B is incorrect), has an onset in adolescence or early adulthood, is stable over time (option C is incorrect), and leads to distress or impairment (option D is incorrect).

18.14—chapter introduction (pp. 733–734)

18.15 Which of the following presentations is characteristic of histrionic personality disorder?

A. A pervasive and excessive need to be taken care of that leads to submissive and clinging behavior and fears of separation.
B. A pervasive pattern of instability in interpersonal relationships, self-image, and affects and marked impulsivity.
C. A pervasive pattern of grandiosity, need for admiration, and lack of empathy.
D. A pervasive pattern of excessive emotionality and attention seeking.

Correct Answer: D. A pervasive pattern of excessive emotionality and attention seeking.

Explanation: The essential feature of histrionic personality disorder is pervasive and excessive emotionality and attention-seeking behavior (option D is correct). The essential feature of borderline personality disorder is a pervasive pattern of instability of interpersonal relationships, self-image, and affects and marked impulsivity (option B is incorrect). The essential feature of narcissistic personality disorder is a pervasive pattern of grandiosity, need for admiration, and lack of empathy (option C is incorrect). The essential feature of dependent personality disorder is a pervasive and excessive need to be taken care of that leads to submissive and clinging behavior and fears of separation (option A is incorrect).

18.15—Histrionic Personality Disorder / Diagnostic Features (pp. 757–758); Borderline Personality Disorder / Diagnostic Features (pp. 753–754); Narcissistic Personality Disorder / Diagnostic Features (pp. 761–762); Dependent Personality Disorder / Diagnostic Features (pp. 768–769)

18.16 Which of the following presentations is characteristic of borderline personality disorder?

A. A pervasive and excessive need to be taken care of that leads to submissive and clinging behavior and fears of separation.
B. A pervasive pattern of instability in interpersonal relationships, self-image, and affects and marked impulsivity.
C. A pervasive pattern of grandiosity, need for admiration, and lack of empathy.
D. Pervasive and excessive emotionality and attention seeking.

Correct Answer: B. A pervasive pattern of instability in interpersonal relationships, self-image, and affects and marked impulsivity.

Explanation: The essential feature of borderline personality disorder is a pervasive pattern of instability of interpersonal relationships, self-image, and affects and marked impulsivity (option B is correct). The essential feature of dependent personality disorder is a pervasive and excessive need to be taken care of that leads to submissive and clinging behavior and fears of separation (option A is incorrect). The essential feature of narcissistic personality disorder is a pervasive pattern of grandiosity, need for admiration, and lack of empathy (option C is incorrect). The essential feature of histrionic personality disorder is pervasive and excessive emotionality and attention-seeking behavior (option D is incorrect).

18.16—Borderline Personality Disorder / Diagnostic Features (pp. 753–754); Histrionic Personality Disorder / Diagnostic Features (pp. 757–758); Narcissistic Personality Disorder / Diagnostic Features (pp. 761–762); Dependent Personality Disorder / Diagnostic Features (pp. 768–769)

18.17 Which of the following presentations is characteristic of dependent personality disorder?

A. A pervasive and excessive need to be taken care of that leads to submissive and clinging behavior and fears of separation.
B. A pervasive pattern of instability in interpersonal relationships, self-image, and affects and marked impulsivity.
C. A pervasive pattern of grandiosity, need for admiration, and lack of empathy.
D. A pervasive pattern of social inhibition, feelings of inadequacy, and hypersensitivity to negative evaluation.

Correct Answer: A. A pervasive and excessive need to be taken care of that leads to submissive and clinging behavior and fears of separation.

Explanation: The essential feature of dependent personality disorder is a pervasive and excessive need to be taken care of that leads to submissive and clinging behavior and fears of separation (option A is correct). The essential feature of borderline personality disorder is a pervasive pattern of instability of interpersonal relationships, self-image, and affects and marked impulsivity (option B is incorrect). The essential feature of narcissistic personality disorder is a pervasive pattern of grandiosity, need for admiration, and lack of empathy (option C is incorrect). The essential feature of avoidant personality disorder is a pervasive pattern of social inhibition, feelings of inadequacy, and hypersensitivity to negative evaluation (option D is incorrect).

18.17—Dependent Personality Disorder / Diagnostic Features (pp. 768–769); Borderline Personality Disorder / Diagnostic Features (pp. 753–754); Narcissistic Personality Disorder / Diagnostic Features (pp. 761–762); Avoidant Personality Disorder / Diagnostic Features (p. 765)

18.18 Which of the following presentations is characteristic of avoidant personality disorder?

A. A pervasive pattern of social inhibition, feelings of inadequacy, and hypersensitivity to negative evaluation.
B. A pervasive pattern of social and interpersonal deficits marked by acute discomfort with, and reduced capacity for, close relationships as well as by cognitive or perceptual distortions, and eccentricities of behavior.
C. A pervasive and excessive need to be taken care of that leads to submissive and clinging behavior and fears of separation.
D. A pervasive pattern of instability in interpersonal relationships, self-image, and affects and marked impulsivity.

Correct Answer: A. A pervasive pattern of social inhibition, feelings of inadequacy, and hypersensitivity to negative evaluation.

Explanation: The essential feature of avoidant personality disorder is a pervasive pattern of social inhibition, feelings of inadequacy, and hypersensitivity to negative evaluation (option A is correct). The essential feature of schizotypal personality disorder is a pervasive pattern of social and interpersonal deficits marked by acute discomfort with, and reduced capacity for, close relationships as well as by cognitive or perceptual distortions and eccentricities of behavior (option B is incorrect). The essential feature of dependent personality disorder is a pervasive and excessive need to be taken care of that leads to submissive and clinging behavior and fears of separation (option C is correct). The essential feature of borderline personality disorder is a pervasive pattern of instability of interpersonal relationships, self-image, and affects and marked impulsivity (option D is incorrect).

18.18—Avoidant Personality Disorder / Diagnostic Features (p. 765); Schizotypal Personality Disorder / Diagnostic Features (pp. 745–746); Borderline Personality Disorder / Diagnostic Features (pp. 753–754); Dependent Personality Disorder / Diagnostic Features (pp. 768–769)

18.19 Which of the following presentations is characteristic of schizotypal personality disorder?

   A. A pervasive pattern of social inhibition, feelings of inadequacy, and hypersensitivity to negative evaluation.
   B. A pervasive pattern of social and interpersonal deficits marked by acute discomfort with, and reduced capacity for, close relationships as well as by cognitive or perceptual distortions, and eccentricities of behavior.
   C. A pervasive and excessive need to be taken care of that leads to submissive and clinging behavior and fears of separation.
   D. A pervasive pattern of instability in interpersonal relationships, self-image, and affects and marked impulsivity.

Correct Answer: B. A pervasive pattern of social and interpersonal deficits marked by acute discomfort with, and reduced capacity for, close relationships as well as by cognitive or perceptual distortions, and eccentricities of behavior.

Explanation: The essential feature of schizotypal personality disorder is a pervasive pattern of social and interpersonal deficits marked by acute discomfort with, and reduced capacity for, close relationships as well as by cognitive or perceptual distortions and eccentricities of behavior (option B is correct). The essential feature of avoidant personality disorder is a pervasive pattern of social inhibition, feelings of inadequacy, and hypersensitivity to negative evaluation (option A is incorrect). The essential feature of dependent personality disorder is a pervasive and excessive need to be taken care of that leads to submissive and clinging behavior and fears of separation (option C is incorrect). The essential feature of borderline personality disorder is a pervasive pattern of instability of interpersonal relationships, self-image, and affects and marked impulsivity (option D is incorrect).

18.19—Schizotypal Personality Disorder / Diagnostic Features (pp. 745–746); Borderline Personality Disorder / Diagnostic Features (pp. 753–754); Avoidant Personality Disorder / Diagnostic Features (p. 765); Dependent Personality Disorder / Diagnostic Features (pp. 768–769)

18.20 Which of the following presentations is characteristic of paranoid personality disorder?

   A. A pervasive pattern of social inhibition, feelings of inadequacy, and hypersensitivity to negative evaluation.
   B. A pattern of pervasive distrust and suspiciousness of others such that their motives are interpreted as malevolent.
   C. A pervasive and excessive need to be taken care of that leads to submissive and clinging behavior and fears of separation.

D. A pervasive pattern of instability in interpersonal relationships, self-image, and affects, and marked impulsivity.

Correct Answer: B. A pattern of pervasive distrust and suspiciousness of others such that their motives are interpreted as malevolent.

Explanation: The essential feature of paranoid personality disorder is a pattern of pervasive distrust and suspiciousness of others such that their motives are interpreted as malevolent (option B is correct). The essential feature of avoidant personality disorder is a pervasive pattern of social inhibition, feelings of inadequacy, and hypersensitivity to negative evaluation (option A is incorrect). The essential feature of dependent personality disorder is a pervasive and excessive need to be taken care of that leads to submissive and clinging behavior and fears of separation (option C is incorrect). The essential feature of borderline personality disorder is a pervasive pattern of instability of interpersonal relationships, self-image, and affects and marked impulsivity (option D is incorrect).

18.20—Paranoid Personality Disorder / Diagnostic Features (pp. 738–739); Borderline Personality Disorder / Diagnostic Features (pp. 753–754); Avoidant Personality Disorder / Diagnostic Features (p. 765); Dependent Personality Disorder / Diagnostic Features (pp. 768–769)

18.21 Which of the following presentations is characteristic of narcissistic personality disorder?

A. A pervasive pattern of social inhibition, feelings of inadequacy, and hypersensitivity to negative evaluation.
B. A pervasive and excessive need to be taken care of that leads to submissive and clinging behavior and fears of separation.
C. A pervasive pattern of instability in interpersonal relationships, self-image, and affects and marked impulsivity.
D. A pervasive pattern of grandiosity, need for admiration, and lack of empathy.

Correct Answer: D. A pervasive pattern of grandiosity, need for admiration, and lack of empathy.

Explanation: The essential feature of narcissistic personality disorder is a pervasive pattern of grandiosity, need for admiration, and lack of empathy (option D is correct). The essential feature of avoidant personality disorder is a pervasive pattern of social inhibition, feelings of inadequacy, and hypersensitivity to negative evaluation (option A is incorrect). The essential feature of dependent personality disorder is a pervasive and excessive need to be taken care of that leads to submissive and clinging behavior and fears of separation (option B is incorrect). The essential feature of borderline personality disorder is a pervasive pattern of instability of interpersonal relationships, self-image, and affects and marked impulsivity (option C is incorrect).

18.21—Narcissistic Personality Disorder / Diagnostic Features (pp. 761–762); Borderline Personality Disorder / Diagnostic Features (pp. 753–754); Avoidant Personality Disorder / Diagnostic Features (p. 765); Dependent Personality Disorder / Diagnostic Features (pp. 768–769)

18.22 Which of the following presentations is characteristic of schizoid personality disorder?

A. A pervasive pattern of social inhibition, feelings of inadequacy, and hypersensitivity to negative evaluation.
B. A pervasive pattern of social and interpersonal deficits marked by acute discomfort with, and reduced capacity for, close relationships, as well as by cognitive or perceptual distortions, and eccentricities of behavior.
C. A pervasive pattern of detachment from social relationships and a restricted range of expression of emotions in interpersonal settings.
D. A pervasive pattern of instability in interpersonal relationships, self-image, and affects and marked impulsivity.

Correct Answer: C. A pervasive pattern of detachment from social relationships and a restricted range of expression of emotions in interpersonal settings.

Explanation: The essential feature of schizoid personality disorder is a pervasive pattern of detachment from social relationships and a restricted range of expression of emotions in interpersonal settings (option C is correct). The essential feature of schizotypal personality disorder is a pervasive pattern of social and interpersonal deficits marked by acute discomfort with, and reduced capacity for, close relationships as well as by cognitive or perceptual distortions and eccentricities of behavior (option B is incorrect). The essential feature of avoidant personality disorder is a pervasive pattern of social inhibition, feelings of inadequacy, and hypersensitivity to negative evaluation (option A is incorrect). The essential feature of borderline personality disorder is a pervasive pattern of instability of interpersonal relationships, self-image, and affects and marked impulsivity (option D is incorrect).

18.22—Schizoid Personality Disorder / Diagnostic Features (p. 742); Schizotypal Personality Disorder / Diagnostic Features (pp. 745–746); Borderline Personality Disorder / Diagnostic Features (pp. 753–754); Avoidant Personality Disorder / Diagnostic Features (p. 765)

18.23 Which of the following presentations is characteristic of antisocial personality disorder?

A. Preoccupation with orderliness, perfectionism, and mental and interpersonal control, at the expense of flexibility, openness, and efficiency.
B. A pervasive pattern of detachment from social relationships and a restricted range of expression of emotions in interpersonal settings.

C. A pattern of pervasive distrust and suspiciousness of others such that their motives are interpreted as malevolent.

D. A pervasive pattern of disregard for, and violation of, the rights of others.

Correct Answer: D. A pervasive pattern of disregard for, and violation of, the rights of others.

Explanation: The essential feature of antisocial personality disorder is a pervasive pattern of disregard for, and violation of, the rights of others (option D is correct). The essential feature of obsessive-compulsive personality disorder is a preoccupation with orderliness, perfectionism, and mental and interpersonal control, at the expense of flexibility, openness, and efficiency (option A is incorrect). The essential feature of schizoid personality disorder is a pervasive pattern of detachment from social relationships and a restricted range of expression of emotions in interpersonal settings (option B is incorrect). The essential feature of paranoid personality disorder is a pattern of pervasive distrust and suspiciousness of others such that their motives are interpreted as malevolent (option C is incorrect).

18.23—Antisocial Personality Disorder / Diagnostic Features (pp. 748–749); Paranoid Personality Disorder / Diagnostic Features (pp. 738–739); Schizoid Personality Disorder / Diagnostic Features (p. 742); Obsessive-Compulsive Personality Disorder / Diagnostic Features (pp. 772–773)

18.24 Which of the following presentations is characteristic of obsessive-compulsive personality disorder?

A. A pervasive pattern of social inhibition, feelings of inadequacy, and hypersensitivity to negative evaluation.

B. A pervasive pattern of social and interpersonal deficits marked by acute discomfort with, and reduced capacity for, close relationships, as well as by cognitive or perceptual distortions, and eccentricities of behavior.

C. Preoccupation with orderliness, perfectionism, and mental and interpersonal control, at the expense of flexibility, openness, and efficiency.

D. A pervasive pattern of detachment from social relationships and a restricted range of expression of emotions in interpersonal settings.

Correct Answer: C. Preoccupation with orderliness, perfectionism, and mental and interpersonal control, at the expense of flexibility, openness, and efficiency.

Explanation: The essential feature of obsessive-compulsive personality disorder is a preoccupation with orderliness, perfectionism, and mental and interpersonal control, at the expense of flexibility, openness, and efficiency (option C is correct). The essential feature of avoidant personality disorder is a pervasive pattern of social inhibition, feelings of inadequacy, and hypersensitivity to negative evaluation (option A is incorrect). The essential feature of schizotypal personality disorder is a pervasive pattern of social and interpersonal deficits marked by acute discomfort with, and reduced capacity for, close relationships as well as by cognitive or perceptual distortions and eccentricities of behavior (option B is incorrect). The essential feature of schizoid personality disorder is a pervasive pattern of detachment from social relationships and a restricted range of expression of emotions in interpersonal settings (option D is incorrect).

18.24—Obsessive-Compulsive Personality Disorder / Diagnostic Features (pp. 772–773); Schizoid Personality Disorder / Diagnostic Features (p. 742); Schizotypal Personality Disorder / Diagnostic Features (pp. 745–746); Avoidant Personality Disorder / Diagnostic Features (p. 765)

CHAPTER 19

Paraphilic Disorders

19.1 Which of the following is not a classification scheme of paraphilic disorders in DSM-5-TR?

A. Anomalous activity preferences.
B. Courtship disorders.
C. Algolagnic disorders.
D. Asynchronous disorders.

Correct Answer: D. Asynchronous disorders.

Explanation: In this chapter, the order of presentation of the listed paraphilic disorders generally corresponds to common classification schemes for these conditions. The first group of disorders is based on anomalous activity preferences. These disorders are subdivided into courtship disorders, which resemble distorted components of human courtship behavior (voyeuristic disorder, exhibitionistic disorder, and frotteuristic disorder), and algolagnic disorders, which involve pain and suffering (sexual masochism disorder and sexual sadism disorder). The second group of disorders is based on anomalous target preferences. These disorders include one directed at other humans (pedophilic disorder) and two directed elsewhere (fetishistic disorder and transvestic disorder). There is no asynchronous disorder classification scheme.

19.1—chapter introduction (p. 779)

19.2 Which of the following is *not* a true statement about paraphilias?

A. The presence of a paraphilia does not always justify clinical intervention.
B. Most paraphilias can be divided into those that involve an unusual activity and those that involve an unusual target.
C. Paraphilias may coexist with normophilic sexual interests.
D. It is rare for an individual to manifest more than one paraphilia.

Correct Answer: D. It is rare for an individual to manifest more than one paraphilia.

Explanation: The term *paraphilia* denotes any intense and persistent sexual interest other than sexual interest in genital stimulation or preparatory fondling with phenotypically normal, physically mature, consenting human partners. In some circumstances, the criteria *intense and persistent* may be difficult to apply, such as in the assessment of persons who are very old or medically ill and who may not have "intense" sexual interests of any kind. In such circumstances, the term *paraphilia* may be defined as any sexual interest greater than or equal to nonparaphilic sexual interests. There are also specific paraphilias that are generally better described as preferential sexual interests than as intense sexual interests.

It is not rare for an individual to manifest two or more paraphilias. In some cases, the paraphilic foci are closely related and the connection between the paraphilias is intuitively comprehensible (e.g., foot fetishism and shoe fetishism). In other cases, the connection between the paraphilias is not obvious, and the presence of multiple paraphilias may be coincidental or else related to some generalized vulnerability to anomalies of psychosexual development. In any event, comorbid diagnoses of separate paraphilic disorders may be warranted if more than one paraphilia is causing suffering to the individual or harm to others.

19.2—chapter introduction (p. 779)

19.3   Which of the following is *not* a paraphilic disorder?

A. Sexual masochism disorder.
B. Transvestic disorder.
C. Transsexual disorder.
D. Voyeuristic disorder.

Correct Answer: C. Transsexual disorder.

Explanation: Transsexualism is not a disorder and is not included in the DSM-5-TR "Paraphilic Disorders" chapter. *Transsexual*, historic term, denotes an individual who seeks, is undergoing, or has undergone a social transition from male to female or female to male, which in many, but not all, cases also involves a somatic transition by gender-affirming hormone treatment and genital, breast, or other gender-affirming surgery (historically referred to as *sex reassignment surgery*).

19.3—Gender Dysphoria chapter introduction (pp. 511–512); Paraphilic Disorders chapter introduction (p. 779)

19.4   Which of the following statements about a person with pedophilic disorder is *true*?

A. Pedophilic disorder is found in 10%–12% of the male population.
B. There is no evidence that neurodevelopmental perturbation in utero increases the probability of development of a pedophilic orientation.

C. Adult males with pedophilia always report that they were sexually abused as children.

D. The individual is at least age 16 years and at least 5 years older than the child or children.

Correct Answer: D. The individual is at least age 16 years and at least 5 years older than the child or children.

Explanation: The population prevalence of individuals whose presentations meet the full criteria for pedophilic disorder is unknown but is likely less than 3% among men in international studies. The population prevalence of pedophilic disorder in women is even more uncertain, but it is likely a small fraction of the prevalence in men.

Because pedophilia is a necessary condition for pedophilic disorder, any factor that increases the probability of pedophilia also increases the risk of pedophilic disorder. There is some evidence that neurodevelopmental perturbation in utero increases the probability of development of a pedophilic interest.

Adult men with pedophilia sometimes report that they were sexually abused as children. It is unclear, however, whether this correlation reflects a causal influence of childhood sexual abuse on adult pedophilia.

19.4—Pedophilic Disorder / diagnostic criteria (pp. 792–793); Prevalence; Development and Course; Risk and Prognostic Factors (pp. 794–795)

19.5 Which of the following statements about pedophilic disorder is *true?*

A. The extensive use of pornography depicting prepubescent or early pubescent children is not a useful diagnostic indicator of pedophilic disorder.

B. Pedophilic disorder is stable over the course of a lifetime.

C. There is an association between pedophilic disorder and antisocial personality disorder.

D. Although normophilic sexual interest declines with age, pedophilic sexual interest remains constant.

Correct Answer: C. There is an association between pedophilic disorder and antisocial personality disorder.

Explanation: There appears to be an interaction between pedophilia and antisocial personality traits such as callousness, impulsivity, and a willingness to take risks without adequate regard for the consequences. Men with pedophilic interest and antisocial personality traits are more likely to act out sexually with children and thus qualify for a diagnosis of pedophilic disorder. Thus, antisocial personality disorder may be considered a risk factor for pedophilic disorder in males with pedophilia.

Laboratory measures of sexual interest, in terms of psychophysiological responses to sexual stimuli depicting children, which are sometimes useful in diagnosing pedophilic disorder in men, are not necessarily useful in diagnosing this disorder in women because there has been very limited research on the assessment of pedophilic sexual interest in women.

Psychophysiological measures of sexual interest may sometimes be useful when an individual's history suggests the possible presence of pedophilic disorder but the individual denies strong or preferential attraction to children. The most thoroughly researched and longest used of such measures is penile plethysmography, although the sensitivity and specificity of diagnosis may vary across sites, which frequently use different stimuli, procedures, and scoring.

Pedophilia per se appears to be a lifelong condition. Pedophilic disorder, however, necessarily includes other elements that may change over time with or without treatment: subjective distress (e.g., guilt, shame, intense sexual frustration, feelings of isolation) or psychosocial impairment or the propensity to act out sexually with children, or both. Therefore, the course of pedophilic disorder may fluctuate, or the intensity might increase or decrease with age.

Adults with pedophilic disorder may report an awareness of sexual interest in children that preceded engaging in sexual behavior involving children or self-identification as an individual with pedophilia. Advanced age is as likely to similarly diminish the frequency of sexual behavior involving children as it does other paraphilically motivated and nonparaphilic sexual behavior.

19.5—Pedophilic Disorder (pp. 794–795)

19.6 A 35-year-old woman tells her therapist that she has recently become intensely aroused while watching movies in which people are tortured and that she regularly fantasizes about torturing people while masturbating. She is not distressed by these thoughts and denies ever having acted on these new fantasies; however, she fantasizes about these activities several times a day. Which of the following best summarizes the diagnostic implications of this patient's presentation?

A. She meets all of the criteria for sexual sadism disorder.
B. She does not meet the criteria for sexual sadism disorder because the fantasies are not sexual in nature.
C. She does not meet the criteria for sexual sadism disorder because she has never acted on the fantasies.
D. She does not meet the criteria for sexual sadism disorder because the interest and arousal began after age 35.

Correct Answer: C. She does not meet the criteria for sexual sadism disorder because she has never acted on the fantasies.

Explanation: The diagnostic criteria for sexual sadism disorder specify the presence of recurrent and intense sexual arousal from the physical or psychological suffering of another person, as manifested by fantasies, urges, or behaviors, over a period of at least 6 months (Criterion A). The individual has acted on these sexual urges with a nonconsenting person, or the sexual urges or fantasies cause clinically significant distress or impairment in social, occupational, or other important areas of functioning (Criterion B).

The diagnostic criteria for sexual sadism disorder are intended to apply both to individuals who freely admit to having such paraphilic interests and to those who deny any sexual interest in the physical or psychological suffering of another individual despite substantial objective evidence to the contrary. Individuals who openly acknowledge intense sexual interest in the physical or psychological suffering of others are referred to as *admitting individuals*. If these individuals also report psychosocial difficulties because of their sexual attractions or preferences for the physical or psychological suffering of another individual, they may be diagnosed with sexual sadism disorder. In contrast, if admitting individuals declare no distress, exemplified by anxiety, obsessions, guilt, or shame, about these paraphilic impulses and are not hampered by them in pursuing other goals, and their self-reported, psychiatric, or legal histories indicate that they do not act on them with nonconsenting persons, then they could be ascertained as having sadistic sexual interest, but their presentation would not meet criteria for sexual sadism disorder.

19.6—Paraphilic Disorders / Sexual Sadism Disorder (pp. 790–791)

19.7   While intoxicated at a Mardi Gras celebration, a 19-year-old woman lifts her blouse and bra as a float goes by to get beads. The event appears on a cable news program watched by friends of her parents, who inform her parents. They insist that she get a psychiatric evaluation 2 months after the vacation. She denies any other similar events in her life but admits that the experience was "sort of sexy." She is currently extremely anxious and distressed about her parents' anger at her and their refusal to allow her to attend parties or go away on vacation until she has an evaluation. She reports that she is unable to attend classes or to focus on her work at college. What is the most appropriate diagnosis?

A. Exhibitionistic disorder.
B. Frotteuristic disorder.
C. Voyeuristic disorder.
D. Adjustment disorder.

Correct Answer: D. Adjustment disorder.

Explanation: This woman's single episode of exposing herself while intoxicated does not qualify for a diagnosis of exhibitionistic disorder because she does not meet the diagnostic criteria—specifically, a 6-month history of recurrent and intense sexual arousal from the exposure of one's genitals to an unsuspecting person, as manifested by fantasies, urges, or behaviors (Criterion A). The diagnostic criteria for exhibitionistic disorder can apply both to individuals who more or less freely disclose this paraphilia and to those who categorically deny any sexual arousal from exposing their genitals to unsuspecting persons despite substantial objective evidence to the contrary. If disclosing individuals also report psychosocial difficulties because of their sexual attractions or preferences for exposing, they may be diagnosed with exhibitionistic disorder. In contrast, if they declare no distress (exemplified by absence of anxiety, obsessions, and guilt or shame about these paraphilic impulses) and are not impaired by this sexual interest in other important areas of functioning, and their self-reported, psychiatric, or legal histories indicate that they do not act on them, they could be ascertained as having exhibitionistic sexual interest but not be diagnosed with exhibitionistic disorder. The population prevalence of individuals whose presentations meet the full criteria for exhibitionistic disorder is unknown, although the disorder is highly unusual in women. Exhibitionistic acts, however, are not uncommon, and single sexually arousing exhibitionistic acts occur up to half as often among women compared with men.

This young woman's current distress is related not to the exhibitionistic act but rather to her parents' attitude and behavior. Her level of distress is out of proportion to the restrictions placed on her by her parents, and it interferes with her functioning. She meets criteria for an adjustment disorder (Criteria A and B).

19.7—Exhibitionistic Disorder / diagnostic criteria; Development and Course; Gender-Related Diagnostic Issues; Differential Diagnosis (pp. 783–785); Adjustment Disorders / diagnostic criteria (p. 319)

19.8   A 16-year-old male tells his therapist that he can see into the bedroom of a woman across the street from his apartment house. He has been watching her since she moved into the apartment 6 months ago. He can see the woman dressing and undressing, which he finds sexually arousing. He has fantasies about the woman compelling him to have sex with her. He expresses no guilt about this because the woman has no shade on the window. The therapist requests a psychiatric consultation to evaluate the patient for a paraphilia. Which of the following is the correct diagnosis?

A. Voyeuristic disorder.
B. Unspecified paraphilic disorder.
C. Other specified paraphilic disorder.
D. Normal adolescent sexual behavior.

Correct Answer: D. Normal adolescent sexual behavior.

Explanation: Adolescence and puberty generally increase sexual curiosity and activity. To reduce the risk of pathologizing normative sexual interest and behavior during pubertal adolescence, the minimum age for the diagnosis of voyeuristic disorder is 18 years (Criterion C).

Individuals with voyeurism experience recurrent, intense sexual arousal from the act of observing an unsuspecting person who is naked, in the process of disrobing, or engaging in sexual activity. Unless the individual acts on these urges with an unsuspecting person (e.g., surreptitiously peeping through a neighbor's window) or unless there is accompanying clinically significant distress or impairment in social, occupational, or other important areas of functioning, a diagnosis of voyeuristic disorder is not warranted.

19.8—Voyeuristic Disorder / Diagnostic Features / Differential Diagnosis (pp. 781–782)

19.9 During an emergency department visit for asthma, a man has indications of being whipped. When asked about the welts, he reports that he self-flagellated during a religious ceremony. A psychiatric consultation is requested, and the man admits that he often fantasizes about being beaten and watches pornography of people being beaten, which is sexually arousing for him. He asks his partner to beat him and cannot achieve an erection if he is not beaten or humiliated. Which of the following describes the situation most accurately?

A. Sexual sadism disorder.
B. Sexual masochism disorder.
C. Voyeuristic disorder.
D. Masochistic personality disorder.

Correct answer: B. Sexual masochism disorder.

Explanation: The diagnostic criteria for sexual masochism disorder are intended to apply to individuals who freely admit to having such paraphilic interests. Such individuals openly acknowledge intense sexual arousal from the act of being humiliated, beaten, bound, or otherwise made to suffer, as manifested by fantasies, urges, or behaviors. If these individuals also report psychosocial difficulties because of their sexual attractions or preferences for being humiliated, beaten, bound, or otherwise made to suffer, they may be diagnosed with sexual masochism disorder.

The term bondage-domination-sadism-masochism (BDSM) is broadly used to refer to a wide range of behaviors that individuals with sexual masochism and/or sexual sadism (as well as other individuals with similar sexual interests) engage in, such as restraints or restriction, discipline, spanking, slapping, sensory deprivation (e.g., using blindfolds), and dominance-submission role-play involving themes such as master/enslaved person, owner/pet, or kidnapper/victim.

The extensive use of pornography involving the act of being humiliated, beaten, bound, or otherwise made to suffer is sometimes an associated feature of sexual masochism disorder.

It is important to distinguish self-harming behaviors that occur during collectively accepted religious and spiritual practices from sadomasochistic behavior conducted for sexual arousal. For example, collective rituals in various religions and societies include suspension from hooks, self-flagellation, self-mortification, and other painful ordeals. The role of sexual arousal or pleasure in these practices remains unknown.

There is no DSM-5-TR diagnosis of masochistic personality disorder.

19.9—Sexual Masochism Disorder / Diagnostic Features / Associated Features / Culture-Related Diagnostic Features (pp. 788–789); Personality Disorders (p. 733)

19.10 Following a syncopal episode, a man is examined in the emergency department and is found to be wearing women's undergarments. He is unable to give a history, and his wife is contacted. When asked about her husband's clothing, she reports that he has worn women's underwear on and off for years, which she finds distressing. She notes that they cannot have sex if he does not cross-dress. Except for wearing the clothing occasionally out of the house, and prior to sex, she states that he is otherwise a "regular guy." Which of the following diagnoses would be most appropriate?

A. Fetishistic disorder.
B. Gender dysphoria.
C. Transvestism.
D. Transvestic disorder.

Correct Answer: D. Transvestic disorder.

Explanation: The diagnosis of transvestic disorder does not apply to all individuals who dress as the opposite sex, even those who do so habitually. It applies to individuals whose cross-dressing or thoughts of cross-dressing are always or often accompanied by sexual excitement (Criterion A) and who are emotionally distressed by this pattern or for whom it impairs their social or interpersonal functioning (Criterion B). The cross-dressing may involve only one or two articles of clothing (e.g., for men, it may pertain only to women's undergarments), or it may involve dressing completely in the inner and outer garments of the other sex and (in men) may include the use of women's wigs and makeup.

In some cases, the course of transvestic disorder is continuous, and in others it is episodic. It is not rare for men with transvestic disorder to lose interest in cross-dressing when they first fall in love with a woman and begin a relationship, but such abatement usually proves temporary. When the desire to cross-dress returns, so does the associated distress.

Transvestic disorder in men is often accompanied by autogynephilia (i.e., a man's paraphilic tendency to be sexually aroused by the thought or image of himself as a woman). Autogynephilic fantasies and behaviors may focus on the idea of exhibiting female physiological functions (e.g., lactation, menstruation), engaging in stereotypically feminine behavior (e.g., knitting), or possessing female anatomy (e.g., breasts).

Some cases of transvestic disorder progress to gender dysphoria. The men in these cases, who may be indistinguishable from others with transvestic disorder in adolescence or early childhood, gradually develop desires to remain in the woman's role for longer periods and to feminize their anatomy. The development of gender dysphoria is usually accompanied by a (self-reported) reduction or elimination of sexual arousal in association with cross-dressing.

Individuals with transvestism experience recurrent and intense sexual arousal from cross-dressing. Unless the fantasies, sexual urges, or behaviors involving cross-dressing are accompanied by clinically significant distress or impairment in social, occupational, or other important areas of functioning, a diagnosis of transvestic disorder is not warranted.

Fetishistic disorder may resemble transvestic disorder, in particular in men with fetishism who put on women's undergarments while masturbating with them. Distinguishing transvestic disorder depends on the individual's specific thoughts during such activity (e.g., are there any ideas of being a woman, being like a woman, or being dressed as a woman?) and on the presence of other fetishes (e.g., soft, silky fabrics, whether they are used for garments or for something else).

Individuals with transvestic disorder do not report an incongruence between their experienced gender and their assigned gender or a desire to be of the other gender; and they typically do not have a history of childhood cross-gender behaviors, which would be present in individuals with gender dysphoria. Individuals with a presentation that meets full criteria for transvestic disorder as well as gender dysphoria should be given both diagnoses.

19.10—Transvestic Disorder / Diagnostic Features / Associated Features / Differential Diagnosis (pp. 799–800)

CHAPTER 20

Medication-Induced Movement Disorders and Other Adverse Effects of Medication

20.1. Which of the following is *not* known to be a consistent risk factor in the development of medication-induced parkinsonism (MIP)?

A. Male sex.
B. Older age.
C. HIV disease.
D. Family history of Parkinson's disease,

Correct Answer: A. Male sex.

Explanation: Consistent risk factors for MIP are female sex, older age, cognitive impairment, other concurrent neurological conditions, HIV infection, family history of Parkinson's disease, and severe psychiatric disease. MIP secondary to antipsychotic use is also reported in children. The risk of MIP is reduced if individuals are taking anticholinergic medications.

20.1—Medication-Induced Parkinsonism / Differential Diagnosis (p. 809)

20.2. Neuroleptic malignant syndrome is a potentially fatal syndrome with an incidence rate of 0.01%–0.02% among individuals treated with neuroleptics. Which of the following is not a sign or symptom of neuroleptic malignant syndrome?

A. Hyperthermia.
B. Generalized rigidity.
C. Elevated creatine kinase.
D. Unchanged mental status.

Correct Answer D: Unchanged mental status.

Explanation: Individuals with neuroleptic malignant syndrome have generally been exposed to a dopamine antagonist within 72 hours prior to symptom development. Hyperthermia (>104°F or >38°C) on at least two occasions, measured orally, associated with profuse diaphoresis, is a distinguishing feature of neuroleptic malignant syndrome, setting it apart from other neurological side effects of other antipsychotic medications and other dopamine receptor blocking agents. Generalized rigidity, described as "lead pipe" in its most severe form and usually unresponsive to antiparkinsonian agents, is a cardinal feature of the disorder and may be associated with other neurological symptoms (e.g., tremor, sialorrhea, akinesia, dystonia, trismus, myoclonus, dysarthria, dysphagia, rhabdomyolysis). Creatine kinase elevation of at least four times the upper limit of normal is commonly seen. Changes in mental status, characterized by delirium or altered consciousness, ranging from stupor to coma, are often an early sign of neuroleptic malignant syndrome.

20.2—Neuroleptic Malignant Syndrome (p. 810)

20.3. A 22-year-old patient with schizophrenia and no comorbid medical issues is admitted to an inpatient unit for treatment of a first episode of psychosis. Risperidone 1 mg is started for paranoia and derogatory auditory hallucinations. Within 24 hours, the patient begins experiencing an oculogyric crisis. The muscle contractions are relieved by an injection of diphenhydramine 50 mg IM. Which of the following is the best explanation for what happened to this patient?

A. Neuroleptic malignant syndrome.
B. Medication-induced acute dystonia.
C. Medication-induced acute akathisia.
D. Tardive dystonia.

Correct Answer: B. Medication-induced acute dystonia.

Explanation: The essential feature of medication-induced acute dystonia is sustained abnormal muscle contractions (increased muscle tone) and postures that develop in association with use of a medication known to cause acute dystonia. Any medication that blocks dopamine D_2-like receptors can induce an acute dystonic reaction (ADR). Most commonly, ADRs occur after exposure to antipsychotics and antiemetic and promotility agents. Dystonic reactions most commonly affect head and neck muscles but can extend to upper and lower limbs or trunk. At least 50% of individuals develop ADR signs and symptoms within 24–48 hours of starting or rapidly raising the dose of antipsychotic medication or other dopamine receptor–blocking agent or reducing a medication being used to treat or prevent acute extrapyramidal symptoms (e.g., anticholinergic agents).

20.3—Medication-Induced Acute Dystonia (p. 812)

20.4. A 55-year-old patient with schizoaffective disorder presents to the emergency department in severe distress. His history includes feeling anxious and edgy for the past week and an inability to unwind at the end of the day. He is unable to sit still and has developed insomnia. The patient is observed to be shifting on the examination table and shaking both legs throughout the examination. His medication history includes risperidone 2 mg PO bid, which was increased from 2 mg daily a week earlier. Which of the following best explains what is happening to the patient?

A. Tobacco withdrawal.
B. Histrionic personality disorder.
C. Medication-induced acute akathisia.
D. Serotonin syndrome.

Correct Answer: C. Medication-induced acute akathisia.

Explanation: The essential features of medication-induced acute akathisia are subjective complaints of restlessness and at least one of the following observed movements: fidgety movements or swinging of the legs while seated, rocking from foot to foot or "walking on the spot" while standing, pacing to relieve the restlessness, or an inability to sit or stand still for at least several minutes. The subjective complaints include a sense of inner restlessness, most often in the legs; a compulsion to move one's legs; distress if one is asked not to move one's legs; and dysphoria and anxiety.

20.4—Medication-Induced Acute Akathisia (p. 813)

20.5. Which of the following is a true statement about tardive dyskinesias?

A. Tardive dyskinesias do not include movements that develop within 1 month after stopping an oral antipsychotic medication.
B. The overall prevalence of tardive dyskinesia in individuals who have been treated with long-term antipsychotic medications is between 10% and 20%.
C. Men are more likely to develop tardive dyskinesia than women.
D. Tardive dyskinesia includes several different types of movements.

Correct answer: D. Tardive dyskinesia includes several different types of movements.

Explanation: The essential features of tardive dyskinesia are abnormal, involuntary movements of the tongue, jaw, trunk, or extremities that develop in association with the use of medications that block postsynaptic dopamine receptors, such as first- and second-generation antipsychotic medications and other medications, such as metoclopramide for gastrointestinal disorders. The movements are present for at least 4 weeks and may be choreiform (rapid, jerky, nonrepetitive), athetoid (slow, sinuous, continual), or semirhythmic (e.g., stereotypies) in nature; however, the movements are distinctly different from the rhythmic (3–6 Hz) tremors commonly seen in medication-induced parkinsonism. Tardive dyskinesia develops during exposure to the antipsychotic medication or other dopamine-blocking agent or within 4 weeks of withdrawal from an oral agent (or within 8 weeks of withdrawal from a long-acting injectable agent). The overall prevalence of tardive dyskinesia in individuals who have received long-term antipsychotic medication treatment ranges from 20% to 30%. There is no obvious gender difference in the susceptibility to tardive dyskinesia, although the risk may be somewhat greater in postmenopausal women.

20.5—Tardive Dyskinesia (pp. 814–815)

20.6. A 41-year-old patient with recurrent depression and anxiety has been taking medication for a year. She has been experiencing "brain zaps," nausea, terrible headaches, and anxiety for the past 3 days. The psychiatrist assesses for any other symptoms and asks about medication adherence, learning that the patient stopped taking her antidepressant "cold turkey" a few days ago. Which of the following medications did the patient likely stop taking?

A. Venlafaxine.
B. Fluoxetine.
C. Thyroid hormone.
D. Lithium.

Correct Answer: A. Venlafaxine.

Explanation: Discontinuation symptoms may occur following treatment with all types of antidepressants. The incidence of this syndrome depends on the dosage and half-life of the medication being taken as well as the rate at which the medication is tapered. The short-acting antidepressants, paroxetine and venlafaxine, are the agents most commonly associated with discontinuation symptoms. Fluoxetine is known to have a long half-life and therefore rarely causes discontinuation symptoms. Both thyroid hormone and lithium are commonly used augmentation strategies when treating depression but are not used as primary agents to treat depression.

20.6—Antidepressant Discontinuation Syndrome (p. 818)

20.7. Which of the following factors does *not* increase the risk of lithium tremor?

A. Anxiety.
B. High serum lithium levels.
C. Personal or family history of tremor.
D. Young age.

Correct answer: D. Young age.

Explanation: A variety of factors may increase the risk of lithium tremor. These factors include increasing age, high serum lithium levels, concurrent use of antidepressant or antipsychotic medication or another dopamine receptor blocking agent, excessive caffeine intake, personal or family history of tremor, presence of alcohol use disorder, and associated anxiety.

20.7—Medication-Induced Postural Tremor (p. 817)

20.8. Which of the following is *not* true about medication-induced postural tremor?

A. The essential feature is a fine tremor occurring during attempts to maintain a posture and developing in association with the use of medication.
B. The tremor is a regular, rhythmic oscillation of the limbs, head, mouth, or tongue with a frequency between 3 and 6 Hz.
C. Medication-induced postural tremor is not diagnosed if the tremor is better accounted for by medication-induced parkinsonism.
D. The tremor can be an early feature of serotonin syndrome.

Correct Answer: B. The tremor is a regular, rhythmic oscillation of the limbs, head, mouth, or tongue with a frequency between 3 and 6 Hz.

Explanation: The tremor associated with medication-induced postural tremor is a regular rhythmic oscillation of the limbs (most commonly hands and fingers), head, mouth, or tongue, most commonly with a frequency between 8 and 12 cycles per second. In contrast, the tremor related to medication-induced parkinsonism is usually lower in frequency (3–6 Hz), is worse at rest, and is suppressed during intentional movement and usually occurs in association with other symptoms of medication-induced parkinsonism (e.g., akinesia, rigidity).

20.8—Medication-Induced Postural Tremor, Differential Diagnosis (p. 817)

CHAPTER 21

Assessment Measures (DSM-5-TR Section III)

21.1 Which of the following factors about traditional categorical diagnosis supports the incorporation of dimensional concepts?

A. Specific treatment guidance.
B. Stable, definitive diagnoses.
C. Low rates of comorbidity.
D. Frequent use of *other* or *unspecified* diagnoses.

Correct Answer: D. Frequent use of *other* or *unspecified* diagnoses.

Explanation: A growing body of scientific evidence favors dimensional concepts in the diagnosis of mental disorders. Limitations of a categorical approach to diagnosis include the failure to find zones of rarity between diagnoses (i.e., delineation of mental disorders from one another by natural boundaries), need for intermediate categories such as schizoaffective disorder, high rates of comorbidity, need for frequent use of *other* or *unspecified* diagnoses, relative lack of utility in furthering identification of unique antecedent validators for most mental disorders, and lack of treatment specificity for the various diagnostic categories.

From both clinical and research perspectives, there is a need for a more dimensional approach that can be combined with DSM-5-TR's set of categorical diagnoses to better capture the heterogeneity in the presentation of various mental and substance use disorders. Such an approach allows clinicians or others to better communicate particular variation of features that apply to presentations that meet criteria for a disorder. Such features include differential severity of individual symptoms (including symptoms that are part of the diagnostic features as well as those that are associated with the disorder) as measured by intensity, duration, and impact on functioning. This combined approach also allows clinicians or others to identify conditions that do not meet criteria for a disorder but are severe and disabling and in need of treatment.

453

21.1—Assessment Measures / chapter introduction (p. 841)

21.2   Which of the following statements accurately describes the World Health Organization Disability Assessment Schedule, Version 2.0 (WHODAS 2.0)?

   A. It focuses only on disabilities due to psychiatric illness.
   B. It assesses a patient's ability to perform activities in six functional areas.
   C. It may not be completed on behalf of a patient with impaired capacity.
   D. It primarily measures physical disability.

   Correct Answer: B. It assesses a patient's ability to perform activities in six functional areas.

   Explanation: The adult self-administered version of the WHODAS 2.0 is a 36-item measure that assesses disability in adults ages 18 years and older. It has been validated across numerous cultures worldwide and has demonstrated sensitivity to change. It assesses disability across six domains, including understanding and communicating, getting around, self-care, getting along with people, life activities (e.g., household, work, and/or school activities), and participation in society. If the adult individual is of impaired capacity and is unable to complete the form (e.g., a patient with major neurocognitive disorder), a knowledgeable informant may complete the proxy-administered version of the measure, which is available at www.psychiatry.org/dsm5.

21.2—World Health Organization Disability Assessment Schedule 2.0 (p. 854)

21.3   What is the function of the DSM-5 Level 1 Cross-Cutting Symptom Measure?

   A. It assesses a patient's ability to perform activities in six areas of daily life functioning.
   B. It assesses the presence and frequency of symptoms in 13 psychiatric domains.
   C. It clarifies symptoms present *at the time of the interview* only.
   D. It is intended primarily as a research tool.

   Correct Answer: B. It assesses the presence and frequency of symptoms in 13 psychiatric domains.

   Explanation: The DSM-5 Level 1 Cross-Cutting Symptom Measure is a patient- or informant-rated measure that assesses mental health domains that are important across psychiatric diagnoses. It is intended to help clinicians identify additional areas of inquiry that may have significant impact on the individual's treatment and prognosis. In addition, the measure may be used to track changes in the individual's symptom presentation over time.

   The adult version of the self-rated DSM-5 Level 1 Cross-Cutting Symptom Measure consists of 23 questions that assess 13 psychiatric domains, including depression, anger, mania, anxiety, somatic symptoms, suicidal ideation, psychosis, sleep problems, memory, repetitive thoughts and behaviors, dissociation, personality functioning, and substance use. Each item inquires about how much (or how often) the individual has been bothered by the specific symptom during the past 2 weeks. If the individual has impaired capacity and is unable to complete the form (e.g., an individual with dementia), a knowledgeable adult informant may complete this measure. The measure was found to be clinically useful and to have good reliability in the DSM-5 field trials that were conducted in adult clinical samples across the United States and in Canada

21.3—Cross-Cutting Symptom Measures / Level 1 Cross-Cutting Symptom Measure (p. 843)

21.4   In clinician review of item scores on the DSM-5 Level 1 Cross-Cutting Symptom Measure for an adult patient, a rating of "slight" would call for further inquiry if found for any item in which of the following domains?

A. Depression.
B. Mania.
C. Anger.
D. Suicidal ideation.

Correct Answer: D. Suicidal ideation.

Explanation: On the adult self-rated version of the DSM-5 Level 1 Cross-Cutting Symptom Measure, each item is rated on a 5-point scale (0=none or not at all; 1=slight or rare, less than a day or two; 2=mild or several days; 3=moderate or more than half the days; and 4=severe or nearly every day). Whereas for most domains, a rating of *mild* (i.e., 2) or greater for any item within the domain is the threshold to guide further inquiry, for the substance use, suicidal ideation, and psychosis domains, a rating of *slight* (i.e., 1) or greater is the threshold for pursuing additional inquiry and follow-up to determine if a more detailed assessment is needed (which may include the Level 2 Cross-Cutting Symptom assessment for that domain).

21.4—Cross-Cutting Symptom Measures / Level 1 Cross-Cutting Symptom Measure / Scoring and Interpretation (pp. 843–846)

21.5   If a parent answers "I don't know" to the question "In the past TWO (2) WEEKS, has your child had an alcoholic beverage (beer, wine, liquor, etc.)?" in the parent/guardian-rated version of the DSM-5 Level 1 Cross-Cutting Symptom Measure, what is the appropriate clinician response?

A. Ask the child questions from the substance use domain of the child-rated Level 2 Cross-Cutting Symptom Measure.
B. Rely on other questions from the substance use domain and do not incorporate this answer into the final score.

C. Ask the parent to ask the child, and schedule a follow-up visit to readminister the questionnaire.

D. Consider reporting the parent to child protective services.

Correct Answer: A. Ask the child questions from the substance use domain of the child-rated Level 2 Cross-Cutting Symptom Measure.

Explanation: On the parent/guardian-rated version of the DSM-5 Level 1 Cross-Cutting Symptom Measure for children ages 6–17, items in 2 of the 12 domains—suicidal ideation/attempts and substance use—are each rated on a "Yes, No, or Don't Know" scale. A parent or guardian's rating of "Don't Know" on the suicidal ideation, suicide attempt, and any of the substance use items, especially for children ages 11–17 years, would warrant additional probing of the issues with the child, including using the child-rated Level 2 Cross-Cutting Symptom Measure for the relevant domain (see Table 2).

21.5—Cross-Cutting Symptom Measures / Level 1 Cross-Cutting Symptom Measure; Table 2 (Parent/guardian-rated DSM-5 Level 1 Cross-Cutting Symptom Measure for child age 6–17) (pp. 849–850); Level 2 Cross-Cutting Symptom Measures (p. 846)

21.6   Which of the following is *not* assessed by the Clinician-Rated Dimensions of Psychosis Symptom Severity measure?

A. Social function.
B. Cognitive function.
C. Depression.
D. Mania.

Correct Answer: A. Social function.

Explanation: The Clinician-Rated Dimensions of Psychosis Symptom Severity measure provides scales for the dimensional assessment of the primary symptoms of psychosis, including hallucinations, delusions, disorganized speech, abnormal psychomotor behavior, and negative symptoms. A scale for the dimensional assessment of cognitive impairment is also included. Many individuals with psychotic disorders have impairments in a range of cognitive domains, which predict functional abilities and prognosis. In addition, scales for dimensional assessment of depression and mania are provided, which may alert clinicians to co-occurring mood pathology. The severity of mood symptoms in psychosis has prognostic value and can guide treatment.

21.6—Clinician-Rated Dimensions of Psychosis Symptom Severity (p. 851)

21.7   When reviewing a patient's responses to items on the World Health Organization Disability Assessment Schedule 2.0 (WHODAS 2.0), the clinician notes that in response to the question "How much time did you spend on your health condition or its consequences?" the patient answered, "Hardly any." The clinician, who has treated the patient for several years, is surprised to see this because she is quite certain that the patient spends most of the day dealing with health concerns. What is the appropriate action for this clinician?

A. Leave the patient's response as is and score accordingly.
B. Indicate on the form that the clinician is making a correction and revise the score.
C. Attempt to obtain additional information from family members in order to clarify the discrepancy.
D. Take the average of the patient's and clinician's differing scores and use that for the final score.

Correct Answer: B. Indicate on the form that the clinician is making a correction and revise the score.

Explanation: The adult self-administered version of the WHODAS 2.0 is a 36-item measure that assesses disability in adults ages 18 years and older. It has been validated across numerous cultures worldwide and has demonstrated sensitivity to change. The clinician is asked to review the individual's response on each item on the measure during the clinical interview and to indicate the self-reported score for each item in the section provided for "Clinician Use Only." If the clinician determines that the score on an item should be different on the basis of the clinical interview and other information available, they may indicate a corrected score in the raw item score box.

21.7—World Health Organization Disability Assessment Schedule 2.0 (p. 854) / Additional Scoring and Interpretation Guidance for DSM-5-TR Users (p. 855)

21.8   The cross-cutting symptom measures in DSM-5 are modeled on which of the following?

A. The International Classification of Functioning, Disability, and Health.
B. The general medical review of systems.
C. The Brief Psychiatric Rating Scale.
D. The Clinical Global Impression Scale.

Correct Answer: B. The general medical review of systems.

Explanation: *Cross-cutting symptom measures* modeled on general medicine's review of systems can serve as an approach for reviewing critical psychopathological domains. The general medical review of systems is crucial to detecting subtle changes in different organ systems that can facilitate diagnosis and treatment. A similar review of various mental systems (or domains), which is the goal of the cross-cutting symptom measures, can aid in a more comprehensive mental status assessment of individuals at the initial evaluation. The review of mental systems can systematically draw attention to signs and symptoms of other domains of mental health and functioning that may be important to the individual's care.

21.8—Assessment Measures/ chapter introduction (pp. 841–842)

21.9   Which of the following is an intended use of severity measures in DSM-5-TR?

A. To evaluate transdiagnostic symptom severity.
B. To quantify treatment-associated side effects.
C. To establish any psychiatric diagnosis.
D. To estimate severity in patients who do not meet full diagnostic criteria for a particular disorder.

Correct Answer: D. To estimate severity in patients who do not meet full diagnostic criteria for a particular disorder.

Explanation: *Severity measures* are disorder-specific, corresponding closely to the criteria that constitute the disorder definition. They may be administered to individuals who have received a diagnosis or who have a clinically significant syndrome that falls short of meeting full criteria for a diagnosis (e.g., use of the Clinician-Rated Dimensions of Psychosis Symptom Severity in individuals whose symptoms meet criteria for schizophrenia). Some of the assessments are self-rated, whereas others are rated by the clinician on the basis of observation of the individual. As with the cross-cutting symptom measures, these measures can be administered both at initial interview and over time to track the severity of the individual's disorder and response to treatment. These assessments help operationalize symptom frequency, intensity, or duration; overall symptom severity; or symptom type (e.g., depression, anxiety, sleep disturbance) for many, although not all, DSM-5-TR diagnoses (e.g., generalized anxiety disorder, social anxiety disorder, psychotic disorders, posttraumatic stress disorder, autism spectrum disorder, social (pragmatic) communication disorder). Data obtained from use of these disorder-specific measures can assist with diagnosis and inform symptom monitoring and treatment planning.

21.9—Assessment Measures / chapter introduction (p. 842)

CHAPTER 22

Culture and Psychiatric Diagnosis (DSM-5-TR Section III)

22.1   Updated in DSM-5-TR, the expanded Outline for Cultural Formulation assesses which of the following items?

A. Cultural preferences in leisure and entertainment choices.
B. Risk factors for specific psychiatric diagnoses.
C. Cultural features of vulnerability and resilience.
D. Definitions of cultural groups and their unified belief structures.

Correct Answer: C. Cultural features of vulnerability and resilience.

Explanation: Although cultural aspects of leisure-time activity may have distal relevance to mental health, leisure activity is not a major category of the DSM-5-TR Outline for Cultural Formulation. *Cultural identity of the individual* includes aspects of ethnic, racial, linguistic, and cultural factors with which the individual identifies. *Cultural conceptualizations of distress* involve culturally specific ways of understanding and coping with distress. *Psychosocial stressors and cultural features of vulnerability and resilience* involve culturally specific stressors and social support systems and related concepts, as well as culturally bound conceptions of work and disability. Approaches to the patient-physician relationship may vary significantly across different cultures. It is essential to understand these differences if one is to establish a helping relationship.

22.1—Outline for Cultural Formulation (pp. 860–862)

22.2   *Cultural identity of the individual* is one of several categories in the DSM-5-TR Outline for Cultural Formulation. Which of the following is a feature of cultural identity of the individual?

A. How cultural constructs influence the individual's experiences of symptoms or psychological problems.
B. Religious affiliation and spirituality.

C. Social determinants of mental health.

D. Prior experiences of racism and discrimination in mental health care.

Correct Answer: B. Religious affiliation and spirituality.

Explanation: In the cultural identity of the individual section of the Outline for Cultural Formulation, the provider is asked to describe the individual's demographic (e.g., age, gender, ethnoracial background) or other socially and culturally defined characteristics that may influence interpersonal relationships; access to resources; and developmental and current challenges, conflicts, or predicaments. Other clinically relevant aspects of identity may include religious affiliation and spirituality, socioeconomic class, caste, personal and family places of birth and growing up, migrant status, occupation, and sexual orientation, among others. Note which aspects of identity are prioritized by the individual and how they interact (intersectionality).

In the cultural concepts of distress section, providers are asked to describe the cultural constructs that influence how the individual experiences, understands, and communicates their symptoms or problems to others. These constructs include cultural idioms of distress, cultural explanations or perceived causes, and cultural syndromes. The psychosocial stressors and cultural features of vulnerability and resilience section describes key stressors, challenges, and supports in the individual's social environment (which may include both local and distant events). These include social determinants of the individual's mental health such as access to resources (e.g., housing, transportation) and opportunities (e.g., education, employment); exposure to racism, discrimination, and systemic institutional stigmatization; and social marginalization or exclusion (structural violence). Levels of functioning, disability, and resilience should be assessed in light of the individual's cultural background. Finally, a section of the Outline for Cultural Formulation is dedicated to considering how the ways that individuals and clinicians are positioned socially and perceive each other in terms of social categories may influence the assessment process. Experiences of racism and discrimination in the larger society may impede establishing trust and safety in the clinical diagnostic encounter.

22.2—Outline for Cultural Formulation (pp. 861–862)

22.3   In what type of clinical setting is the Cultural Formulation Interview (CFI) meant to be used?

A. Any setting.

B. Outpatient clinic.

C. Emergency department.

D. Inpatient hospital.

Correct Answer: A. Any setting.

Explanation: The "Cultural Formulation" section presents an outline for a systematic person-centered cultural assessment that is designed to be used by any clinician providing services to any individual in any care setting. This section also includes an interview protocol, the Cultural Formulation Interview, that operationalizes these components. Symptom presentations, interpretations of the illness or predicament that precipitates care, and help-seeking expectations are always influenced by individuals' cultural backgrounds and sociocultural contexts. A person-centered cultural assessment can help improve the care of every individual, regardless of their background. Cultural formulation may be especially helpful for individuals who are affected by health care disparities driven by systemic disadvantage and discrimination.

22.3—Culture and Psychiatric Diagnosis / chapter introduction (p. 859)

22.4 In which of the following clinical situations is the Cultural Formulation Interview (CFI) meant to be helpful?

A. The clinician and patient have a shared belief system regarding the nature of the problem and the appropriate therapeutic approach.
B. The patient presents with a symptom complex that is distressing but does not fit any DSM-5-TR diagnosis.
C. The clinician and the patient speak different languages.
D. The clinician is finding it difficult to identify the correct code for the patient's primary clinical diagnosis.

Correct Answer: B. The patient presents with a symptom complex that is distressing but does not fit any DSM-5-TR diagnosis.

Explanation: The CFI can be used in the initial assessment of individuals of any age, in any clinical setting, regardless of the cultural background of the individual or of the clinician. Individuals and clinicians who appear to share the same cultural background may nevertheless differ in ways that are relevant to care. The CFI may be used in its entirety, or components may be incorporated into a clinical evaluation as needed. The CFI may be especially helpful in clinical practice when any of the following occur: difficulty in diagnostic assessment owing to significant differences in the cultural, religious, or socioeconomic backgrounds of the clinician and the individual; uncertainty about the fit between culturally distinctive symptoms and diagnostic criteria; difficulty in judging illness severity or impairment; divergent views of symptoms or expectations of care based on previous experience with other cultural systems of healing and health care; disagreement between the individual and clinician on the course of care; potential mistrust of mainstream services and institutions by individuals with collective histories of trauma and oppression; and limited engagement in and adherence to treatment by the individual.

When the clinician and patient have a shared belief system regarding the nature of the problem and the appropriate therapeutic approach, there may be less of a need to administer the CFI—not because cultural factors are not playing a role but because the clinician and patient are embedding these factors in their shared cultural assumptions and are therefore already addressing these issues even without a formal questionnaire. Note that this answer stresses a shared belief system and an agreed-on approach to the current problem; however, one should not assume a shared belief system just because the patient is from the same ethnic or religious group.

22.4—Cultural Formulation Interview (CFI) (pp. 862–863)

22.5   Which of the following accurately distinguishes the concept of race from that of ethnicity?

    A. Race is based on superficial physical attributes, whereas ethnicity is based on culturally constructed group identity.
    B. Race is a biological construct, whereas ethnicity is socially constructed.
    C. Race is generally region-specific, whereas ethnicity is a construct generally carried across societies.
    D. Race tends to be self-assigned by the identified group, whereas ethnicity is attributed by outsiders.

Correct Answer: A. Race is based on superficial physical attributes, whereas ethnicity is based on culturally constructed group identity.

Explanation: Race is a social, not a biological, construct that divides humanity into groups on the basis of a variety of superficial physical traits such as skin color that have been falsely viewed as indicating attributes and capacities assumed to be inherent to the group. Racial categories and constructs have varied over history and across societies and have been used to justify systems of oppression, slavery, and genocide. The construct of race is important for psychiatry because it can lead to racial ideologies, racism, discrimination, and social oppression and exclusion, which have strong negative effects on mental health. There is evidence that racism can exacerbate many psychiatric disorders, contributing to poor outcome, and that racial biases can affect diagnostic assessment.

Ethnicity is a culturally constructed group identity used to define peoples and communities. It may be rooted in a common history, ancestry, geography, language, religion, or other shared characteristics of a group, which distinguish that group from others. Ethnicity may be self-assigned or attributed by outsiders. Increasing mobility, intermarriage, and intermixing of cultural groups have defined new mixed, multiple, or hybrid ethnic identities. These processes may also lead to the dilution of ethnic identification.

22.5—Culture and Psychiatric Diagnosis / Key Terms (pp. 859–860)

22.6   In DSM-5-TR, which of the following is included in *cultural concepts of distress*?

A. Culturally specific alternative names for DSM-5-TR psychiatric disorders.
B. Culturally specific subtypes of psychiatric disorders.
C. Culturally influenced explanations of symptoms.
D. A unifying explanation of variable symptom expression in psychiatric disorders.

Correct Answer: C. Culturally influenced explanations of symptoms.

Explanation: *Cultural concepts of distress* describe the ways individuals express, report, and interpret experiences of illness and distress. Cultural concepts of distress include idioms, explanations or perceived causes, and syndromes. Symptoms are expressed and communicated using cultural idioms of distress—behaviors or linguistic terms, metaphors, phrases, or ways of talking about symptoms, problems, or suffering that are commonly used by individuals with similar cultural backgrounds to convey a wide range of concerns. Such idioms may be used for a broad spectrum of distress and may not indicate a psychiatric disorder. Common contemporary idioms in the United States include *burnout*, *feeling stressed*, *nervous breakdown*, and *feeling depressed*, in the sense of experiencing dissatisfaction or discouragement that does not meet criteria for any psychiatric disorder. Culturally specific explanations and syndromes are also common and are distributed widely across populations. This section also provides some illustrative examples of idioms, explanations, and syndromes from diverse geographic regions. The examples were chosen because they have been well studied, and their lack of familiarity to many U.S. clinicians highlights their specific verbal and behavioral expressions and communicative function.

22.6—Culture and Psychiatric Diagnosis / chapter introduction (p. 859)

22.7   Which of the following best defines *cultural idioms of distress*?

A. Idiosyncratic clusters of symptoms restricted to specific geographic regions.
B. Collective, shared ways of experiencing and discussing concerns.
C. Perceived causes or explanatory models regarding distress.
D. Culturally specific terms that correspond to specific DSM-5-TR diagnoses.

Correct Answer. B. Collective, shared ways of experiencing and discussing concerns.

Explanation: The term *cultural concepts of distress* refers to ways that individuals experience, understand, and communicate suffering, behavioral problems, or troubling thoughts and emotions. Three main types of cultural concepts of distress may be distinguished. *Cultural idioms* of distress are ways of expressing distress that may not involve specific symptoms or syndromes but that provide collective, shared ways of experiencing and talking about personal or social concerns. For example, everyday talk about "nerves" or "depression" may refer to widely varying forms of suffering without mapping onto a discrete set of symptoms, a syndrome, or a disorder. *Cultural explanations* or perceived causes are labels, attributions, or features of an explanatory model that indicate culturally recognized meaning or etiology for symptoms, illness, or distress. *Cultural syndromes* are clusters of symptoms and attributions that tend to co-occur among individuals in specific cultural groups, communities, or contexts and that are recognized locally as coherent patterns of experience.

These three cultural concepts of distress—cultural idioms of distress, cultural explanations, and cultural syndromes—are more relevant to clinical practice than the older formulation *culture-bound syndrome*. Specifically, the term *culture-bound syndrome* ignores the fact that clinically important cultural differences often involve explanations or experience of distress rather than culturally distinctive configurations of symptoms. Furthermore, the term *culture-bound* overemphasizes the extent to which cultural concepts of distress are characterized by highly idiosyncratic experiences that are restricted to specific geographic regions.

22.7—Cultural Concepts of Distress / Relevance for Diagnostic Assessment (pp. 871–873)

22.8   Which of the following accurately characterizes *ataque de nervios*?

A. Intense emotional upset, including acute anxiety, anger, and grief, and crying or screaming and shouting uncontrollably.
B. Intense anxiety about and avoidance of interpersonal situations for fear of inadequacy or offensiveness.
C. A frightening event perceived to cause the soul to leave the body, resulting in illness or sadness.
D. A general state of vulnerability to stressful life events.

Correct Answer: A. Intense emotional upset, including acute anxiety, anger, and grief, and crying or screaming and shouting uncontrollably.

Explanation: *Ataque de nervios* ("attack of nerves") is a syndrome found in Latinx cultural contexts, characterized by symptoms of intense emotional upset, including acute anxiety, anger, or grief; screaming and shouting uncontrollably; attacks of crying; trembling; heat in the chest rising into the head; and becoming verbally and physically aggressive. Attacks frequently occur as a direct result of a stressful event relating to the family, such as news of the death of a close relative, conflicts with a spouse or children, or witnessing an accident involving a family member.

Taijin kyofusho ("interpersonal fear disorder") is a syndrome found in Japanese cultural contexts that is characterized by anxiety about and avoidance of interpersonal situations due to the thought, feeling, or conviction that the individual's appearance and actions in social interactions are inadequate or offensive to others. *Susto* is an illness in some Latinx cultural contexts that is attributed to a frightening event that causes the soul to leave the body and results in unhappiness and sickness, as well as difficulties functioning in key social roles. *Nervios* refers to a general state of vulnerability to stressful life experiences and to difficult life circumstances.

22.8—Examples of Cultural Concepts of Distress (pp. 873–879)

22.9   What is the term for a cultural concept of distress, coined in South Asia, involving an individual's fear that various symptoms may be attributed to semen loss?

A. *Kufungisisa.*
B. *Dhat syndrome.*
C. *Maladi dyab.*
D. *Shenjing shuairuo.*

Correct Answer: B. *Dhat syndrome.*

Explanation: *Dhat syndrome* is a term that was coined in South Asia little more than half a century ago to account for common clinical presentations of young men who attributed their various symptoms to semen loss. Despite the name, it is not a discrete syndrome but rather a cultural explanation of distress for individuals who refer to diverse symptoms, such as anxiety, fatigue, weakness, weight loss, erectile dysfunction, other multiple somatic complaints, and depressed mood. The cardinal feature is anxiety and distress about the loss of *dhat* in the absence of any identifiable physiological dysfunction. *Dhat* was identified by individuals as a white discharge that was noted on defecation or urination. Ideas about this substance are related to the concept of *dhatu* (semen) described in the Hindu system of medicine, Ayurveda, as one of seven essential bodily fluids whose balance is necessary to maintain health. Although *dhat syndrome* was formulated as a clinical category to help inform local clinical practice, related ideas about the harmful effects of semen loss have been shown to be widespread in the general population, suggesting a cultural disposition for explaining health problems and symptoms with reference to *dhat*-related concepts.

22.9—Examples of Cultural Concepts of Distress / *Dhat syndrome* (pp. 874–875)

22.10   Which of the following does the term *kufungisisa* represent?

A. Idiom of distress.
B. Cultural explanation.
C. Both.
D. Neither.

Correct Answer: C. Both.

Explanation: *Kufungisisa* ("thinking too much") is an idiom of distress and a cultural explanation among the Shona of Zimbabwe. As an explanation, it is considered to be causative of anxiety, depression, and somatic problems (e.g., "My heart is painful because I think too much"). As an idiom of psychosocial distress, it is indicative of interpersonal and social difficulties (e.g., marital problems, having no money to take care of children, unemployment). *Kufungisisa* involves ruminating on upsetting thoughts, particularly worries, including concerns about chronic physical illness, such as HIV-related disorders. *Kufungisisa* is associated with a range of psychopathology, including anxiety symptoms, excessive worry, panic attacks, depressive symptoms, irritability, and posttraumatic stress disorder.

22.10—Examples of Cultural Concepts of Distress / *Kufungisisa* **(pp. 876)**

22.11 Which of the following psychiatric disorders is associated with *hikikomori*?

A. Obsessive-compulsive disorder.
B. Alcohol use disorder.
C. Schizophrenia.
D. Attention-deficit/hyperactivity disorder.

Correct Answer: C. Schizophrenia.

Explanation: *Hikikomori* (a Japanese term composed from the words *hiku* [to pull back] and *moru* [to seclude oneself]) is a syndrome of protracted and severe social withdrawal observed in Japan that may result in complete cessation of in-person interactions with others. The typical picture in *hikikomori* is an adolescent or young adult male who does not leave his room within his parents' home and has no in-person social interactions. This behavior initially may be ego-syntonic but usually leads to distress over time; it is often associated with high intensity of internet use and virtual social exchanges. Other features include no interest in or willingness to attend school or work. The 2010 guideline of the Japan Ministry of Health, Labor, and Welfare requires 6 months of social withdrawal for a diagnosis of *hikikomori*. The extreme social withdrawal seen in *hikikomori* may occur in the context of an established DSM-5-TR disorder ("secondary") or may manifest independently ("primary"). *Hikikomori* is associated with social anxiety disorder, major depressive disorder, generalized anxiety disorder, posttraumatic stress disorder, autism spectrum disorder, schizoid personality disorder, avoidant personality disorder, and schizophrenia or other psychotic disorder. The condition also may be associated with internet gaming disorder and, in adolescents, with school refusal.

22.11—Examples of Cultural Concepts of Distress / *Hikikomori* **(p. 875)**

22.12 Which of the following accurately describes *Khyâl cap*?

A. Social withdrawal involving the complete cessation of in-person interaction with others.
B. Physical or mental illness, distress, or dysfunction caused by another's ill will toward the sufferer.
C. A general vulnerability to stressful life events and difficult experiences.
D. A sudden onset of dizziness, palpitations, shortness of breath, anxiety, or autonomic arousal.

Correct Answer: D. A sudden onset of dizziness, palpitations, shortness of breath, anxiety, or autonomic arousal.

Explanation: "*Khyâl* attacks" (*khyâl cap*), or "wind attacks," is a syndrome found in Cambodian cultural contexts. Common symptoms include those of panic attacks, such as dizziness, palpitations, shortness of breath, and cold extremities, as well as other symptoms of anxiety and autonomic arousal (e.g., tinnitus, neck soreness). *Khyâl* attacks include catastrophic cognitions centered on the concern that *khyâl* (a windlike substance) may rise in the body—along with blood—and cause a range of serious effects (e.g., compressing the lungs to cause shortness of breath and asphyxia; entering the cranium to cause tinnitus, dizziness, blurry vision, and a fatal syncope). *Khyâl* attacks may occur without warning but are frequently brought about by triggers such as worrisome thoughts, standing up (i.e., orthostasis), specific odors with negative associations, and agoraphobic-type cues such as going to crowded spaces or riding in a car. *Khyâl* attacks usually meet panic attack criteria and may shape the experience of other anxiety and trauma- and stressor-related disorders. *Khyâl* attacks may be associated with considerable disability.

22.12—Examples of Cultural Concepts of Distress / *Khyâl cap* (pp. 875–876)

22.13 How do cultural concepts of distress relate to DSM-5-TR nosology?

A. One-to-one correspondence.
B. Providing specific diagnostic criteria.
C. Static correspondence across time and geography.
D. May apply to multiple disorders.

Correct Answer: D. May apply to multiple disorders.

Explanation: Cultural concepts of distress arise from local folk or professional diagnostic systems for mental and emotional distress, and they may also reflect the influence of biomedical concepts. Cultural concepts of distress have four key features in relation to the DSM-5-TR nosology: 1) There is seldom a one-to-one correspondence of any cultural concept of distress with a DSM diagnostic entity; the correspondence is more likely to be one-to-many in either direction. 2) Cultural concepts of distress may apply to a wide range of symptom and functional severity, including presentations that do not meet DSM-5-TR criteria for any mental disorder. 3) In common usage, the same cultural term frequently denotes more than one type of cultural concept of distress (e.g., "depression" may be used to describe a syndrome, an idiom of distress, or an explanation or perceived cause). 4) Like culture and DSM itself, cultural concepts of distress may change over time in response to both local and global influences.

22.13—Cultural Concepts of Distress / Relevance for Diagnostic Assessment (pp. 871–872)

CHAPTER 23

Alternative DSM-5 Model for Personality Disorders (DSM-5-TR Section III)

23.1   Which of the following terms best describes the diagnostic approach proposed in the Alternative DSM-5 Model for Personality Disorders?

A. Categorical.
B. Dimensional.
C. Hybrid.
D. Developmental.

Correct Answer: C. Hybrid.

Explanation: Provided as an alternative to the extant personality disorders classification in Section II, this hybrid dimensional-categorical model in Section III defines personality disorder in terms of impairments in personality functioning and pathological personality traits (option C is correct; options A and B are incorrect). On some occasions, what appears to be a personality disorder may be better explained by another mental disorder, the physiological effects of a substance or another medical condition, or a normal developmental stage (option D is incorrect).

23.1—chapter introduction (p. 881); Criteria E, F, and G: Alternative Explanations for Personality Pathology (Differential Diagnosis) (p. 883)

23.2   In the Alternative DSM-5 Model for Personality Disorders, personality disorders are characterized by pathological personality traits and which of the following?

A. Impairments in personality functioning.
B. Impairments in identity.
C. Impairments in self-direction.
D. Impairments in empathy.

Correct Answer: A. Impairments in personality functioning.

Explanation: In the Alternative DSM-5 Model for Personality Disorders, personality disorders are characterized by impairments in personality *functioning* and pathological personality *traits* (option A is correct). A diagnosis of a personality disorder requires two determinations: 1) an assessment of the level of impairment in personality functioning, which is needed for Criterion A, and 2) an evaluation of pathological personality traits, which is required for Criterion B. Identity, self-direction, and empathy are all considered elements of personality functioning; self functioning involves identity and self-direction; interpersonal functioning involves empathy and intimacy.

23.2—chapter introduction (p. 881); General Criteria for Personality Disorder (p. 881); Criterion A: Level of Personality Functioning (p. 882); Table 1 (p. 883)

23.3   Which of the following is a domain of the Alternative DSM-5 Model for Personality Disorders?

   A. Emotional lability.
   B. Intimacy avoidance.
   C. Disinhibition.
   D. Cognitive and perceptual dysregulation.

Correct Answer: C. Disinhibition.

Explanation: Pathological personality traits are organized into five broad domains: negative affectivity, detachment, antagonism, disinhibition, and psychoticism (option C is correct). Emotional lability is considered a facet of negative affectivity (option A is incorrect). Intimacy avoidance is considered a facet of detachment (option B is incorrect). Cognitive and perceptual dysregulation is considered a facet of psychoticism (option D is incorrect).

23.3—Criterion B: Pathological Personality Traits (p. 882); Table 3 (Definitions of DSM-5 personality disorder trait domains and facets) (pp. 899–901)

23.4   In addition to negative affectivity, which of the following maladaptive trait domains is most associated with avoidant personality disorder?

   A. Detachment.
   B. Antagonism.
   C. Disinhibition.
   D. Psychoticism.

Correct Answer: A. Detachment.

Explanation: Typical features of avoidant personality disorder are avoidance of social situations and inhibition in interpersonal relationships related to feelings of ineptitude and inadequacy, anxious preoccupation with negative evaluation and rejection, and fears of ridicule or embarrassment. Characteristic difficulties are apparent in identity, self-direction, empathy, and/or intimacy, along with specific maladaptive traits in the domains of negative affectivity and detachment (option A is correct). Characteristic difficulties in other personality disorders are apparent in identity, self-direction, empathy, and/or intimacy, along with specific maladaptive traits in the domain of negative affectivity (borderline personality disorder), antagonism (antisocial, borderline, and narcissistic personality disorders), and/or disinhibition (antisocial and borderline personality disorders); options B and C are incorrect. Characteristic difficulties in schizotypal personality disorder include specific maladaptive traits in the domains of psychoticism and detachment (option D is incorrect).

23.4—Antisocial Personality Disorder (pp. 884–885); Avoidant Personality Disorder (pp. 885–886); Borderline Personality Disorder (pp. 886–887); Schizotypal Personality Disorder (pp. 889–890)

23.5   Which of the following is included in the Section III personality trait system?

A. The Personality Psychopathology Five (PSY-5).
B. The Level of Personality Functioning Scale (LPFS).
C. The Five Factor Model of personality (FFM).
D. The Personality Inventory for DSM-5 (PID-5).

Correct Answer: C. The Five Factor Model of personality (FFM).

Explanation: The Section III personality trait system includes five broad domains of personality trait variation—negative affectivity (vs. emotional stability), detachment (vs. extraversion), antagonism (vs. agreeableness), disinhibition (vs. conscientiousness), and psychoticism (vs. lucidity)—comprising 25 specific personality trait facets. These five broad domains are maladaptive variants of the five domains of the extensively validated and replicated personality model known as the Five Factor Model of personality (FFM) or Big Five (option C is correct) and are also similar to the domains of the Personality Psychopathology Five (PSY-5; option A is incorrect). The specific level of impairment in personality functioning and the pathological personality traits that characterize the individual's personality can be specified for personality disorder—trait specified (PD-TS), using the Level of Personality Functioning Scale (LPFS) and the pathological trait taxonomy. The LPFS may also be used as a global indicator of personality functioning without specification of a personality disorder diagnosis or in the event that personality impairment is subthreshold for a disorder diagnosis (option B is incorrect). The personality trait model is operationalized in the Personality Inventory for DSM-5 (PID-5), which can be completed in its self-report form by patients and in its informant-report form by those who know the patient well (option D is incorrect).

23.5—The Personality Trait Model (p. 893); Personality Disorder Diagnosis (p. 891); Rating Level of Personality Functioning (p. 892); Assessment of the DSM-5 Section III Personality Trait Model (p. 894)

23.6   Disturbances in self and interpersonal functioning constitute the core of personality psychopathology, and in the alternative DSM-5-TR diagnostic model for personality disorders they are evaluated on a continuum. Which of the following is a characteristic of healthy self functioning?

    A. Comprehension and appreciation of others' experiences and motivations.
    B. Variability of self-esteem.
    C. Fluctuating boundaries between self and others.
    D. Experience of oneself as unique.

Correct Answer: D. Experience of oneself as unique.

Explanation: Elements of healthy self functioning include identity (experience of oneself as unique, with clear boundaries between self and others [option D is correct and option C is incorrect]; stability of self-esteem and accuracy of self-appraisal [option B is incorrect]; and capacity for, and ability to regulate, a range of emotional experience) and self-direction (pursuit of coherent and meaningful short-term and life goals; utilization of constructive and prosocial internal standards of behavior; and ability to self-reflect productively). Elements of healthy interpersonal functioning include empathy (comprehension and appreciation of others' experiences and motivations [option A is incorrect], tolerance of differing perspectives, and understanding of the effects of one's own behavior on others) and intimacy (depth and duration of connection with others, desire and capacity for closeness, and mutuality of regard reflected in interpersonal behavior).

22.6—Criterion A: Level of Personality Functioning (p. 882); Table 1 (Elements of personality functioning) (p. 883)

23.7   Which of the following is a general criterion for personality disorder in the Alternative DSM-5-TR Model for Personality Disorders?

    A. The individual experiences mild impairment in personality (self/interpersonal) functioning.
    B. The individual demonstrates two or more pathological personality traits.
    C. The impairments in personality functioning and the individual's personality trait expression may fluctuate over time.
    D. The impairments in personality functioning and the individual's personality trait expression are not better explained by another mental disorder.

Correct Answer: D. The impairments in personality functioning and the individual's personality trait expression are not better explained by another mental disorder.

Explanation: In the Alternative DSM-5 Model for Personality Disorders, the essential features of a personality disorder are as follows: moderate or greater impairment in personality (self/interpersonal) functioning (option A is incorrect); one or more pathological personality traits (option B is incorrect); the impairments in personality functioning and the individual's personality trait expression are relatively inflexible and pervasive across a broad range of personal and social situations; the impairments in personality functioning and the individual's personality trait expression are relatively stable across time, with onsets that can be traced back to at least adolescence or early adulthood (option C is incorrect); the impairments in personality functioning and the individual's personality trait expression are not better explained by another mental disorder (option D is correct); the impairments in personality functioning and the individual's personality trait expression are not solely attributable to the physiological effects of a substance or another medical condition (e.g., severe head trauma); and the impairments in personality functioning and the individual's personality trait expression are not better understood as normal for an individual's developmental stage or sociocultural environment.

23.7—General Criteria for Personality Disorder (pp. 881–882)

23.8 In order to meet the proposed diagnostic criteria for antisocial personality disorder in the Alternative DSM-5 Model for Personality Disorders, an individual must have maladaptive personality traits in which of the following domains?

A. Negative affectivity.
B. Detachment.
C. Antagonism.
D. Psychoticism.

Correct Answer: C. Antagonism.

Explanation: In antisocial personality disorder, characteristic difficulties are apparent in identity, self-direction, empathy, and/or intimacy, along with specific maladaptive traits in the domains of antagonism and disinhibition (option C is correct). In avoidant personality disorder and obsessive-compulsive personality disorder, characteristic difficulties are apparent in identity, self-direction, empathy, and/or intimacy, along with specific maladaptive traits in the domains of negative affectivity and detachment (options A and B are incorrect). In borderline personality disorder, characteristic difficulties are apparent in identity, self-direction, empathy, and/or intimacy, along with specific maladaptive traits in the domains of negative affectivity, and also antagonism and/or disinhibition (option A is incorrect). In schizotypal personality disorder, characteristic difficulties are apparent in identity, self-direction, empathy, and/or intimacy, along with specific maladaptive traits in the domains of psychoticism and detachment (options B and D are incorrect).

23.8—Antisocial Personality Disorder (pp. 884–885); Avoidant Personality Disorder (pp. 885–886); Borderline Personality Disorder (pp. 886–887); Obsessive-Compulsive Personality Disorder (pp. 888–889); Schizotypal Personality Disorder (pp. 889–890).

23.9   Which of the following statements best characterizes the relationship between severity of personality dysfunction—as rated on the Level of Personality Functioning Scale (LPFS)—and presence of a personality disorder?

A. A moderate level of impairment in personality functioning is required for the diagnosis of a personality disorder.
B. Impairment in personality functioning is unrelated to the presence of a personality disorder.
C. The severity of impairment in personality functioning is unrelated to the number of personality disorders.
D. The severity of impairment in personality functioning is unrelated to the severity of the personality disorder.

Correct Answer: A. A moderate level of impairment in personality functioning is required for the diagnosis of a personality disorder.

Explanation: In the LPFS, impairment in personality functioning predicts the presence of a personality disorder (option B is incorrect), and the severity of impairment predicts whether an individual has more than one personality disorder or one of the more typically severe personality disorders (options C and D are incorrect). A moderate level of impairment in personality functioning is required for the diagnosis of a personality disorder (option A is correct); this threshold is based on empirical evidence that the moderate level of impairment maximizes the ability of clinicians to accurately and efficiently identify personality disorder pathology.

23.9—Criterion A: Level of Personality Functioning (p. 882)

23.10 Which of the following statements about the Level of Personality Functioning Scale (LPFS) is most accurate?

A. A rating of moderate or greater impairment is necessary for the diagnosis of a personality disorder.
B. A rating of mild impairment is necessary for the diagnosis of a personality disorder.
C. The LPFS can be used only with specification of a personality disorder diagnosis.
D. To use the LPFS, the clinician selects the level that captures the person's lowest lifetime level of impairment.

Correct Answer: A. A rating of moderate or greater impairment is necessary for the diagnosis of a personality disorder.

Explanation: To use the LPFS, the clinician selects the level that most closely captures the individual's *current overall* level of impairment in personality functioning (option D is incorrect). The rating is necessary for the diagnosis of a personality disorder (moderate or greater impairment) and can be used to specify the severity of impairment present for an individual with any personality disorder at a given point in time (option A is correct and option B is incorrect). The LPFS may also be used as a global indicator of personality functioning without specification of a personality disorder diagnosis or in the event that personality impairment is subthreshold for a disorder diagnosis (option C is incorrect).

23.10—Rating Level of Personality Functioning (p. 892)